# UNDERSTANDING ANESTHESIA

**Robert M. Julien, M.D., Ph. D.**
St. Vincent's Hospital and Medical Center
Portland, Oregon

**Addison-Wesley Publishing Company**
Medical Division
Menlo Park, California
Reading, Massachusetts / London / Amsterdam
Don Mills, Ontario / Sydney

*Sponsoring Editor:* Katherine Pitcoff
*Production Editor:* Ron Newcomer
*Book and Cover Designer:* Lisa S. Mirski
*Copy Editor:* Perry Ewell
*Illustrator:* Gerald A. Harper



Library of Congress Cataloging in Publication Data

Julien, Robert M.
Understanding anesthesia.

Includes bibliographical references and index.
1. Anesthesia. 2. Medical assistants. I. Title.
[DNLM: 1. Anesthesia. WO 200 J94u]
RD82.J85 1984 617'.96 84-18616
ISBN 0-201-11601-4

BCDEFGHIJK-HA-898765

The author and publishers have exerted every effort to ensure that drug selection and dosage formulations and composition of formulas set forth in this text are in accord with current recommendations and practice at the time of publication. However, in view of ongoing research, changes in government regulations, the reformulation of nutritional products, and the constant flow of information relating to drug therapy and drug reactions, the reader is urged to check product information on composition or the package insert for each drug for any change in indications of dosage and for added warnings and precautions. This is particularly important where the recommended agent is a new and/or infrequently employed drug.

Addison-Wesley Publishing Company
Medical/Nursing Division
2725 Sand Hill Road
Menlo Park, California 94025

# Contents

# Preface

This textbook is written as an introduction to anesthesia for health science students with little or no previous exposure to the field. It presents to the reader discussions of preoperative evaluation, anesthesia equipment and monitoring, techniques of intubation, regional anesthesia and vascular cannulation, anesthetic pharmacology (including autonomic and vascular pharmacology), choice of anesthesia techniques, postanesthetic recovery, fluid management, and special considerations relevant to pediatric and obstetrical anesthesia. It is my hope that through this book the student will come to appreciate not only the techniques involved in anesthesia, but the thought processes that accompany the design of a specific anesthetic for a specified surgical procedure in a particular patient. The fact that each anesthetic is viewed as a unique entity designed specifically for each patient demonstrates the continuing evolution of anesthesiology as an art and science.

To appreciate the specialty of anesthesiology it is necessary to look at the progress it has made within the past three or four decades. Anesthesia has rapidly progressed from a poorly developed subdivision of surgery into a highly sophisticated art and scientific medical discipline.

The perioperative responsibilities of the anesthesiologist are multi-fold and include (1) insuring that the patient is in optimal physical condition for surgery, (2) providing a safe and effective anesthetic for the patient during surgery, and (3) leaving the patient postoperatively in stable condition without anesthetic complication or residual.

In a broader sense, the American Society of Anesthesiology defines anesthesiology as:

"a practice of medicine dealing with but not limited to the

a. management of procedures for rendering a patient insensible to pain and emotional stress during surgical, obstetrical, and certain other medical procedures;
b. support of life functions during the stress of anesthetic and surgical manipulations;

c. clinical management of the patient unconscious from whatever cause;
d. management of problems in pain relief;
e. management of problems in cardiac and respiratory resuscitation;
f. application of specific methods of respiratory therapy;
g. clinical management of various fluid, electrolyte, and metabolic disturbances."

It is the purpose of this book to introduce the reader to the many roles in which the anesthesiologist must be skilled in order to fulfill these responsibilities. These include the competent clinician well versed in patient evaluation and pathophysiology; the clinical pharmacologist able to use a wide range of anesthetics and other drugs including barbiturates, tranquilizers, opiates, opiate antagonists, vasoactive substances, cardiotonics, antihypertensives, neuromuscular agents, antibiotics, and steroids; and the technician skilled in the placement of regional nerve blocks and invasive monitoring devices. The anesthesiologist needs to have a broad knowledge of surgery and surgical techniques, and their specific anesthetic requirements, and must be able to use and correctly interpret a variety of monitoring devices.

The rapid and continuing advancement of anesthesiology into a sophisticated medical discipline has been accompanied by a new awareness of anesthesia as a desirable medical specialty, attracting increased professional respect, public awareness, and student interest. It is my hope that this book will communicate my own sense of excitement and will stimulate yours.

## Acknowledgments

The preparation of this manuscript has involved many individuals who truly deserve my heartfelt thanks: Mrs. Janice Reigel, Ms. Lynn Magnusen, and my son, Scott Julien, for the preparation of the manuscript; Mrs. Susan Mosedale and Dr. Jack Elder for their review of the early manuscript; Dr. Gerald Harper for his illustrations; and, most importantly, my wife, Judi, for her self-sacrificing support and encouragement.

Robert M. Julien, M.D., Ph. D.

# Introduction to the Student

## Anesthesiology—The Specialty

The dynamics of anesthesia practice are just now being clarified and widely appreciated. Anesthesia encompasses not only the interoperative care of the surgical patient, but also includes preoperative consultation, decision making in evaluating and preparing patients for surgery, choosing and performing anesthesia techniques, postoperative management, care of the critically ill patient, pulmonary and respiratory care, and consultation on and treatment of patients with pain syndromes.

## Role of the Anesthesiologist

To fulfill these needs, today's anesthesiologist must be a highly trained clinician as well as a skilled technician. Indeed, this amalgamation of clinical acumen with the ability to perform highly skilled technical duties provides unique opportunities filled with excitement and challenge.

Anesthesia also demands highly refined skills in interpersonal relationships. Hospitalization is traumatic, bringing patients into a close awareness of their own frailty, humanity, vulnerability, and limited life-span. Hospitalization can also be a depersonalizing experience for a patient, one in which self-dignity, self-direction, and self-determination may be compromised. The "system" often requires that patients give up control over their very lives to individuals whom they have never met and yet must unquestionably trust. Personal interactions therefore become equally important as diagnostic and technical skills. The anesthesiologist must be able to develop rapport with the patient and family rapidly, and to work with them to design an anesthetic plan appropriate for the surgery, yet consistent with the patient's and the family's needs and desires. These interpersonal skills must also be extended to the medical and nursing staffs since the professionals with whom the anesthesiologist interacts must trust, support, respect, and regularly consult the anesthesiologist so that all involved in patient care may work as a skilled medical-surgical "team" to provide optimal and appropriate care.

## The Anesthesiology Rotation

As you begin your first anesthesia experiences, all the background you have accumulated to date will be called upon. One of the major skills you will need to acquire is the proper preoperative evaluation and preparation of patients for anesthesia and surgery. Many of the preoperative concerns of the anesthesiologist are not intuitively obvious to practitioners outside the specialty. Examples might include control of hypertension, discontinuation of heparin or warfarin (Coumadin) if regional anesthesia is a possibility, control of reactive airway diseases with therapeutically effective levels of drugs, and continuation of chronically injested medications (anticonvulsants, for example) through the perioperative fasting periods when plasma levels of medications might fall to subtherapeutic levels. The importance of "tuning up" a patient for surgery, appreciating and controlling a patient's medical problems, cannot be overstated. This knowledge is essential for all students, not just those planning a career in anesthesiology.

In addition to heightening your appreciation of the perioperative medical management of a patient, anesthesiology exposure should help teach you some commonly needed technical skills such as airway evaluation and management, care of the apneic and unresponsive patient, skills of intravascular cannulation, interpretation of data recorded from invasive and noninvasive monitors, limitations of mechanical and electronic monitoring, principles of ventilator management, and use of potent pharmacologic agents to modulate body functions.

Finally, I hope that through this exposure to anesthesia, you, the student, may share in the excitement and challenge of anesthesia, possibly providing some of you with new insights into career possibilities.

# I

# THE PREANESTHETIC PERIOD

# 1. Preoperative Evaluation of the Patient

## Introduction

Every patient scheduled to receive an anesthetic for surgery should ideally be examined by an anesthesiologist the evening before surgery. The purposes of the preoperative visit are to evaluate the patient's current physical condition, establish rapport and confidence, and decide on the anesthetic procedure to be used.

The anesthesiologist seeks to determine whether the patient is in an optimal state of health, and whether the patient's physical condition can be improved prior to surgery. Such determination involves review of the patient's hospital charts and previous anesthesia records, patient history, physical examination, laboratory profile, and ordering of any additional tests that might provide important information. The anesthesiologist discusses with the patient the upcoming surgery and addresses any concerns about it.

## The Chart Review

Before interviewing the patient, the anesthesiologist should thoroughly review the available records and compile a list of past and present medical problems, current pharmacologic management, untoward reactions to drugs, and allergies. Records of previous anesthetics are invaluable sources of information: they indicate a patient's responses to drugs previously used for premedication; they detail the anesthetic agents and techniques employed; and they describe any problems that were encountered. Such problems might have included difficult intubations, adverse responses to anesthetics, any cardiac arrhythmias and their treatment, and any postanesthetic complications necessitating treatment.

If the patient has a history of chronic illness such as hypertension, diabetes, or epilepsy, the anesthesiologist should review the current status of the disease and the drugs used in its management. Progress notes may offer details of the present diagnosis and the surgical plan.

Known or suspected disease necessitates laboratory evaluation. For example, infection or bleeding requires complete blood counts, possibly including evaluation of coagulation. Patients with pulmonary disease may require preoperative pulmonary function and arterial blood gas tests. Patients taking diuretics should have a recent assay for serum potassium. Certain chronically administered medications may necessitate assay of their concentrations in plasma. Examples include assay of digitalis preparations, anticonvulsants, and aminophylline. The readings at the end of this chapter detail anesthetic considerations for specific disorders.

In contrast, the laboratory evaluation of healthy surgical patients is undergoing critical evaluation, primarily due to the expense of possibly unnecessary studies. Critical analysis of broad-spectrum testing has revealed that many studies are of minimal value in the asymptomatic patient undergoing elective surgery, and they contribute little information that influences either the choice or the conduct of the anesthetic. Thus, in many centers, only minimal testing is performed on healthy, asymptomatic patients in whom neither the history nor the physical examination indicate systemic dysfunction. Required testing may include only a recent hemoglobin or hematocrit.

In what situations, therefore, might additional laboratory or diagnostic information be necessary or useful? First, and most obviously, additional evaluation is essential in patients whose history or physical examination is suggestive of systemic disorder or dysfunction, as previously mentioned. Second, the perioperative period may be one of the few times an otherwise healthy patient may seek medical attention. If this is the case, relatively few tests will screen for potentially serious disorders which may be asymptomatic in their early stages and which may necessitate decisions to al-

**TABLE 1-1**
**Suggested Screening Tests for Asymptomatic Healthy Patients Scheduled to Undergo "Peripheral" Procedures Involving No Blood Loss**

| Age (yr) | Men | Women |
|---|---|---|
| Under 40 | | Hemoglobin or hematocrit, pregnancy test* |
| 40–59 | Electrocardiogram, BUN/glucose | Hemoglobin or hematocrit, electrocardiogram, BUN/glucose |
| Over 60 | Hemoglobin or hematocrit, electrocardiogram, chest x-ray, BUN/glucose | Hemoglobin or hematocrit, electrocardiogram, chest x-ray BUN/glucose |

*Test that might be (but probably is not) indicated for medicolegal reasons.

Table reproduced from Roizen, M.F. 1984. Preoperative preparation for a healthy patient for anesthesia: What laboratory tests are necessary?, *1984 refresher course lectures.* Fifty-eighth Congress of the International Anesthesia Research Society, Cleveland. p. 138.

ter the anesthetic management of the patient. Such tests might include: serum glucose (screen for diabetes mellitus); SGOT and BUN (screen for hepatitis and liver disease); urinalysis for glucose and protein (screen for diabetes and renal disease); ECG (for patients over 40 years of age); and chest x-ray (for patients over 50 and cigarette smokers over 40 years of age). Even though these tests will likely be normal, they serve well as baselines for tests at a later age.

Roizen (1984) has compiled recommendations for preoperative testing in healthy patients, based upon patient age and sex (Table 1-1). He argues that asymptomatic disease (as determined by careful history and physical examination) is rare, and that extensive testing may not be cost-effective in light of limited resources for health care. He states: ". . . for healthy patients, one should probably do less laboratory testing rather than more. We all have a responsibility to provide optimum care within the bounds of finite resources."

Finally, the anesthesiologist should note any information concerning the patient's personality and mental state that might be useful when conducting the interview or when prescribing preoperative medications, or that might indicate any concerns that might be troubling the patient.

## The Patient Interview

Following the chart review, the patient is interviewed. Important points to cover include: cardiovascular symptoms; hypertension; pulmonary, renal, and liver diseases; diabetes; bleeding disorders; symptoms of neurologic abnormalities; and smoking and alcohol habits. A listing of questions designed to screen for abnormalities in these areas is presented in Table 1-2.

Next, the anesthesiologist performs a physical examination, concentrating on the heart, the lungs, the peripheral pulses, and on the skin at points where needles may be inserted, and making a careful evaluation of mouth and airway. A suggested outline for such examination is listed in Table 1-3. The results of the history and physical examination can be summarized on Table 1-4 for reference and for consultation with colleagues and faculty. This table may be reproduced and completed for each patient to whom an anesthetic will be administered.

The anesthesiologist should discuss the range of anesthetic techniques appropriate for use during the surgery (Chapter 10). Advantages and disadvantages for each technique should be outlined. If possible, the patient should be allowed to participate in the decision, since this helps preserve the patient's dignity and control of self. Discussion of preanesthetic medication (Chapter 2) can follow. The patient should be informed of possible complications of anesthesia, the alternatives available, and what to expect during recovery from anesthesia.

At all points in the interview, there should be time for the patient to express his concerns freely. The anesthesiologist should relax and listen closely. If family members are present, they should be allowed to express their concerns also, and to ask questions.

**TABLE 1-2**
**Screening Questionnaire for Preoperative Organ-System Review**

| | Yes | No |
|---|---|---|
| *Hepato-renal* | | |
| Have you ever had hepatitis or yellow jaundice? | ☐ | ☐ |
| Have you ever been told that you have liver or gall bladder disease? | ☐ | ☐ |
| Have you had an anesthetic within the last few months? | ☐ | ☐ |
| Have you had kidney disease? | ☐ | ☐ |
| Have you ever had kidney stones? | ☐ | ☐ |
| Have you had any bladder or urinary infections? | ☐ | ☐ |
| Have you seen blood in your urine? | ☐ | ☐ |
| *Cardiovascular* | | |
| Have you ever had chest pain? | ☐ | ☐ |
| Have you ever had a heart attack? | ☐ | ☐ |
| Have you ever had rheumatic fever? | ☐ | ☐ |
| Have you ever had high blood pressure? | ☐ | ☐ |
| Have you ever had a heart murmur? | ☐ | ☐ |
| Have you ever taken medicine for your heart? | ☐ | ☐ |
| Have you ever taken digitalis? | ☐ | ☐ |
| Have you ever taken medicine for high blood pressure? | ☐ | ☐ |
| How many pillows do you sleep on? ________________ | | |
| Do you wake up at night short of breath? | ☐ | ☐ |
| How many stairs can you climb? ________________ | | |
| Are you able to keep up with your gardening or housework? | ☐ | ☐ |
| What is the most vigorous thing you have done lately? ________________ | | |
| *Pulmonary* | | |
| How many cigarettes do you smoke per day? ________________ | | |
| How many years have you smoked cigarettes? ________________ | | |
| Have you had a cold or cough in the past month? | ☐ | ☐ |
| Have you ever had asthma? | ☐ | ☐ |
| Have you ever had difficulty breathing? | ☐ | ☐ |
| Have you ever been told that you have any problems with your lungs? | ☐ | ☐ |
| Do you have a morning cough? | ☐ | ☐ |
| Do you ever cough up anything? How much? ________________ | ☐ | ☐ |
| Have you ever had pneumonia? | ☐ | ☐ |
| *Neurologic* | | |
| Have you ever had any problems with your nervous system? | ☐ | ☐ |
| Have you ever lost consciousness? | ☐ | ☐ |
| Have you ever had a convulsion or a seizure? | ☐ | ☐ |
| Have you ever lost your vision? | ☐ | ☐ |
| Have you ever had difficulty talking? | ☐ | ☐ |
| Do you have headaches? | ☐ | ☐ |
| Do you have backaches? | ☐ | ☐ |
| Do you have any problems with aches and pains? | ☐ | ☐ |
| *General* | | |
| Are you an easy bruiser? | ☐ | ☐ |
| Do you bleed easily? | ☐ | ☐ |

**TABLE 1-2**
**(continued)**

| | Yes | No |
|---|---|---|
| When you cut yourself, does it continue to bleed? | ☐ | ☐ |
| Do your gums bleed? | ☐ | ☐ |
| If female, are you pregnant? | ☐ | ☐ |
| Is there a possibility that you might be pregnant? | ☐ | ☐ |
| List your allergies below, not listed above. | | |
| Do you take any drugs or medicine? What for? ____________ | ☐ | ☐ |
| Had you ever had a bad reaction to a medicine? | ☐ | ☐ |
| Have you ever had an anesthetic? | ☐ | ☐ |
| Have you or your family members had problems with anesthetics? | ☐ | ☐ |
| Are there any other problems with your health that I should know about? | ☐ | ☐ |
| How much wine or beer do you drink per day? ____________ | | |
| How much hard liquor do you drink per day? ____________ | | |

Please list the medicines you take:

____________________________________________
____________________________________________
____________________________________________
____________________________________________
____________________________________________

Please list your allergies:

____________________________________________
____________________________________________
____________________________________________
____________________________________________
____________________________________________

## Humanistic Considerations

Few experiences in life are as traumatic to an individual as surgery. Fear of death, pain, disability, and disfigurement may be overwhelming. Patients often muster all coping mechanisms known to them, but even then, they may be unable to cope, and they need the assistance of a concerned and compassionate physician. Indeed, compassion is a major part of medical competence.

In arguing that medical care need not suffer as a result of compassion, Glick (1981) states: "In the field of medicine . . . there is no inherent contradiction between the scientific and the compassionate." And further, "both technology and compassion have as a goal healing the patient; we can ignore either, only at the peril of producing poor medicine. We need physicians who are both compassionate and competent."

The presurgical patient enters a world of strangers, becomes emotionally vulnerable, and is asked to place complete trust in a medical team that, though professional, is for the most part unknown. Although the patient has little basis for evaluating the physicians' competence, they necessarily become the focus of trust.

The vulnerability and dependency generate considerable preoperative anxiety in the patient. Indeed, anxiety is normal and to be expected. This section will discuss several ways in which the medical staff can assist patients in reducing their level of anxiety.

## Interview Tone

As discussed above, the patient interview should be conducted with concern and compassion. The tone that is set must be professional, but not detached.

## Honesty

All interviews must be conducted in an atmosphere of complete honesty. The patient should be told the relative risks involved in the anesthetic procedure and any alternatives that are consistent with the requirements of the proposed surgery. Such honesty often helps alleviate preoperative anxiety.

**TABLE 1-3**
**Preanesthetic Physical Examination**

Supine and standing blood pressure and pulse rate
Temperature and body weight and height
Auscultation and percussion examination of the heart and lungs
Palpation and auscultation of the carotid pulse
Skin examination in areas of anticipated needle punctures
Neck mobility and range of motion
Airway examination
- Size of the mouth and tongue
- Ability to open the mouth widely
- Size of the mandible relative to the maxilla (i.e., overbite, receding chin)
- Patency of the nasal passages
- Length of the neck
- Presence of dentures; loose, chipped, or missing teeth; protruding teeth; bridges or caps; extent of dental disease

If history suggests possible cardiac failure:
- Jugular veneous distension
- Ability to walk up a flight of stairs

If radial artery catheterization is planned:
- Bilateral Allen test (Chapter 4) for ulnar artery patency

Further organ system examination as dictated by patient history

## TABLE 1-4
## Suggested Format for Summarizing Patient History, Physical Examination, Laboratory Studies, and Anesthetic Plan

| **NAME** **UNIT #** | | **ROOM #** **DATE** **TIME** |
|---|---|---|
| **Preoperative diagnosis:** | | **Proposed surgery:** |
| Family history (MH, anesthesia problems, prolonged paralysis) | HISTORY | Neurologic history (seizures, strokes, neuropathy) |
| Prior anesthetics (dates, agents, problems) | | Alcohol and tobacco |
| Cardiovascular (infarcts, angina, CHF, HTN) | | Musculoskeletal (arthritis, neck and joint mobility, ROM) |
| Pulmonary (asthma, cough, sputum, dyspnea) | | Hepatorenal (jaundice, hepatitis, uremia, last dialysis) |
| Medications (steroids, tricyclics, MAO inhibitors, cardiac drugs, ASA, anticoagulant, eye drops) | | Bleeding history (transfusion reactions) |
| Other (metabolic and endocrine, infectious disease) | | Recent respiratory infections |
| Vital signs and gross appearance<br>BP____ HR____ Temp____<br>Ht____ Wt____<br>Jaundice ☐ Cyanosis ☐<br>Pallor ☐ Dehydration ☐ | EXAMINATION | Neck<br>Eyes IOP<br>Extremities (pulses, clubbing, edema, Allen test, mobility) |
| Upper airway | | Abdomen (ascites, organomegally) |
| Heart | | Spine |
| Lungs | | Neurologic (mental status, motor, sensory, cranial nerves, ICP) |
| Hematology | LABORATORY | Urinalysis |
| Chemistries (electrolytes, glucose, BUN, creatinine) | | Pulmonary function tests |
| Coagulation values (PT, PTT, platelets, bleeding time) | | ECG |
| Arterial blood gases | | Other |
| Blood products needed?<br>Yes____ No____ Available?____ | | |

***General Assessment and Anesthetic Plan***

Include special position requirements, monitoring needs, patient preferences, regional vs. general anesthesia

Full explanation of procedures, alternatives, and risks conducted with patient?
Yes____ No____

ASA classification____
NPO? Yes____ No____
Ordered from:____

Premedication ordered?
Yes____ No____
Drugs ordered:

Interviewer:____

## Pain

It is inevitable that most patients will feel some pain following surgery, a fact that should not be withheld. The patient should be allowed to voice concerns about postoperative pain, and these concerns should be acknowledged. The anesthesiologist should reassure the patient that appropriate measures will be taken to provide comfort without sacrificing the safety of the patient (i.e., the patient will not be sedated so heavily as to not be able to ventilate adequately).

One should never say that something that will probably be painful will not be so. Later, after experiencing pain, a patient might remember such statements, and the attitude provoked may make future surgical experiences more frightening. This is especially true of children.

## Education

An excellent method of reducing patient anxiety is to spend a few minutes describing the operating room and its equipment. Explaining what will be done before the induction of anesthesia (e.g., application of ECG pads and a blood pressure cuff, starting an intravenous infusion, etc.) may lessen anxiety.

## Positive Focus

As a general rule, the anesthesiologist should focus on the positive effects of surgery, reassuring the patient that the anxieties and the pain will be counterbalanced by an improvement in well-being. The risk of anesthesia is less than the risk of no surgery at all.

## Spiritual Concerns

As surgery approaches, patients often become acutely aware of their own frailty and frequently think of the nearness of death. Such reflections often bring them into a deep emotional and spiritual relationship with God. Spiritual concerns need attention and affirmation. A demonstration of understanding—in words, a touch, a holding of hands, or a prayer, if the physician and patient feel thus moved—can help sustain the patient. The patient can be encouraged to talk to clergy if this seems appropriate.

## Perioperative Considerations

On the morning of surgery, the anesthesiologist should warmly greet the patient in the preoperative holding area. The patient should be asked about any concerns and whether additional sedative is desired before going to the operating room. Ideally, the intravenous catheter (Chapter 4) should be placed and the intravenous infusion started in the holding area so that antianxiety agents can be administered (Chapter 2). This also reduces the anxiety-producing delay between the time the patient enters the operating room and the time when anesthesia is induced.

## The Preanesthetic Note

After the patient interview, the anesthesiologist writes a detailed note on the patient's current hospital record, summarizing the results of the consultation and detailing the proposed anesthetic management. The anesthesiologist should record that the chosen anesthetic procedure, the anesthetic alternatives, and the risks of anesthesia were explained and accepted by the patient.

The anesthesiologist assigns to the patient one of five *physical status categories,* defined by the American Society of Anesthesiologists (ASA) to indicate the patient's relative risk from the anesthesia and the probable need for invasive monitoring and postoperative intensive care.

An *ASA Class I* patient has no organic, physiologic, biochemical, or psychiatric disturbance, and the pathologic condition prompting the operation is localized and not part of a systematic disturbance.

An *ASA Class II* patient has mild to moderate systematic disease caused either by the condition prompting surgery or by other processes. The systemic disturbance is usually under good medical control.

An *ASA Class III* patient has severe systematic disease, usually under incomplete medical control, which places the patient at higher than normal risk for perioperative complications. Such diseases include poorly controlled hypertension, diabetes, coronary artery insufficiency, previous myocardial infarction, and emphysema.

An *ASA Class IV* patient has one or more severe systematic disorders that are life-threatening. Examples include recent myocardial infarction or stroke, and advanced pulmonary, hepatic, or renal diseases.

An *ASA Class V* patient has little chance of survival but is submitted to surgery in desperation.

Finally, for a patient in any of the five classes who undergoes emergency surgery and is not considered to be in optimal physical condition, the letter *E* is placed after his numerical classification. Thus, the classification of *IE* might be assigned to an otherwise healthy patient who presents with acute appendicitis for an emeregency appendectomy.

The final aspect of the preoperative visit is the writing of orders for laboratory studies (discussed previously) or preanesthetic medications (Chapter 2) as needed.

## Preoperative Visits with Outpatients

One of the most difficult problems an anesthesiologist faces is the preoperative evaluation of outpatients. Ideally, the patient should be seen the day prior to surgery and the interview handled in the manner already described. For a variety of reasons, however, outpatients are often not seen by the anesthesiologist until only shortly before surgery.

If a patient cannot be classified as ASA Class I or II, the surgery should probably be delayed until the patient can be more completely evaluated and prepared. The anesthesiologist must also be convinced that the patient has taken nothing by mouth on the day of the surgery, since vomiting with aspiration of vomitus can result in disastrous complications (see Chapter 2). Whatever records are available should be reviewed. Results of laboratory tests should be available and within normal limits. As with any surgical patient, chewing gum, dentures, and all prosthetic devices (such as contact lenses) must be removed.

Outpatients often express extreme anxiety, since they have not become accustomed to the hospital environment and are not pharmacologically premedicated. Therefore, the anesthesiologist must rapidly establish rapport and confidence. The anesthesia procedures should be explained before premedication, if any, is given, and before the patient is taken to the operating room; possible complications should be clearly described. Any patient who feels rushed or impersonally handled may develop hostile attitudes later, if complications arise.

## Preoperative Evaluation of Emergency Patients

Patients who present with a condition requiring immediate surgery provide numerous problems for the anesthesiologist. Decisions about such a patient must be made in rapid sequence. Preoperative evaluation and laboratory studies may be incomplete. The patient may have eaten recently and have a full stomach, and may be suffering from such conditions as dehydration, blood loss, active bleeding, increased intracranial pressure, or have a perforated internal organ.

The preoperative visit in emergency patients is necessarily brief and conducted in an atmosphere of anxiety and urgency, and occasionally not until the patient has arrived in the operating room. There may be little time to question either the patient or the family. The primary objectives of this visit are to determine the patient's state of health and hydration, and to arrange for fluids, monitoring equipment, and drugs for cardiovascular support. If the patient's condition is unstable, decision is made whether to stabilize before moving or to rapidly transport the patient directly to the operating room where attempts will be made to stabilize vital signs and proceed immediately with surgery.

### *Readings and References*

Glick, S.M. 1981. Humanistic medicine in a modern age. *N.Eng. J. Med.* 304:1036–1038.

Guerra, F., and Aldrete, J.A., editors. 1980. *Emotional and psychological responses to anesthesia and surgery.* New York: Grune & Stratton.

Molitch, M.E., editor. 1982. *Management of medical problems in surgical patients.* Philadelphia: F.A. Davis Co.

Roizen, M.F. 1981. Routine preoperative evaluation. In: *Anesthesia.* Miller, R.D., editor. New York: Churchill Livingstone, pp. 1–19.

Roizen, M.F. 1981. Preoperative evaluation of patients with diseases that require special preoperative evaluation and intraoperative management. In: *Anesthesia.* Miller, R.D., editor. New York: Churchill Livingstone, pp. 20–93.

———. 1984. Preoperative preparation of a healthy patient for anesthesia: what laboratory tests are necessary? *1984 review course lectures:* Fifty-Eighth Congress of the International Anesthesia Research Society, Cleveland. pp. 133–139.

Stoelting, R.K., and Dierdorf, S.F. 1983. *Anesthesia and co-existing disease.* New York: Churchill Livingstone.

Vandam, L.D., editor. 1984. *To make the patient ready for anesthesia: medical care of the surgical patient.* 2nd ed. Menlo Park, Calif.: Addison-Wesley.

Vickers, M.D., editor. 1982. *Medicine for anaesthetists.* Boston: Blackwell Scientific. 2nd ed.

Yao, F.F., and Artusio, J.F. 1983. *Anesthesiology: problem-oriented patient management.* Philadelphia: J.B. Lippincott.

# 2. Preanesthetic Medication for Adults

Few subjects in anesthesia generate greater controversy than surgical premedication. Some anesthesiologists advocate sedating patients very heavily before taking them to the operating room. At the other extreme are those who hold that premedication is rarely necessary. While most anesthesiologists would agree that the patient's preoperative apprehension should be lessened, they do not agree on how this should be accomplished. Chapter 1 discussed psychological approaches to reduce anxiety. This chapter will discuss current philosophies about the need for pharmacologic premedication in adults, will encourage a critical examination of these philosophies, and will encourage individualization of premedication for each patient. Premedication for children is a separate topic and will be discussed in Chapter 13.

## The Origin of Premedication

From the mid-nineteenth century until the mid-twentieth century, anesthesia was usually induced with inhaled ether vapor. This technique resulted in a slow and tumultuous induction, accompanied by excitement, anxiety, struggling, and delirium. The patient suffered an outpouring of bronchial and salivary secretions, marked increases or decreases in heart rate were common, and hypertension was often profound. Laryngospasm, respiratory tract irritability, nausea, and vomiting occurred frequently. Aspiration of vomitus with subsequent pulmonary complications was dreaded.

In those early days, electrocardiographic monitoring and drugs for resuscitation and for the preoperative control of hypertension, arrhythmias, heart disease, diabetes, etc., were unknown. Intravenous lines and fluids were unavailable. Thus, to shorten and smooth the induction of ether anesthesia, patients were often brought to the operating room heavily medicated or narcotized. To achieve this end, patients were premedicated with anticholinergic drugs (drying agents) and narcotics. While complete discussion of these drugs will be presented in Chapter 6, the pharmacology relevant to their use as premedication is presented in this chapter.

Intramuscular atropine was used to prevent salivary and bronchial secretions and to blunt the slowing of the heart rate that often accompanied ether inductions. The side effects of atropine administrations (discussed later) were considered a small price to pay for the increased safety it brought to surgery.

The narcotic, morphine, was used to relieve preoperative pain and provide preoperative sedation. Patients who received it appeared sleepy and unconcerned about the upcoming surgery. Although morphine-premedicated patients experienced depressed respiration and remained relatively unresponsive for prolonged periods after surgery, these effects, too, were considered a small price to pay for a safer and smoother ether induction. The effects of morphine on arterial blood gas measurements were unknown.

With the advent of the nonexplosive anesthetics, halothane (in 1956), enflurane (in 1972), and isoflurane (in 1981), the use of ether in the U.S. has virtually ceased. Inductions are usually accomplished quickly with intravenous agents, and the outpouring of secretions seen with ether seldom occurs. Rapid-acting muscle relaxants, such as succinylcholine, have reduced the occurrence of laryngospasm. Finally, routine electrocardiographic monitoring and intravenous infusions allow the early detection and treatment of complications. Thus, the need for generous premedication to avoid the problems caused by ether has virtually disappeared. Today, the primary objective of premedication is relief from preoperative anxiety. Secondary goals may include analgesia, amnesia, sedation, reduced gastric acidity, or reduction of salivary gland secretions.

Egbert and co-workers (1963) compared the effects of pentobarbital (Nembutal) with the effects of a reassuring, informative preoperative visit by an anesthesiologist. Their data (Table 2-1) demonstrated that the preoperative visit was the more effective premedication, and that the effects of the pentobarbital were relatively minor. Subsequent studies have confirmed this original observation, repeatedly demonstrating that the preoperative visit with frank discussion on the anesthetic procedure, the surgery, and the patient's fears remains the most effective way to allay anxiety.

**TABLE 2-1**
**Premedication versus Preoperative Visit by Anesthesiologist***

| | No Visit, No Drug | Visit Alone | Drug Alone | Drug and Visit |
|---|---|---|---|---|
| | | *Percent* | | |
| Feel nervous | 58 | 40 | 61 | 38 |
| Feel drowsy | 18 | 26 | 30 | 38 |
| Judged adequately sedated | 35 | 65 | 48 | 71 |

*Comparison of effects of pentobarbital 2 mg/kg IM, 1 hour before induction of anesthesia, with those of a reassuring, informative preoperative visit by the anesthetist.

Modified from Egbert, L.D.; Battit, G.E.; Turndorf, H.; et al. 1963. The value of the preoperative visit by an anesthetist. *J. Am. Med. Assoc.* 185:553.

# Pharmacology of Premedications

## Anticholinergic (Antimuscarinic) Agents

Table 2-2 lists the major body organs innervated by cholinergic neurons of the muscarinic type, and the organs' responses to cholinergic block. Drugs used to produce muscarinic blockade include atropine, scopolamine, and glycopyrrolate (Robinul). It can be seen that, while cholinergic blockade decreases salivary secretions, it markedly affects the eyes, the sweat and lacrimal glands, the heart, smooth muscle, and the central nervous system. Indeed, premedication with anticholinergic drugs can lead to significant patient discomfort. As a general rule, these drugs should be used only when their specific effects are desired; for example, to prevent succinylcholine-induced bradycardia and salivation during anesthesia induction.

## Opiate Narcotics

The effects of opiate narcotics include dose-related analgesia, sedation, indifference to external stimuli, and respiratory depression. Narcotic premedication may be important for patients who are in pain, or who must undergo painful procedures before anesthesia induction (procedures such as introducing arterial or central venous catheters). Narcotic premedication may also be useful for producing a basal level of

**TABLE 2-2**
**Effects of Cholinergic Blockade on Several Organ Systems**

| Organ | Response to Cholinergic Block* |
|---|---|
| *Eye* | Pupillary dilatation with photophobia<br>Blurred vision<br>Increased intraocular pressure (may be a problem in patients with glaucoma) |
| *Glands* | |
| Sweat | Decreased ability to sweat, secondary increase in body temperature |
| Salivary | Decreased secretions and dry mouth |
| Lacrimal | Decreased ability to tear |
| *Heart* | Increased heart rate |
| *Smooth muscles* | Increased gastric emptying time<br>Urinary retention<br>Bronchial dilatation |
| *Central nervous system*† | Sedation<br>Amnesia<br>Disorientation and hallucinations |

*Respones are to atropine, scopolamine, and glycopyrrolate.
†Effects on the central nervous system are seen primarily with scopolamine, much less with atropine, and not with glycopyrrolate, which does not cross the blood-brain barrier.

**TABLE 2-3**
**Major Effects of Narcotic Analgesics on Several Organ Systems**

| Organ | Response to Narcotic Analgesics |
|---|---|
| Eye | Pupillary constriction |
| Gastrointestinal tract | Constipation<br>Colic and abdominal pain<br>Nausea and vomiting |
| Cardiovascular system | Orthostatic hypotension |
| Central nervous system | Sedation and analgesia<br>Euphoria/dysphoria |
| Respiratory system | Respiratory depression<br>Reduced cough reflexes |

anesthesia before using the "balanced" technique of general anesthesia (Chapter 10), and for the anxious patient who has angina.

The *routine* use of opiates for premedication can be questioned, primarily because of the effects listed in Table 2-3. Accidental overdosage can jeopardize patient safety (Chapter 1). Respiratory depression, along with decreased coughing ability, predisposes to postoperative pulmonary complications. Abdominal cramping, nausea, and vomiting can result and can simulate the pain of angina pectoris. Postoperative constipation can be bothersome. Although the behavioral effects of narcotics are usually pleasant, patients occasionally experience unpleasant feelings and mental depression. Many patients report narcotic "allergies." Close questioning may differentiate true allergic responses (e.g., rashes, hives, etc.) from expected pharmacologic responses (e.g., abdominal cramps and nausea).

## Sedative-Hypnotic Agents

The sedative-hypnotic agents comprise a large number of varied compounds whose primary effect is a progressive depression of the central nervous function. Most widely used of these compounds are the barbiturates and benzodiazepines. The effects of these drugs occur along a continuum as the dose is increased: relief from anxiety, disinhibition, sedation, hypnosis, general anesthesia, and coma. Low doses (discussed later) are commonly used for premedication; the antianxiety and sedative effects being the ones desired. However, the young and the elderly may respond to these drugs with disorientation, delirium, agitation, increased anxiety, and other manifestations resembling a state of intoxication—effects the opposite of those intended.

Barbiturates used as premedication include pentobarbital and secobarbital, in doses of approximately 1–2 mg/kg administered orally, intramuscularly, or rectally. Their duration of action is about 4–6 hours.

Benzodiazepines commonly used as premedications include diazepam (Valium) and lorazepam (Ativan). It should be noted that their half-lives are quite long, 16 hours or more, and persistent effects should be expected, especially in elderly patients where the half-lives are even longer. Their premedication doses are approximately 0.12 mg/kg (diazepam) and 0.04 mg/kg (lorazepam), administered orally.

Chloral derivatives, such as chloral hydrate, chloral betaine, and triclofos sodium, are useful sedative-hypnotics, especially in children and the elderly in whom excitement reactions seem to occur less frequently than with barbiturate or benzodiazepine premedication. Orally administered, these drugs have a rapid onset of action (about 30 minutes) and a fairly short duration of action (about 4–6 hours).

All the sedatives discussed cause the same depressant effects as alcohol and can substitute for alcohol in alcohol-dependent patients.

## Tranquilizers and Antihistamines

Since the early 1950s, tranquilizers and antihistamines have been widely used as components of preanesthetic mixtures. These drugs and their adult doses include the phenothiazines (e.g., promethazine, 25–50 mg IM), the butyrophenones (e.g., droperidol, 2.5–5.0 mg IM), and hydroxyzine (50–100 mg IM). All have sedative, anti-nausea, antivomiting, anticholinergic, and sympathetic blocking properties, the latter being responsible for the occasional reduction in blood pressure which can accompany their use. Their wide margin of safety and their antiemetic properties have made them useful. However, their use is limited by long durations of action, postoperative sedation, and occasional dysphoria.

Promethazine (Phenergan) produces prominent antihistiminic and anticholinergic effects. It is used for its sedative, antimetic, and drying properties. Hydroxyzine (Vistaril) is an antihistamine with properties similar to promethazine. Intramuscular injections of hydroxyzine can be painful if not properly performed. Droperidol (Inapsine) produces sedative and antiemetic effects. Dysphoria caused by excessive doses of droperidol can be quite bothersome.

## Cimetidine

Gastric contents in the fasting preoperative patient are routinely quite acidic (i.e., pH less than 2.5). Should a patient vomit during the induction of anesthesia, and such vomitus be aspirated into the lungs, severe pneumonitis can result and can lead to respiratory failure. A mortality rate of about 28% will result from aspiration of gastric secretions with a pH value of less than 2.5 (James et al., 1984). Anticholinergics do little to increase acidity. Antacids have inconsistent effects on gastric acidity and tend to increase gastric volume. Antacid particles can cause severe pulmonary complications if they are vomited and aspirated.

The drug cimetidine (Tagamet) is a histamine $H_2$-receptor antagonist which reduces the ability of histamine to produce secretions of gastric juice with a low pH. It therefore reliably increases gastric pH to above 5.0 if given at least 2 hours before anesthesia. Aspiration of gastric contents at this more neutral pH level results in a much milder pneumonitis, with decreased morbidity and mortality. The current recommended dose of cimetidine is 300 mg orally the evening before surgery plus 300 mg intramuscularly 2 hours preoperatively (Figure 2-1). See Hodgkinson et al. (1983), Moir (1983), and Solanki et al. (1984) for further discussion of cimetidine.

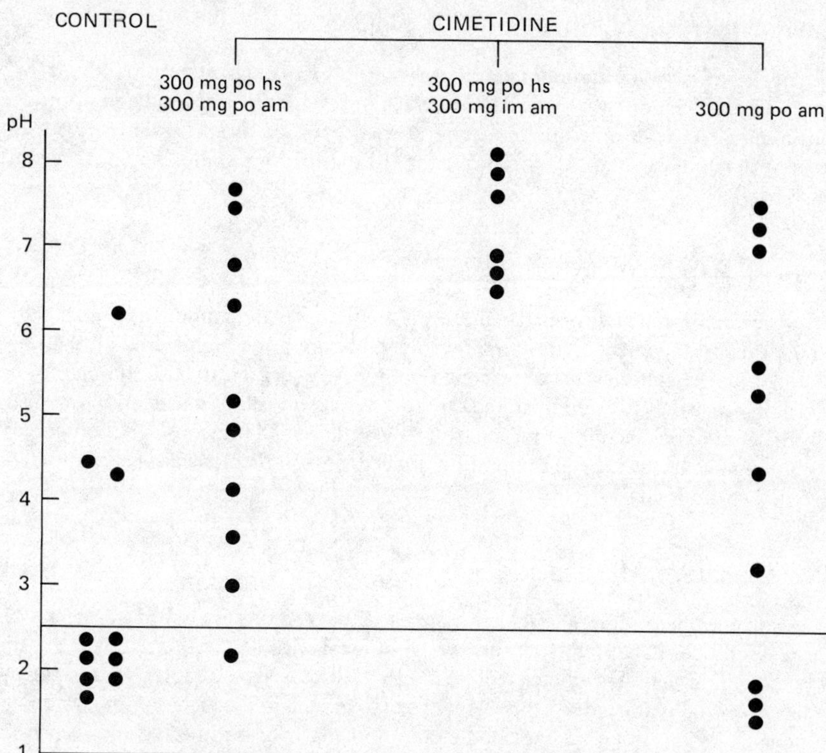


**Figure 2-1.** Distribution of gastric aspirate pH values in control and cimetidine-treated patients. Note that patients receiving cimetidine orally at bedtime and intramuscularly had the most consistent elevations in gastric pH.
(From Weber, L., and Hirschman, C.A. *Anesth. Analg.* 58:426–27, 1979).

## Timing of Premedication

Although "premedication" usually refers to a drug administered approximately 1 hr before surgery, premedication may be administered at other times before anesthesia is induced.

### Bedtime Sedative

The night before surgery, patients are usually apprehensive about their upcoming surgery, and their apprehension may induce wakefulness. In addition, hospital surroundings tend to make normal sleep difficult. During the preanesthetic visit, the anesthesiologist should discuss this with the patient; such discussion often has a calming effect. In addition, a bedtime sedative can be ordered according to the patient's desires. An orally administered benzodiazepine, such as flurazepam (15–30 mg), may help alleviate insomnia.

### Early Morning Medication

Sedatives are often administered early on the morning of surgery, about 1–2 hours before the induction of anesthesia. Such orally administered sedatives produce a calming effect with only minimal respiratory depression or anticholinergic side effects. A benzodiazepine, such as diazepam (10 mg) or lorazepam (2 mg), is recommended.

### On-call Medication

The traditional view of premedications are that they are administered "on call." Under this arrangement, drugs are preordered but are not administered until an operating nurse telephones, usually about 1 hour before surgery, to request that they be given. Because they are administered on short notice, on-call premedications are usually ordered to be given intramuscularly. As was discussed previously, the efficacy of such premedications is open to question. Indeed, on-call premedications can often be avoided without adverse effect.

### Perioperative Medication

The anesthesiologist should greet the patient in the surgery holding area and offer reassurances (Chapter 1). A skin wheal of local anesthetic is placed over the site where the intravenous catheter will be inserted (discussed in Chapter 4), and the intravenous fluid is started. At this point, a sedative such as diazepam (5 mg) or a narcotic such as morphine (5 mg) or fentanyl (50 mg) can be injected intravenously before the patient is taken to the operating room. These drugs should be injected slowly and the patient observed continuously thereafter by the anesthesiologist. Intravenous diazepan can sometimes be painful; a small dose of intravenous lidocaine (1–2 mL of 1%) preceding the diazepan may reduce the pain.

## Summary and Conclusions

1. Pharmacologic agents need not be prescribed routinely as premedications for all patients.
2. Anticholinergic agents are not indicated for the vast majority of patients. Their use is accompanied by significant patient discomfort. If needed, they can be given intravenously shortly before the induction of anesthetia.
3. Narcotics can produce respiratory depression, which may place the patient at risk. Patients given opiates should be closely observed, and narcotic antagonists should be readily available.
4. Sedative-hypnotic drugs have little significant advantage over a placebo in relieving patient anxiety. However, they are antiepileptic and substitute for alcohol in alcohol-dependent patients. When used, the oral route of administration is preferred.

5. Cimetidine premedication is effective in neutralizing gastric acid and decreasing gastric volume, thereby reducing the risk of pulmonary complications if vomitus is aspirated.
6. When a patient requires medications prior to the induction of anesthesia, they can easily and safely be administered intravenously just prior to surgery.
7. A concerned, informative, reassuring preoperative visit by the anesthesiologist is the best way to reduce anxiety.
8. A convenient protocol for pharmacologic premedication for an adult patient is as follows:
   (a) Cimetidine, 300 mg orally at bedtime the night before surgery.
   (b) Flurazepam, 15–30 mg orally at bedtime if needed for sleep.
   (c) Diazepam (10 mg) or lorazepam (2 mg) orally 1–2 hours before anesthesia.
   (d) Cimetidine, 300 mg intramuscularly 2 hours before anesthesia.
   (e) Morphine (0.05–0.1 mg/kg) and/or scopolamine (0.3–0.5 mg) intramuscularly "on call" if profound preoperative analgesia and amnesia are desired.

## *Readings and References*

Bynum, L.J., and Pierce, A.K. 1976. Pulmonary aspiration of gastric contents. *Am. Rev. Resp. Dis.* 114:1229.

Egbert, L.D.; Battit, G.E.; Turndorf, H., et al. 1963. The value of the preoperative visit by an anesthetist. *J. Am. Med. Assoc.* 185:553.

Forrest, W.H.; Brown, C.R.; and Brown, B.W. 1977. Subjective responses to six common preoperative medications. *Anesthesiology* 47:241–47.

Hodgkinson, R.; Glassenberg, R.; Joyce, T.H., et al. 1983. Comparison of cimetidine (Tagamet) with antacid for safety and effectiveness in reducing gastric acidity before elective cesarean section. *Anesthesiology* 59:86–90.

James, C.F.; Modell, J.H.; Gibbs, C.P., et al. 1984. Pulmonary aspiration—effects of volume and pH in the rat. *Anesth. Analg.* 63:665–68.

Leigh, J.M.; Walker, J.; and Janaganathan, P. 1977. Effect of preoperative anesthetic visit on anxiety. *Br. Med. J.* 2:987–89.

Mirakhur, R.K. 1979. Anticholinergic drugs. *Br. J. Anaesth.* 51:671.

Moir, D.D. 1983. Cimetidine, antacids, and pulmonary aspiration (editorial). *Anesthesiology* 59:81–83.

Ominsky, A.J. 1979. Premedication in the anxious patient (lecture 131). In: *Thirtieth annual refresher course lectures.* 1979 Annual Meeting of the American Society of Anesthesiologists. Park Ridge, Ill.: American Society of Anesthesiologists.

Solanki, D.R.; Suresh, M.; and Ethridge, H.C. 1984. The effects of intravenous cimetidine and metoclopramide on gastric volume and pH. *Anesth. Analg.* 63:599–602.

Stoelting, R.K. 1978. Gastric fluid pH in patients receiving cimetidine. *Anesth. Analg.* 57:675.

———. 1981. Psychological preparation and preoperative medication. In: *Anesthesia.* Miller, R.D., editor. New York: Churchill Livingstone, pp. 95–105.

# II

# PREPARATION FOR ANESTHESIA

# 3. Introduction to the Operating Room

## Organization of an Operating Room

Suites of operating rooms (ORs) are arranged in several ways. A currently popular and quite efficient design is a suite with the operating rooms arranged in a cluster pattern around a central core area (Figure 3-1). A patient-staff corridor is located on the outer perimeter. Before entering the OR suite, all personnel should be properly attired. Shoes and all exposed hair should be covered. A face mask must be worn whenever one enters either an OR or the central core area.

Individual ORs have physical layouts which vary little from hospital to hospital. Most are about 400 square feet in size. Other rooms requiring bulky equipment (such as heart-lung machines for cardiac surgery) may be up to 800 square feet in size. The equipment setup of a general surgical suite is illustrated in Figure 3-2. Note the position of the anesthesia machine and anesthesia equipment cart, both located at the head of the operating table, with intravenous (I.V.) support poles and suction bottles in close proximity. (The operation of the table is discussed later in this chapter; the anesthesia machine is discussed in Chapter 4.)

## Patient Transport

The patient should be brought from the ward to the holding area of the operating suite by an attendant skilled in the handling of pharmacologically premedicated patients who might be anxious and frightened, and who might also be quite ill. In his or her hospital room, the patient should be carefully transferred from the bed to the litter, have his or her identity verified, and then be transported to the surgical holding area with all available medical records.

In the holding area, a nurse or the anesthesiologist should greet the patient with compassionate reassurance. The patient's identity should again be verified and, if possible, the patient should be challenged with questions designed to eliminate any risk of mistake (name of surgeon, planned procedure, etc.). The chart should be ex-

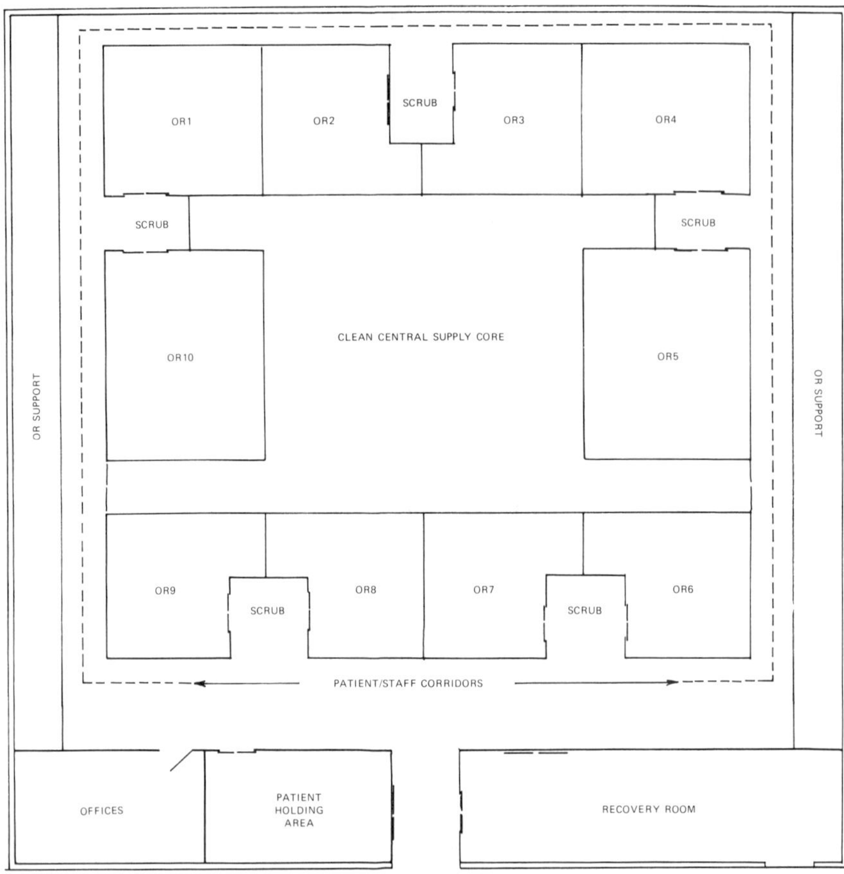


**Figure 3-1.** Schematic of a proposed suite of operating rooms (ORs).

amined for a signed surgical consent, laboratory results, completed history and physical examination, preoperative surgical and anesthesia notes, and the availability of blood products. The patient should be asked about the preoperative fasting period (6 hours of fasting is usually minimal). The mouth should be clear of all prostheses or chewing gum. All jewelry should be removed or covered.

If the patient appears apprehensive, and if time allows, the intravenous catheter (Chapter 4) can be inserted while the patient is in the holding area and sedative (i.e., diazepam, 2.5 mg increments) administered intravenously.

## The Anesthesia Record

While the patient is in the holding area, the anesthesiologist should start preparation of an anesthesia record (Figure 3-3) by writing on it the date, patient's name,

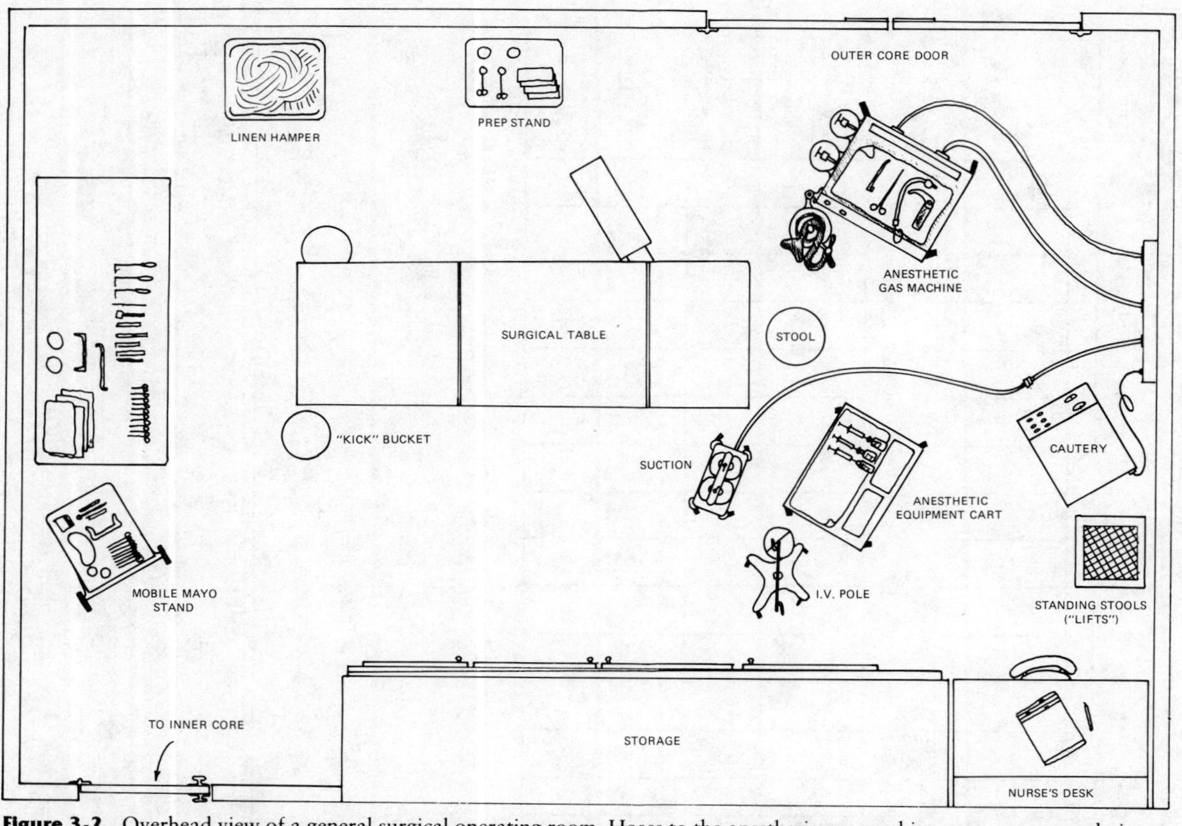


**Figure 3-2.** Overhead view of a general surgical operating room. Hoses to the anesthesia gas machine carry oxygen and nitrous oxide from central supply tanks through the wall-mounted gas outlet.

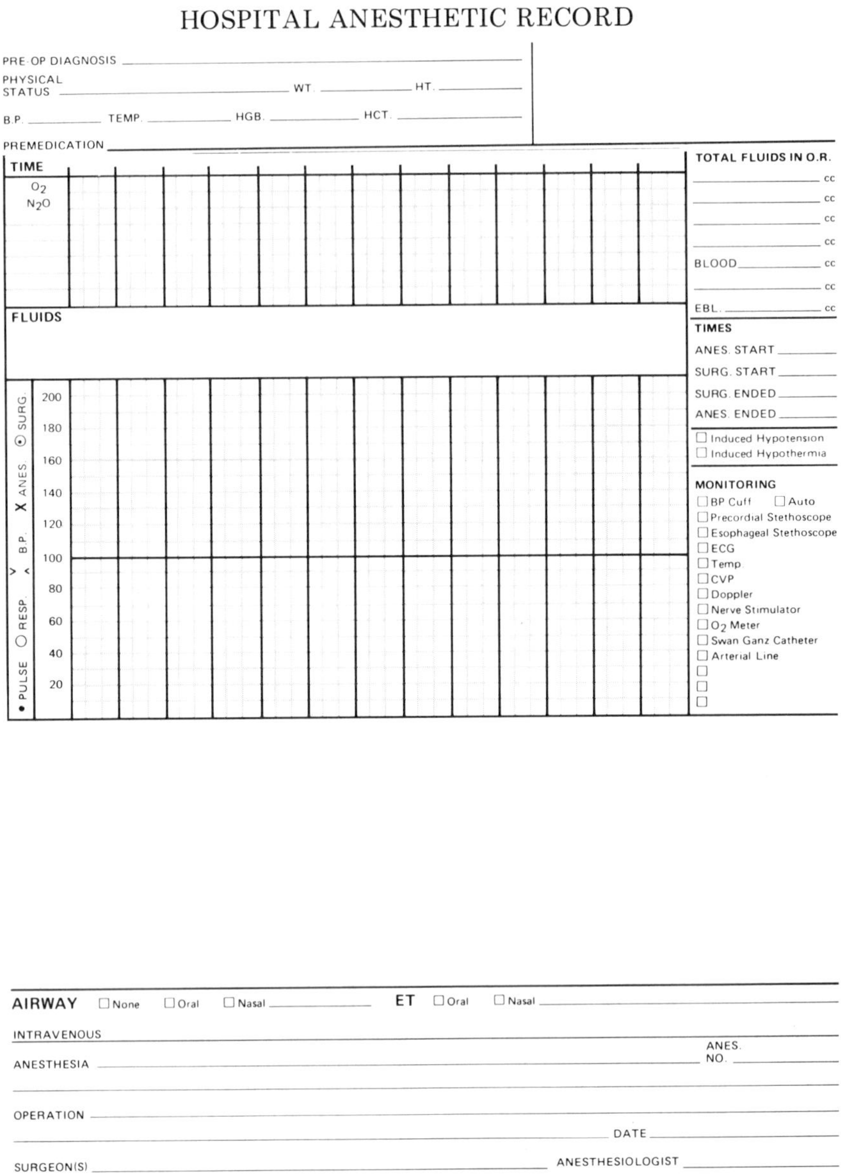

HOSPITAL ANESTHETIC RECORD

PRE-OP DIAGNOSIS ______
PHYSICAL STATUS ______ WT. ______ HT. ______
B.P. ______ TEMP. ______ HGB. ______ HCT. ______
PREMEDICATION ______

TIME
$O_2$
$N_2O$

FLUIDS

• PULSE ○ RESP. ∨ ∧ B.P. X ANES. ⊙ SURG.
200
180
160
140
120
100
80
60
40
20

TOTAL FLUIDS IN O.R.
______ cc
______ cc
______ cc
______ cc
BLOOD ______ cc
______ cc
EBL. ______ cc

TIMES
ANES. START ______
SURG. START ______
SURG. ENDED ______
ANES. ENDED ______

☐ Induced Hypotension
☐ Induced Hypothermia

MONITORING
☐ BP Cuff ☐ Auto
☐ Precordial Stethoscope
☐ Esophageal Stethoscope
☐ ECG
☐ Temp
☐ CVP
☐ Doppler
☐ Nerve Stimulator
☐ $O_2$ Meter
☐ Swan Ganz Catheter
☐ Arterial Line
☐
☐
☐

AIRWAY ☐ None ☐ Oral ☐ Nasal ______ ET ☐ Oral ☐ Nasal ______
INTRAVENOUS ______
ANESTHESIA ______ ANES. NO. ______
OPERATION ______
DATE ______
SURGEON(S) ______ ANESTHESIOLOGIST ______

**Figure 3-3.** A "typical" blank anesthesia record.

birth date, medical record identification number, any previous medications and their effects, the anesthesiologist's name, the surgeon's name, preoperative laboratory values of anesthesia significance, the preoperative diagnosis, concise but significant medical history (e.g., heart or lung disease, allergies, etc.), the planned surgical procedure, and the patient's preoperative ASA classification. Table 1-4 (Chapter 1) may fulfill these requirements if there is not sufficient room on the anesthesia record. The patient is then transported to an OR previously prepared by the anesthesiologist (an "Anesthesia Checklist" is presented in Chapter 4).

Following placement of appropriate monitors, including blood pressure cuff, ECG electrodes, and precordial stethescope (Chapter 5), preinduction vital signs are recorded on the anesthesia record, such recording continues at a maximum interval of 5 minutes until the patient leaves the OR after surgery. More frequent recording is done if the patient's condition so dictates. Commonly used symbols on the record are as follows:

| | | |
|---|---|---|
| V | Systolic blood pressure | |
| Λ | Diastolic blood pressure | |
| × | Mean blood pressure | |
| ● | Pulse rate | |
| ○ | Respiratory rate | |
| T | Body temperature | |
| × | Start of anesthesia | (indicated on bottom of record) |
| ʘ | Surgical incision | (indicated on bottom of record) |

The record shown in Figure 3-3 has two areas intended for listing the drugs administered. The space at the bottom of the page is for summarizing the drugs and anesthesia technique used, while the spaces on the left side of the page are used to list the doses and times of administration of all drugs and fluids administered. All drug doses, fluids, and the patient's vital signs continue in a time sequence across the page. Therefore, reviewing the chart, one can correlate alterations in vital signs with anesthesia induction, surgical incision, fluid alterations, or depth of anesthesia. There should also be ample space on the record to add other information about the surgery or the anesthetic that might be of importance.

One should be aware that the anesthetic record is the single most important legal and historical document recording intraoperative events. The record must be legible, complete, accurate, dynamic, and unaltered. Except in rare instances, the record should be completed as events occur rather than in an after-the-fact, retrospective fashion. Obviously, should one be in a crisis situation, the needs of the patient come first. Even then, the record should be completed as soon as possible.

An example of a completed record is shown in Figure 3-4. Review of this record may clarify some of the points discussed above. The patient whose record is shown is a male, about 23 years old (birthdate: March 14, 1959), classified by the anesthesiologist as ASA Class I. The patient had previously fractured his left ankle, undergone prior surgical repair, and is brought to surgery for removal of screws previously placed in the ankle. Premedication (diazepam, 10 mg orally) was judged satisfactory. Two anesthesiologists (staff and resident) and three surgeons (staff, senior resident, and junior resident) are listed. The lower section of the page indicates that the technique was that of inhalation anesthesia (halothane, nitrous oxide [Chapter 10]) administered through a semiclosed anesthesia circle with carbon dioxide absorber (SCCA) (see Chapter 4). Sodium thiopental (Pentothal) was used for induction of anesthesia. The details of the technique indicate that the patient was preoxygenated with 100% oxygen, then given two doses of thiopental, a 40 mg "test dose," followed by a 360 mg "sleep dose." Anesthesia was then maintained with 2% halothane in a mixture of nitrous oxide (3 L/min flow rate) and oxygen (2 L/min flow rate), all ad-

HOSPITAL ANESTHETIC RECORD

PRE-OP DIAGNOSIS S/P FRACTURED LEFT ANKLE

PHYSICAL STATUS ASA I WT. 85 kg HT. 5'-11"

B.P. 130/70 TEMP. 36.6 HGB. 14.3 HCT. 44.1

23 yo w ♂
PT. NO. 78 16 86
DATE OF BIRTH 03-14-59

PREMEDICATION DIAZEPAN 10mg p.o.

| TIME | $14^{15}$ | $14^{30}$ | X | $15^{00}$ | X | $15^{30}$ |
|---|---|---|---|---|---|---|
| $O_2$ | 5ℓ-2 | | | 5 | | |
| $N_2O$ | 3ℓ | | | 1 | | |
| Haloth. | 2% | | 1% | 0.8 | 1 | |
| Thio. | 40/360 | | | | | |

FLUIDS $D_5LR$

B.P. ∨ ∧ X ANES. ⊙ SURG. • PULSE ○ RESP. — 200, 180, 160, 140, 120, 100, 80, 60, 40, 20

X ⊙

TOTAL FLUIDS IN O.R.
Crystaloid 400 cc
BLOOD NONE cc
EBL 50 cc

TIMES
ANES. START $14^{15}$
SURG. START $14^{45}$
SURG. ENDED $15^{07}$
ANES. ENDED $15^{15}$

☐ Induced Hypotension
☐ Induced Hypothermia

MONITORING
☒ BP Cuff ☐ Auto
☒ Precordial Stethoscope
☐ Esophageal Stethoscope
☒ ECG
☒ Temp.
☐ CVP
☒ Doppler
☐ Nerve Stimulator
☒ $O_2$ Meter
☐ Swan Ganz Catheter
☐ Arterial Line

X = Pre oxygenate - thiopent 40/360
Mask with Halothane 2%/
$N_2O$ 3ℓ/$O_2$ 2ℓ.

Meds: NONE
Allergies: NONE
ROS: NON-SIG.

PAR
B.P. 140/90
P. 60/min.
R. 12/min.
COND. Satisfac.

AIRWAY ☐ None ☒ Oral ☐ Nasal ET ☐ Oral ☐ Nasal MASK - SCCA

INTRAVENOUS 18G Ⓛ arm - Thiopental

ANESTHESIA Halothane - $N_2O$ - $O_2$ / Spontaneous Ventilation ANES. NO. 2-670

OPERATION Removal of Screws from Ⓛ Ankle

DATE 11-7-82

SURGEON(S) D. Smith / B. Thompson / J. D'Niel ANESTHESIOLOGIST Chuu / Julien

**Figure 3-4.** A well-prepared and completed anesthetic record (see text for discussion).

ministered by face mask. At approximately 2:45 P.M., the halothane concentration was reduced to 1.0%. Monitors consisted of an ECG, blood pressure cuff with Doppler flowmeter probe, a precordial stethescope, and an oxygen analyzer (all discussed in Chapter 5). Anesthesia started at 2:15 P.M., with surgical incision at 2:45 P.M. Vital signs (blood pressure and heart rate) remained stable throughout the 1-hour anesthetic. Fluids administered consisted of 400 mL of $D_5LR$ (5% dextrose in lactated Ringer's solution). Estimated blood loss (EBL) was minimal. The patient's condition in the recovery room postoperatively was satisfactory, with blood pressure of 140/90 mm Hg, pulse of 60 beats/min, and respiratory rate of 12 breaths/min.

# Preparation and Positioning

## The Operating Table

Several types of operating tables may be found within a suite of operating rooms. These include the general operating table, an orthopedic table, and a urology table. Of these, the general operating table is most common, as use of the other two tables is restricted to special purposes which will not be elaborated upon here.

The general operating table is adjustable for height, and the top is usually divided into four sections to support the major body parts: head, back, thighs, and feet (Figure 3-5). A fifth section, the kidney rest, is located between the back and thigh sections. The head section is usually removable for situations where the patient is positioned further towards the foot of the bed and when the presence of the section might impede the anesthesiologist's access to the patient.

The position of each section is controlled by levers located at the head of the bed (Figure 3-6). The head section is moved up or down by means of the lever-lock located under the head section, while the remaining sections are controlled by a lever on the right side of the table (as viewed by an anesthesiologist standing at the head of the

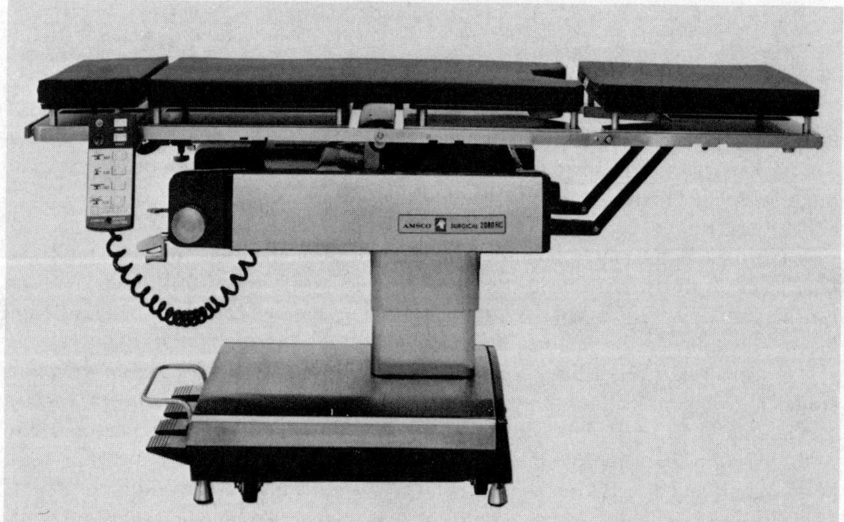

**Figure 3-5.** Surgical operating table (Photograph courtesy of American Sterilizer Company).

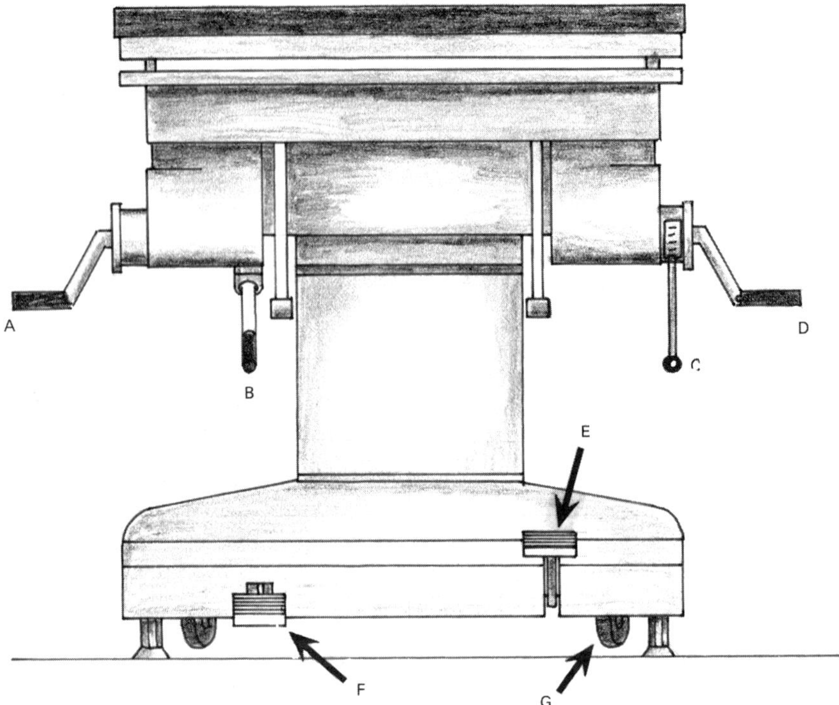


**Figure 3-6.** The surgical operating table as viewed from the head of the table. **A**, Lever controlling horizontal tilt of the table. **B**, Lever controlling elevation of the kidney rest. **C**, Multiselector bar for activating foot, lateral (side-to-side) rotation, back, and flex of the table. **D**, Lever regulating range of movement of multisector bar. **E**, Foot-operated lever for table elevation. **F**, Floor lock. **G**, Wheels, shown elevated off floor in table-lock situation.

bed). This lever allows the back and foot sections to be raised or lowered independently. The lever also allows the table to be "flexed" at the junction of the back and thigh sections. Finally, it permits the anesthesiologist to rotate the entire tabletop either to the right or to the left. A third lever, located on the left side of the table, controls the angle of the tabletop, allowing patient position to be varied from Trendelenburg's (head down) position to reverse Trendelenburg's (head up) position over a range of at least +20° to -20°. A ratchet located under the head of the bed raises and lowers the kidney rest. Finally, a floor lock is located near the floor.

Since surgical procedures are performed with the patient resting on the back, stomach, or side, there are three basic positions: supine (dorsal recumbent), prone, and lateral (Figure 3-7). Modifications of these positions are shown in Figures 3-8 to 3-10. It is important to note that each position results in a unique redistribution of body weight and affects circulation, tissue perfusion, and alveolar ventilation.

The supine position is most common. The patient is usually anesthesized while lying in this position and postural modification is made after the induction of anesthesia. Patients with masses in the abdomen (i.e., tumors, pregnant uterus) may experience hypotension when supine, due to compression of the inferior vena cava. Vena caval obstruction can often be relieved by placing a pad or roll under the right hip to shift the mass to the left (left lateral displacement). Obese patients may experience respiratory difficulties because of the tissue weight on the chest and the abdomen, compressing the thorax and displacing the diaphragm cephalad.

Placing a supine patient in Trendelenburg's position further displaces the diaphragm cephalad, increasing intrathoracic pressure, and decreasing functional residual capacity. Thus, alveolar ventilation may become inadequate in the anesthetized, spontaneously breathing patient, necessitating controlled ventilation (Chapter 10).

Patients in reverse Trendelenburg's position have respiratory function more like that in the sitting or the erect position. However, anesthetic-induced decreases in venous tone, together with the lack of muscle movement in the legs during anesthesia, may result in pooling of blood in both the legs and the pelvis, with decreased venous

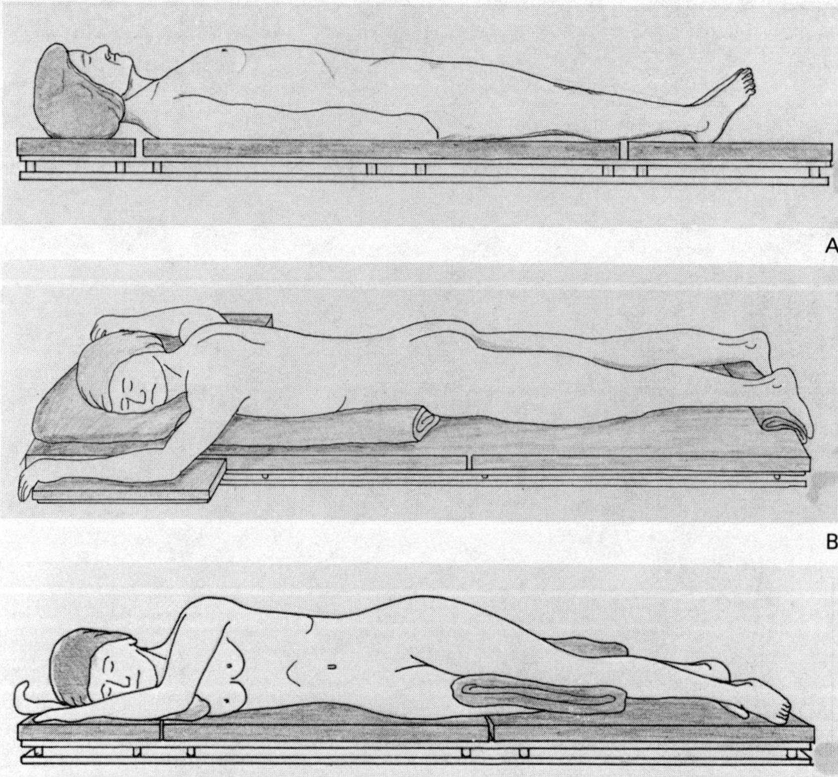


**Figure 3-7.** Positions on general surgical table.
**A,** Supine (dorsal recumbent).
**B,** Prone position (unsafe if arms above 90°).
**C,** Lateral position.

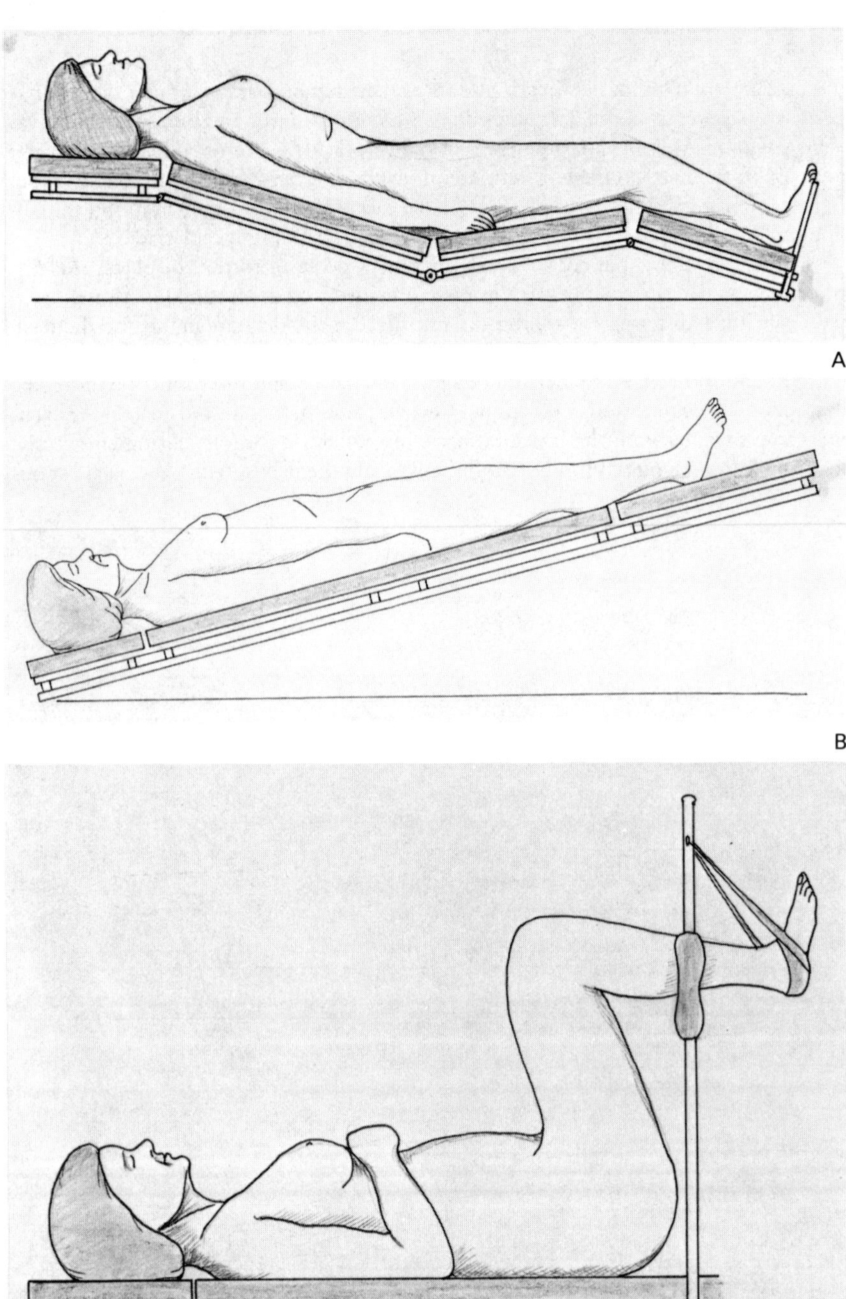


**Figure 3-8.** Modifications of the supine position. **A,** Reverse Trendelenburg's position with table flexed in a modified "lawn-chair" position. **B,** Trendelenburg's position. **C,** Lithotomy position.

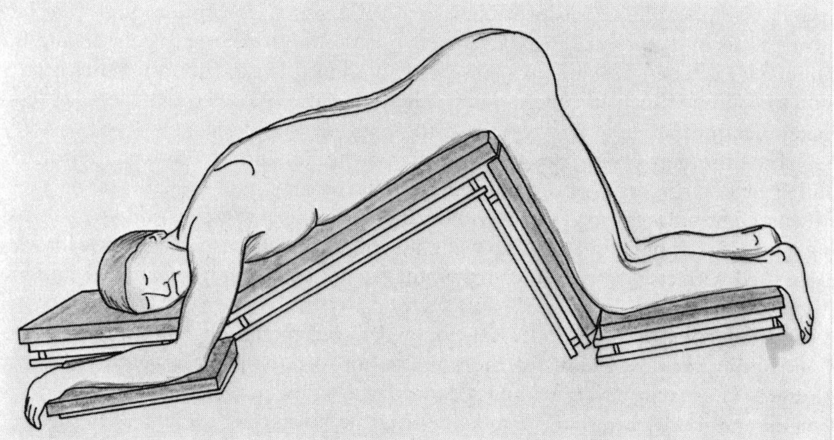

**Figure 3-9.** The "jackknife" modification of the prone position for ano-rectal surgery.

return to the heart. Venous return can be aided by the preoperative placement of support hose.

The sitting position (not illustrated) is associated with several problems, including peripheral pooling of blood and anesthetic-induced hypotension. More important, however, are problems associated with the surgery for which this position is commonly used (i.e., neurosurgery for posterior fossa craniotomies). The most wor-

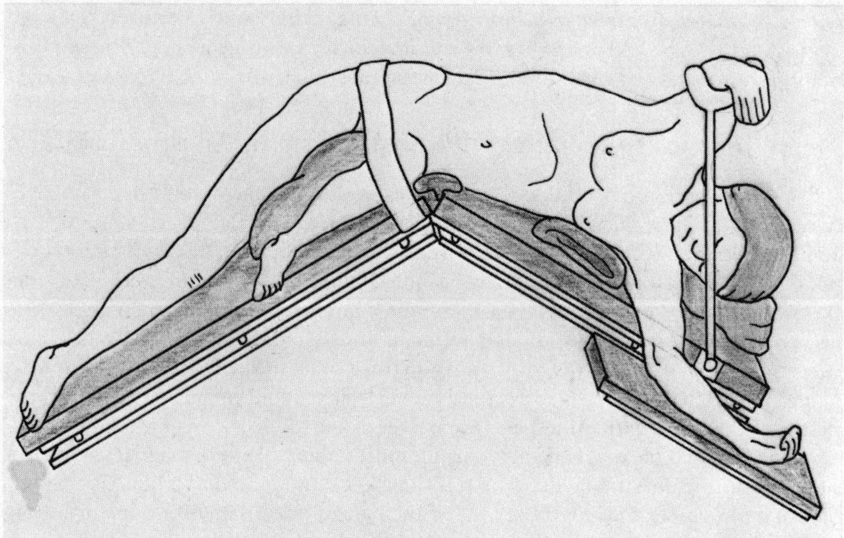

**Figure 3-10.** Modification of the lateral position for kidney surgery. Note the elevated kidney rest, axilliary and thigh pads, head support, and the support of the right arm to reduce brachial plexus stretching.

rysome complication of this procedure involves vascular absorption of air into lacerated veins in the posterior fossa. The air is carried into the right ventricle and the pulmonary arteries (air embolus). Severe ventilation:perfusion abnormalities can result. Detection of such air emboli is best achieved by use of a precordial Doppler flowmeter (Chapter 5).

The lithotomy position is widely used in obstetrics and gynecology, in urology, and in general surgery for procedures around the rectum. In obese patients, the pressure of the flexed legs forces intraabdominal contents against the diaphragm, increasing intrathoracic pressure and decreasing functional residual capacity. Nerve injuries associated with the legs pressing against the leg holders are not uncommon and are discussed later.

Patients placed in the prone position experience chest and abdominal compression. Respiratory excursions of the ribs are impeded, as is movement of the diaphragm. Thus, ventilation is impaired and respiration should be controlled during general anesthesia. Body rolls extending lengthwise from the shoulders to the iliac crest elevate the chest and abdomen and permit better diaphragmatic excursion. Nerve injuries associated with malpositioning of the armrest are discussed below. One must be careful of pressure on an eye when the patient's head is turned to the side. Compression of the optic nerve can result in blindness. Finally, salivary secretions freely roll out of the mouth, tending to moisten and loosen adhesive tape holding the endotracheal tube in place. Intraoperative, accidental extubation of patients lying prone can be disastrous, especially since reintubating a prone patient is extremely difficult.

In the lateral position, vena caval compression can follow positioning with the right side down, especially if the kidney rest is elevated. In addition, there is a marked increase in ventilation-perfusion mismatch, since the lower lung is well perfused but poorly ventilated and the upper lung is well ventilated but poorly perfused. Such patients should not be allowed to breathe spontaneously during general anesthesia; ventilation should be controlled by the anesthesiologist.

## Nerve Injuries Associated with Positioning in Anesthesia

The prevention of peripheral nerve injuries during general anesthesia involves two steps: (a) *awareness* that nerve injuries can occur as a result of stretching or compression, and (b) *inspection* to insure that nerve stretching or compression does not occur. Should injury occur, it may become obvious soon after anesthesia, or a delay of several days may be involved. Common complaints include pain, hyperesthesias, paresthesias, numbness, altered reflexes, and sympathetic loss. Recovery may occur over weeks or months, or damage may be permanent. Discussion of specific nerve injuries will be oriented to the bracheal plexus and its terminal nerves, the nerves of the lower extremities, and the nerves of the face.

The brachial plexus is the nerve trunk most vulnerable to damage from malpositioning during anesthesia. Stretching is the chief cause of injury. Abduction, external rotation, and extension of the arm to an angle of more than 60° to the operating table places the brachial plexus at risk for injury. Turning the head away from such an outstretched arm causes further stretching (Figure 3-11). Suspending the arm from an "ether screen" with the patient in the lateral position can stretch the brachial plexus around the clavicle and the pectoralis minor tendon. Finally, Trendelenburg's position (with shoulder braces used to prevent the patient from sliding down the operating table) can injure the plexus by pinching it between the clavicle and the first rib, especially if the arm is outstretched. Such patients should be positioned with the head in a neutral position, with the arms at the sides, and with any shoulder braces placed over the acromia (not over the clavicles); and these braces should be well padded.

The radial nerve may be injured as it traverses the forearm if the arm sags off the side of the operating table, or it may be injured in the midhumerus if it is pinched between the humerus and an ether screen (Figure 3-12).

The ulnar nerve can be injured when it is compressed between the edge of the

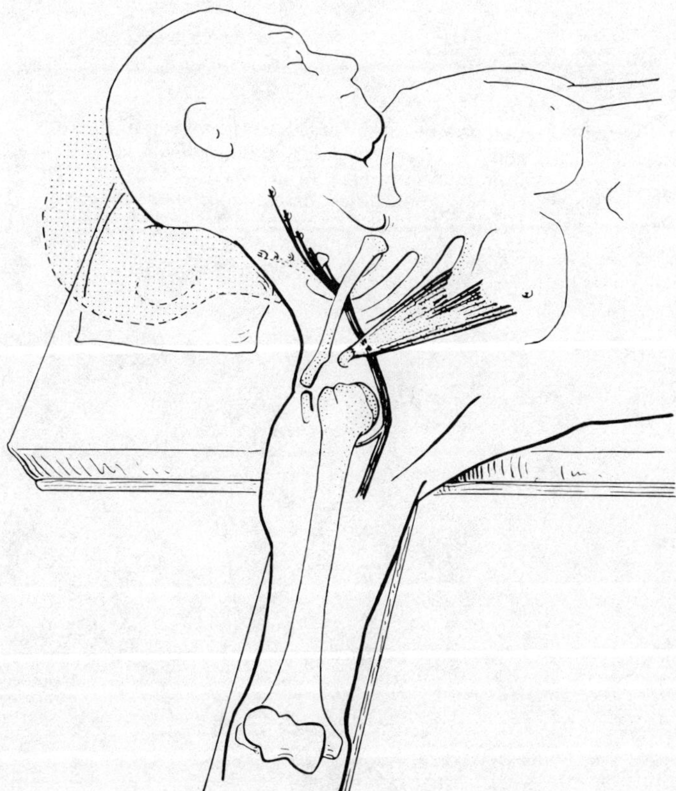

**Figure 3-11.** The brachial plexus is stretched when the arm is abducted, extended, and externally rotated, and the head is deviated to the opposite side. (Reproduced with permission from Britt, B. A.; Joy, N., and Mackay, M. B. 1983. Positioning trauma. In: *Complications in anesthesiology.* Orkin, F. K., and Cooperman, L. H., editors. Philadelphia: J. B. Lippincott, pp. 646–70.)

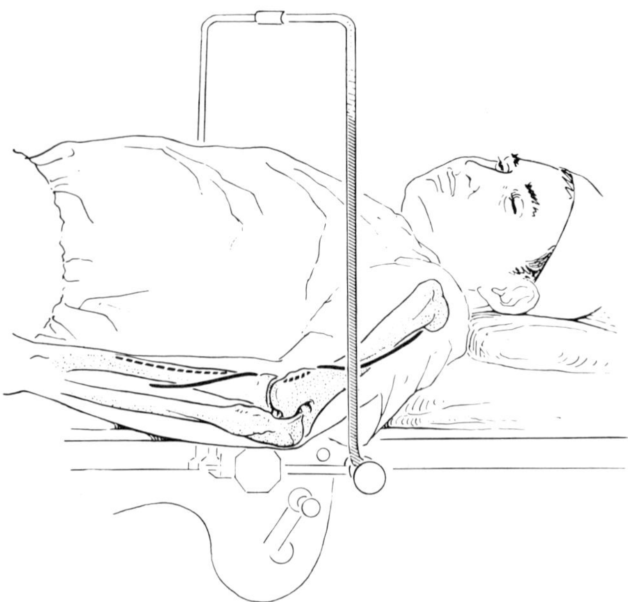

**Figure 3-12.** Compression of the radial nerve between the humerus and an "ether screen." (Reproduced with permission from Britt, B.A.; Joy, N.; and Mackay, M.B. 1983. Positioning trauma. In: *Complications in anesthesiology.* Orkin, F.K., and Cooperman, L.H., editors. Philadelphia: J. B. Lippincott, pp. 646–70.

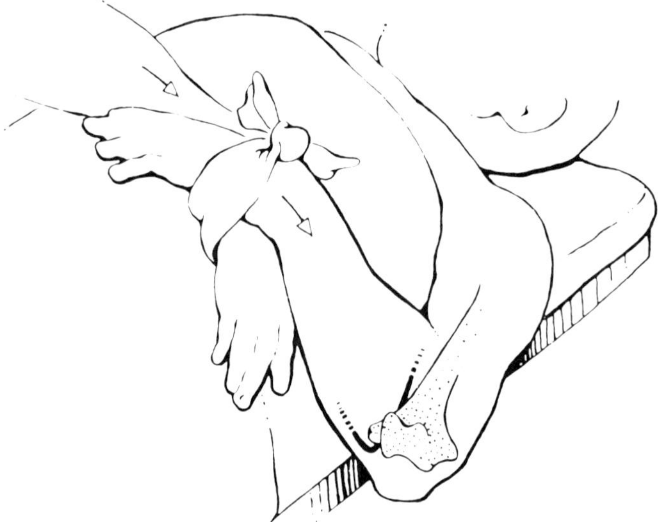

**Figure 3-13.** Ulnar nerve injury by compression of the medial epicondyle of the humerous and the edge of the operating table. (Reproduced with permission from Britt, B. A.; Joy, N.; and Mackay, M. B. 1983. Positioning trauma. In: *Complications in anesthesiology.* Orkin, F. K., and Cooperman, L. H., editors. Philadelphia: J. B. Lippincott, pp. 646–70.)

operating table and the medial epicondyle of the humerus. Such can occur when the elbow is allowed to sag off the table (Figure 3-13).

In the lower limbs, any of several nerves can be damaged when the patient is in the lithotomy position. The common peroneal nerve can be compressed as it travels around the head of the fibula at the tibial condyle and is pressed against a laterally placed leg brace. The saphenous nerve may be pinched between the leg brace and the medial aspect of the tibia if the foot is suspended lateral to the brace. The femoral nerve may be damaged by excessive external rotation of the leg, but, more commonly, by compression by the self-retaining retractors used during a pelvic laparotomy.

On the head, damage to the optic nerve can result from pressure on the eye when the patient is in the prone position with the eye pressing against the table or head-holder. Other nerves subject to injury include the supraorbital nerve (injured by pressure from endotracheal tube connectors) and the facial nerve (injured by excessive traction on the angle of the mandible).

When patients are placed in the lateral position, the head should be well supported on a pillow, pads should be placed between the knees (as well as between the feet), a roll should be placed below the axilla (an axillary roll), and the elbows should be well padded.

## *Readings and References*


Britt, B.A., and Gordon, R.A. 1964. Peripheral nerve injuries associated with anesthesia. *Can. Anesth. Soc. J.* 11:514–36.

Britt, B.A.; Joy, N.; and Mackay, M.B. 1983. Positioning trauma. In: *Complications in anesthesiology.* Orkin F.K., and Cooperman, L.H., editors. Philadelphia: J.B. Lippincott, pp. 646–70.

Martin, J.T. 1978. *Positioning in anesthesia and surgery.* Philadelphia: W.B. Saunders.

Miller, R.D. 1981. The immediate preinduction period. In: *Anesthesia.* Miller, R.D., editor. New York: Churchill Livingstone, pp. 107–14.

# 4. Anesthesia Apparatus

Anesthesiology requires certain specialized equipment. The important equipment used in anesthesia consists of:

1. The anesthesia machine
2. Intubation apparatus
3. Equipment for inserting intravenous and intraarterial lines
4. Patient-monitoring equipment

The first three of these are discussed in this chapter. Equipment for patient monitoring is discussed in Chapter 5.

## The Anesthesia Machine

The anesthesia machines commonly used in operating rooms all function in much the same way, although they do not all look alike, and their principles of operation can be easily understood. A typical machine is illustrated in Figure 4-1.

The anesthesia machine consists of two parts: a system for metering and mixing anesthetic gases and vapors, and a system for delivering this mixture to the patient.

The basic elements of gas-metering and gas-mixing systems are as follows:

1. A source of gases
2. A source of the volatile liquid anesthetics
3. A means of metering and controlling the delivery of gases and vapors
4. Safety devices
5. A common outlet for delivery of gases and vapors to the breathing circuit

The two gases commonly used in anesthesia are nitrous oxide ($N_20$) and oxygen ($0_2$). In most hospitals, these two gases are piped into each operating room from central storage cylinders located outside the operating suites. They are usually supplied at a pressure of about 50 pounds per square inch (psi) and are connected to the

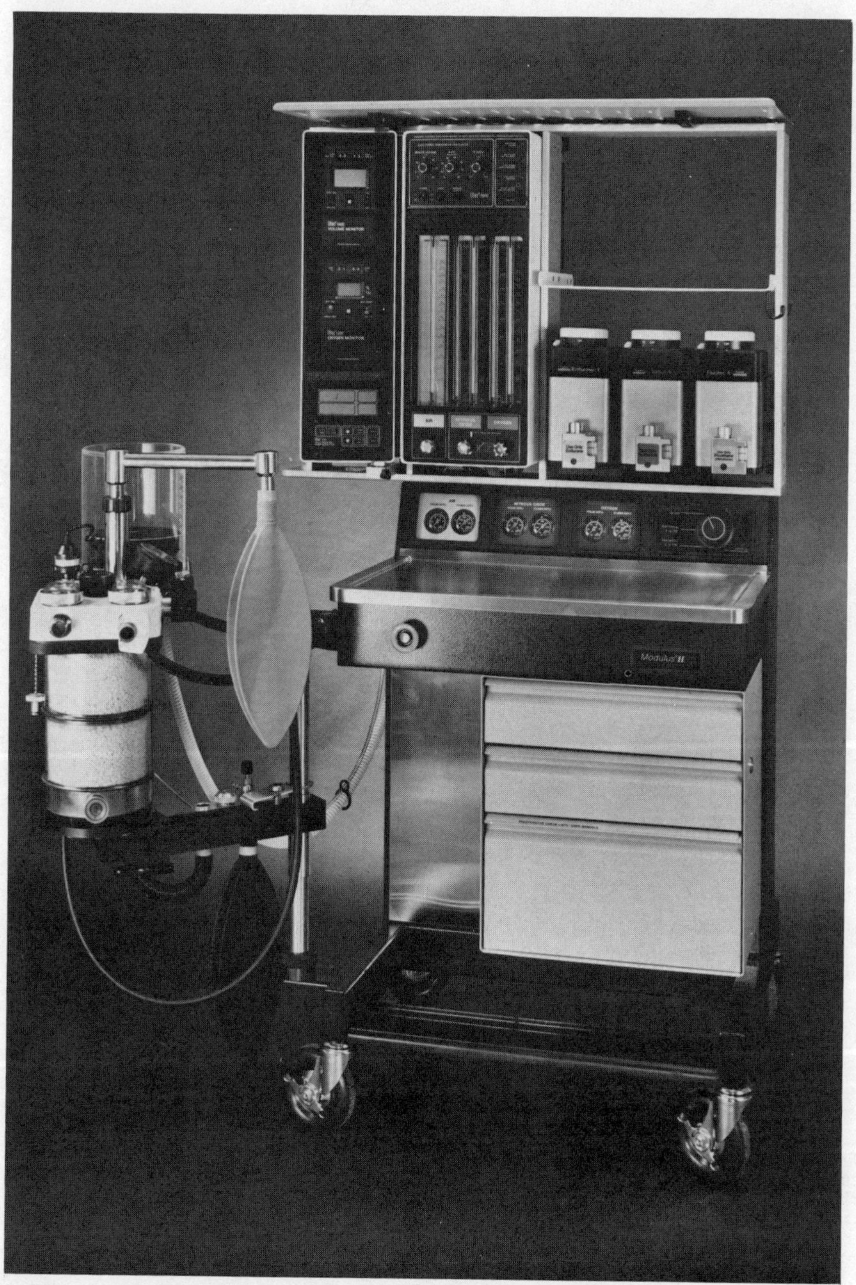

**Figure 4-1.** The Modulus II Anesthesia Machine (courtesy of Ohio Medical Products, a division of the BOC Group, Inc.).

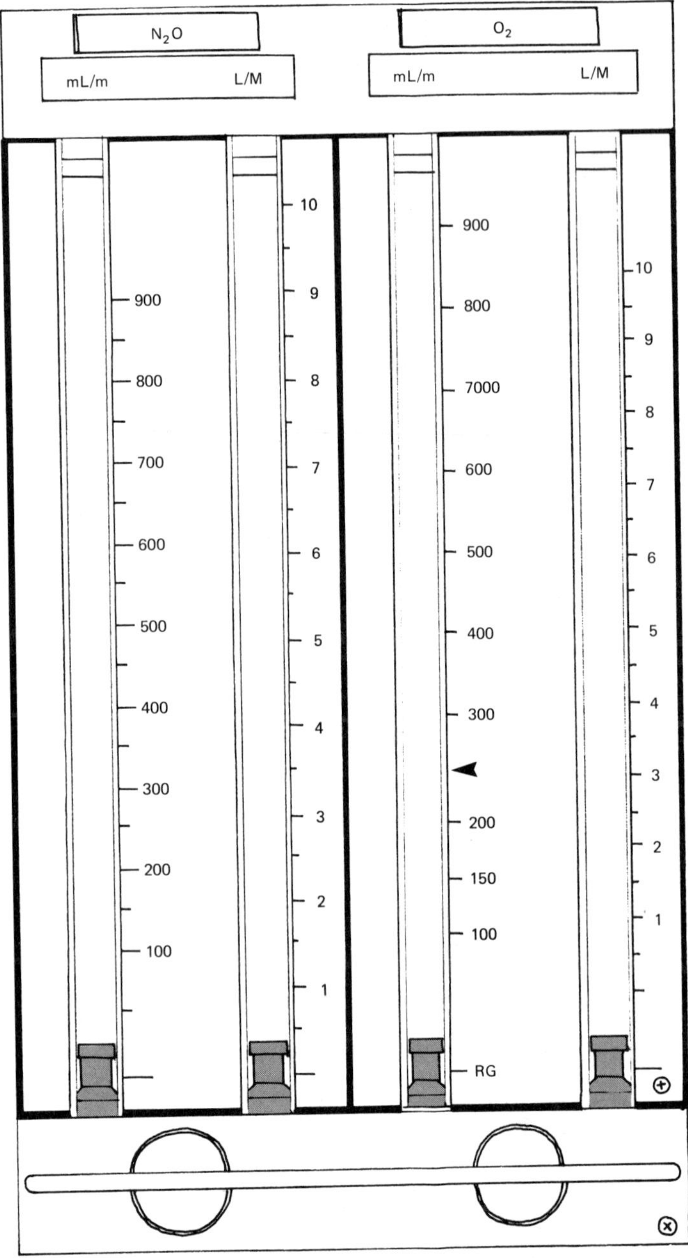


**Figure 4-2.** A, Drawing of nitrous oxide ($N_2O$) and oxygen ($O_2$) flowmeters, each with dual fine and course flowtubes.

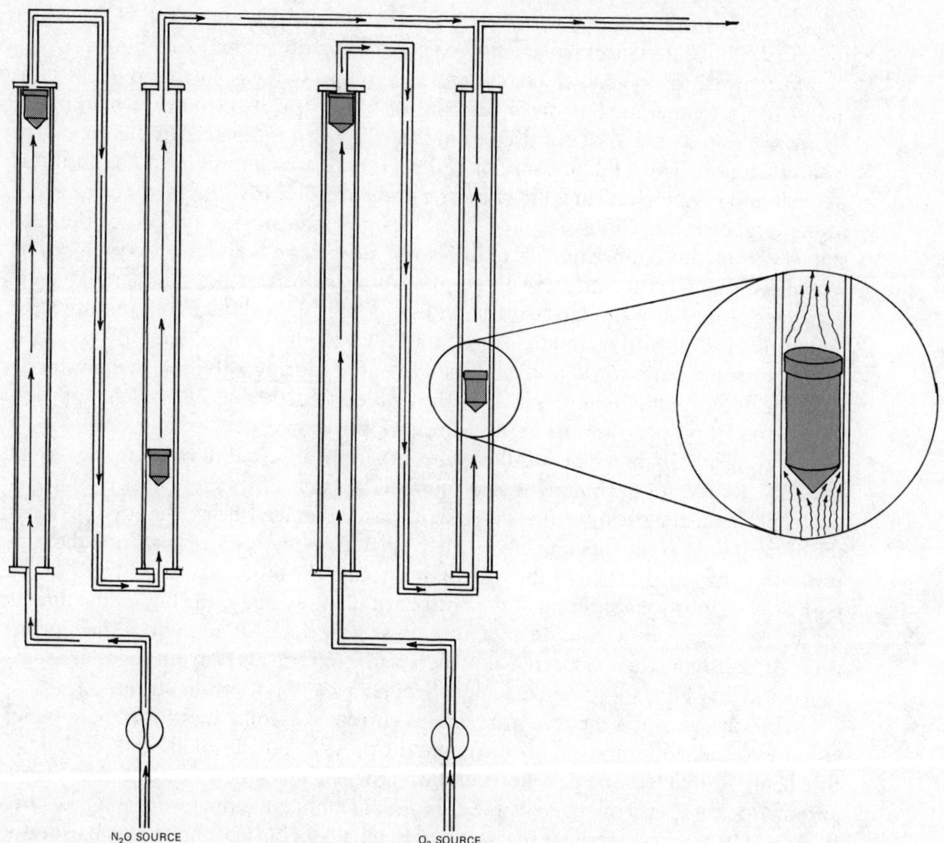


**Figure 4-2. *(continued)*** B, Schematic diagram of the series function of each dual flow-tube. In operation, the left, or fine tube, records low flows (usually up to about 1 L/min) until the float in the tube reaches the upper limit of the tube. Flows above this amount cause the float in the right, or course flow tube, to rise in proportion to the rate of gas flow. The flows through the $N_2O$ and $O_2$ flow-meters then combine before delivery to the patient.

anesthesia machine by hoses fitted with a non-interchangeable connector that is specific for each gas.

Because central supplies of the gases may occasionally fail, auxillary cylinders of oxygen and nitrous oxide are mounted on the sides or back of the anesthesia machine for emergency use. The auxillary cylinders are usually of the "E" type. Oxygen-containing "E" cylinders are painted green (in the U.S.A.) and, when full, contain 625 L of compressed oxygen, with a tank pressure of 2200 psi. The student should note that in the case of oxygen, the gauge pressure is proportional to the volume of oxygen in the cylinder. As oxygen is used, the pressure falls proportionately. Thus, when the cylinder is half-full, it contains 312.5 L. At a flow rate of 2 L/min, a full "E" cylinder (625 L, 2200 psi pressure) will supply oxygen for slightly more than 5 hours.

In contrast to oxygen, which is stored as a compressed gas, nitrous oxide is a liquid at room temperature under a pressure of 750 psi in its cylinder, which in the U.S.A. is painted blue. As gas is used from the cylinder, it is replaced by gas vaporized from the liquid. Thus, the pressure of 750 psi is maintained until most (about 80%) of the liquid is vaporized, at which time the pressure falls rather rapidly. The pressure in the nitrous oxide cylinders, therefore, does not indicate the amount of the substance within. Since more nitrous oxide can be stored as a liquid than oxygen can be stored as a gas, there is a greater volume of nitrous oxide in an "E" cylinder than there is oxygen stored in a similar cylinder. Indeed, a full "E" cylinder contains approximately 1600 L of nitrous oxide. Thus, at a flow rate of 3 L/min, one "E" tank will supply nitrous oxide for about 9 hours. Pressure-reducing valves in the anesthesia machine decrease the high pressures in the cylinders (2200 and 750 psi) to approximately the 50 psi pressures from the central supply source.

The anesthesia machine has flowmeters that are adjusted to regulate the rate of gas flow desired for each patient (see Figure 4-2). Each flowmeter consists of a vertically positioned glass tube. It is tapered, its inside diameter being slightly smaller at the bottom than at the top, and it contains a float. Anesthetic gases pass from the supply source into the bottom of the tube, exit through the top, and are delivered to the patient. The more gas entering at the bottom of the flowmeter, the higher the float is pushed by the gas flow, and the more gas flows past the float and out of the tapered tube. After leaving their respective flowmeters, the oxygen and nitrous oxide are combined and leave the anesthesia machine through a small port on the front.

The vapors of the three volatile liquids currently used in anesthesia, halothane, enflurane, and isoflurane (Figure 4-3), join the flows of nitrous oxide and oxygen before being supplied to the patient from the anesthesia machine. Although the volatile anesthetics are stored on the machine as liquids at ambient temperature and pressure, they must be vaporized before the patient can inhale them. The anesthesia machine is therefore equipped with vaporizers in which gas comes into intimate contact with the volatile liquid anesthetic. The gas exiting from the vaporizer is nearly saturated with anesthetic. Two types of anesthetic vaporizers are in common use: the copper kettle and the precalibrated, temperature-compensated vaporizer.

In the *copper kettle vaporizer* (Figure 4-4), one of the volatile anesthetics is added through a filling spout on the kettle, and the kettle is tightly capped. A measured amount of oxygen is delivered through a separate flowmeter to the kettle, and is bubbled through the anesthetic liquid. Intimate gas-liquid contact is achieved by passing the gas through a sintered bronze (Porex) disk to form very small bubbles that produce maximal vaporization efficiency by providing a large surface for the gas-liquid interface.

The concentration of anesthetic vapor can be calculated from the vapor pressure of the anesthetic at the temperature divided by the atmospheric pressure. Thus:

$$\%\ \text{vapor} = \frac{\text{vapor pressure}}{\text{atmospheric pressure}} \times 100$$

Note that vapor pressure is dependent on temperature, since heat is required for the change of a liquid to its gaseous state.

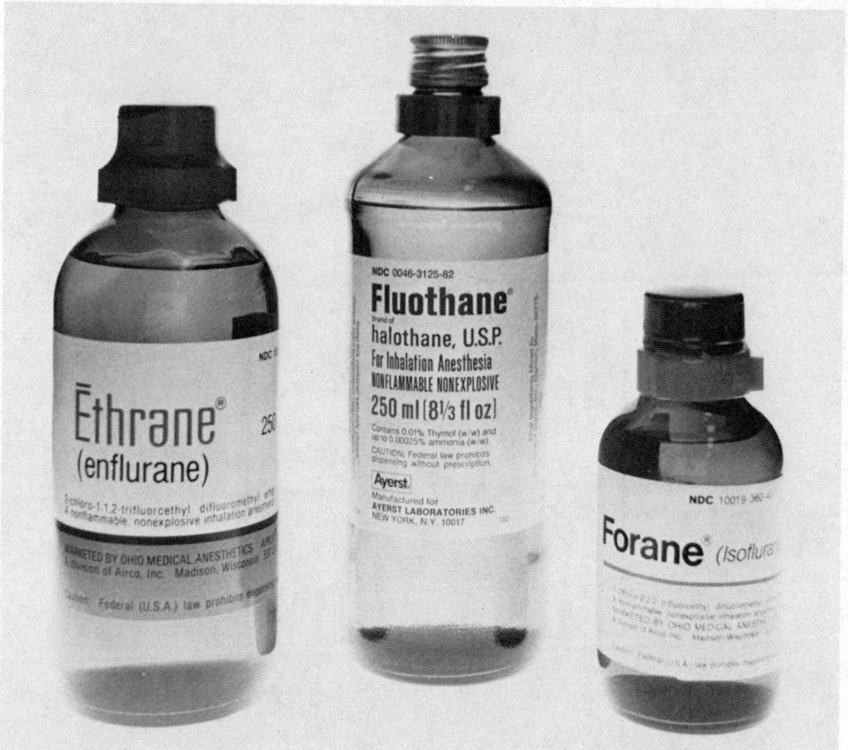


**Figure 4-3.** The three volatile liquid anesthetics currently used in the U.S.

The vapor pressure of both halothane and isoflurane at room temperature is approximately 240 mm Hg, or about 33% of atmospheric pressure. Thus, 33% of the gas leaving the copper kettle is halothane or isoflurane and 67% is oxygen. For example, if 100 mL/min of oxygen is passed through a copper kettle vaporizer, the mixture exiting the kettle will be two-third oxygen and one-third vapor (i.e., 100 mL of oxygen and 50 mL of vapor). Thus, each 100 mL of oxygen entering the kettle will add 50 mL of vapor, delivering 150 mL of gas.

The concentration of volatile anesthetic vapor exiting from the gas machine and delivered to the patient is calculated as the volume of vapor delivered per minute divided by the total gas flow. The latter includes the flow through the kettle plus the direct flow of oxygen and nitrous oxide. Thus:

$$\text{\% vapor delivered} = \frac{\text{mL of vapor}}{\text{total gas flow}} \times 100$$

If oxygen and nitrous oxide from the flowmeters total 5 L/min, the bubbling of 100 mL/min of oxygen through the vaporizer will yield a vapor concentration of approximately 1% halothane or isoflurane.

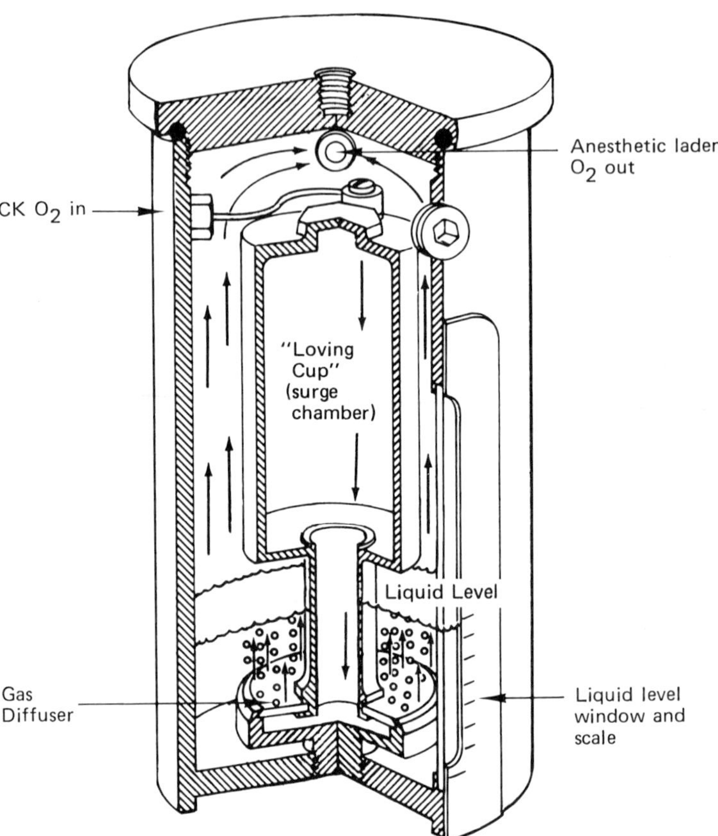


**Figure 4-4.** Schematic diagram of the copper kettle vaporizer. Oxygen enters the inlet on the side of the kettle (CK $O_2$ in), travels to a "loving cup," which dissipates the effect of sudden surges of gas, passes downwards then up through a sintered bronze disk (gas diffuser). The resultant bubbles of oxygen rise through the anesthetic liquid and the saturated vapor which results exits through the exhaust port (anesthetic laden $O_2$ out). This vapor is eventually diluted by joining the $N_2O$ and $O_2$ gas flows from the flowmeter (Figure 4-2B) before delivery to the patient (drawing courtesy of the Foregger Company).

Thus, for halothane and isoflurane:

$$\% \text{ vapor delivered} = \frac{50 \text{ mL}}{5150 \text{ mL}} \times 100 \cong 1\%$$

The vapor pressure of enflurane at room temperature is approximately 180 mm Hg, or about 25% atmospheric pressure. Bubbling 100 mL/min of oxygen through a copper kettle filled with enflurane will yield a mixture that is 25% enflurane (i.e.,

33.3 mL/min). Thus, each 100 mL of oxygen entering the kettle will add 33.3 mL of enflurane vapor, delivering 133.3 mL of gas. Adding this 133.3 mL to a 3 L/min total gas flow would yield approximately a 1% concentration of enflurane inhaled. Thus:

$$\% \text{ enflurane delivered} = \frac{33.3 \text{ mL}}{3/33 \text{ mL}} \times 100 \cong 1\%$$

Therefore, beginners in anesthesia might find it convenient to use a total gas flow of 5 L of oxygen and nitrous oxide (2 L and 3 L respectively) when using halothane or isoflurane in order to simplify calculation of delivered concentrations of these potent anesthetic agents. Similarly, when using enflurane, a total gas flow of 3 L of oxygen and nitrous oxide (1 L and 2 L respectively) will simplify calculations for this agent. Since the partial pressure is dependent on temperature, increases in temperature will increase the partial pressure, and thus the amount of liquid entering the gaseous phase. At a temperature of 30 C, the vapor pressure of these volatile anesthetics is approximately double that at 20 C, and thus their concentration in the inspired mixture will double.

The *precalibrated, agent specific, temperature-compensated vaporizers* (Figure 4-5) do not require making the above calculations. With these devices, the desired percentage of anesthetic vapor is obtained by turning a knob that alters the amount of gas flowing either through the vaporizer or through a bypass directly to the patient. These vaporizers are specific for individual volatile anesthetics, and provide relatively constant concentrations of vapor over wide variations in flow rate and over fairly wide extremes in room temperature. The settings on the vaporizer are calibrated in volume percent, with a temperature-compensating device insuring accurate output over commonly used flow rates.

After the mixture of oxygen, nitrous oxide, and anesthetic vapor leaves the anesthetic machine, it is delivered to an anesthesia breathing circuit. There are several

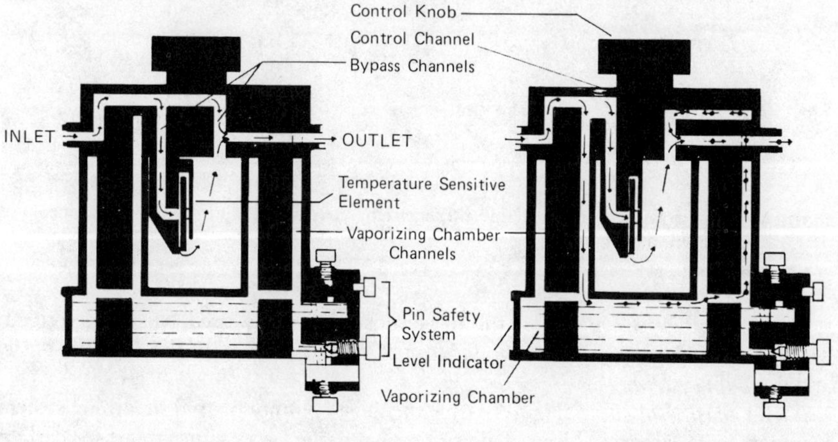


**Figure 4-5.** Schematic drawing of a precalibrated, temperature-compensated, agent-specific (halothane) vaporizer, the Fluotee Mark III. (Figure from Dorsch, J. A. and Dorsch, S. E. 1975. *Understanding Anesthesia Equipment*. Baltimore: Williams & Wilkins.)

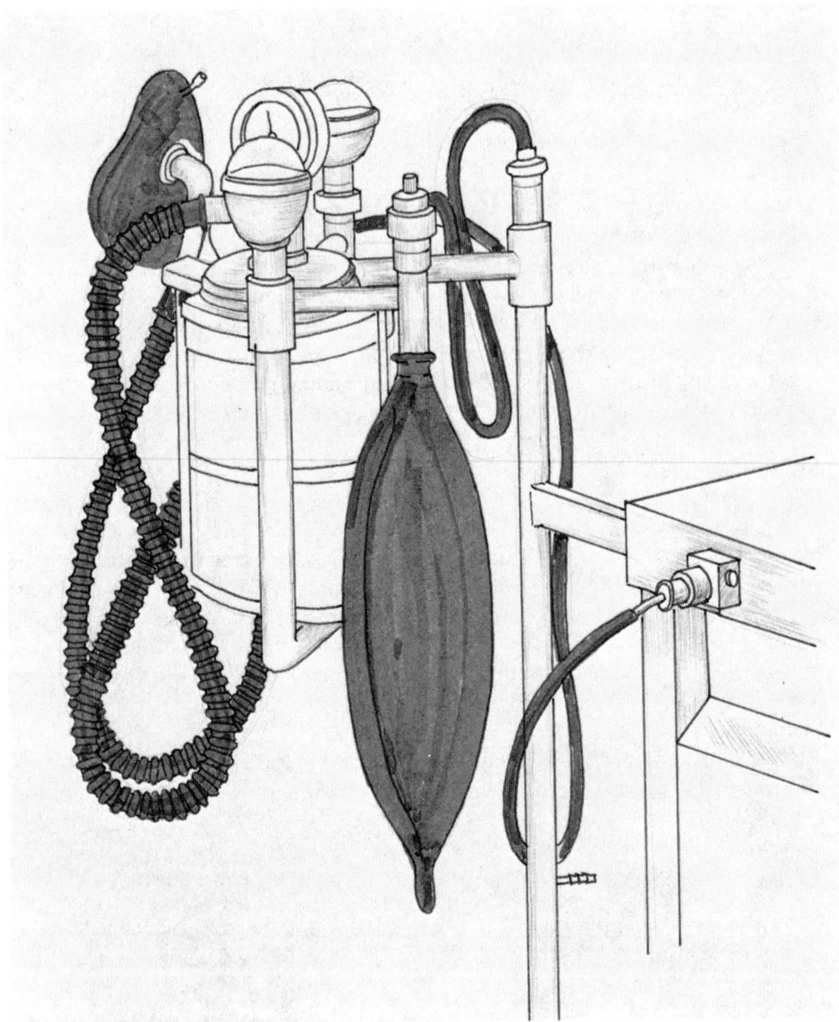

**Figure 4-6.** Illustration of a typical anesthesia circle (see text and Figure 4-7 for description of components).

types of breathing circuits, but the three most commonly used will be described. These are the *anesthesia circle, the Jackson-Rees modification of the Ayre's T-piece,* and the *Bain system.*

The *anesthesia circle* (Figure 4-6) is the most commonly used breathing system for adults and larger children. This system is unique because it contains a carbon dioxide absorber which allows for the partial rebreathing of expired gases. Such rebreathing would not be possible without the absorber since carbon dioxide would accumulate and be toxic.

Figure 4-7 illustrates the design of the anesthesia circle. As shown, the anesthesia

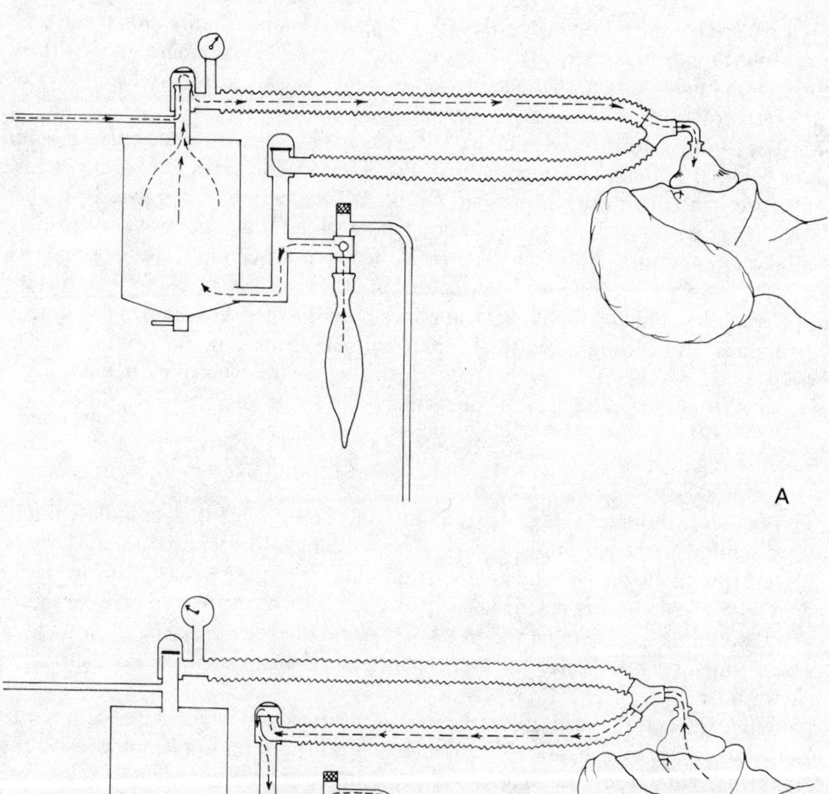


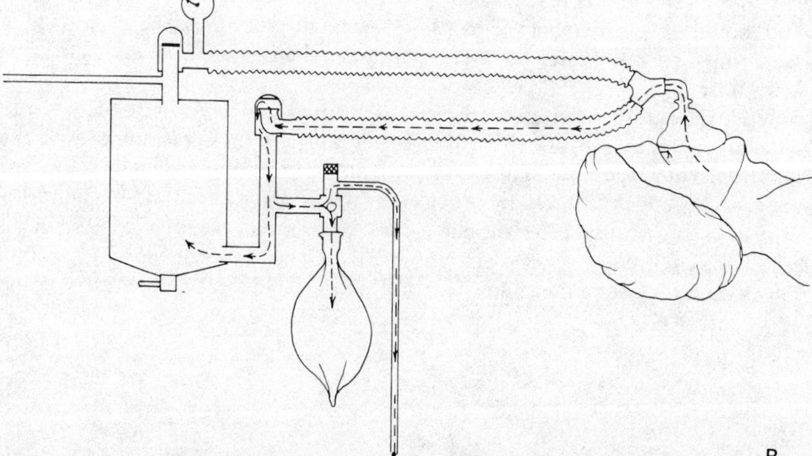


**Figure 4-7.** Design of the anesthesia circle. **A**, Inhalation cycle. As the patient inspires, gas is drawn from both the reservoir bag (through the $CO_2$ absorber and the inhalation one-way valve) and the fresh gas flow from the outlet of the anesthesia machine. The exhalation one-way valve is closed and prevents rebreathing of $CO_2$-containing gases. **B**, Exhalation cycle. On expiration, gases pass through the exhalation one-way valve into both the $CO_2$ absorber and the reservoir bag. Excess gas is exhausted through a "pop-off" valve to the scavenging system. The inhalation one-way valve is closed and prevents $CO_2$ accumulation in the inspiratory hose, thereby minimizing rebreathing of $CO_2$.

circle consists of the following parts: (a) a fresh gas inlet, (b) unidirectional valves, (c) a carbon dioxide absorber, (d) a pressure relief valve, (e) a pressure gauge, (f) two corrugated hoses, (g) a Y-piece connected to a face mask or endotracheal tube, and (h) a reservoir bag.

The fresh gas inlet is the point at which the gas mixture from the anesthesia machine enters the circle. The two one-way valves ensure foreward movement of gases in the circle and minimize rebreathing of expired gases before $CO_2$ is absorbed. These valves offer resistance in the circle, limiting its use in infants. They are also subject to malfunction and must be checked carefully before use (see the "Anesthesia Checklist," Table 4-6). The reservior bag is added in order to compensate for variations in respiratory demand and to allow the anesthesiologist to assist or control the patient's ventilation. The carbon dioxide absorber contains soda lime (a mixture of 95% $Ca(OH)_2$ and 5% NaOH), a substance which reacts with exhaled carbon dioxide to remove it from the circuit. The chemical reactions are as follows:

1. $CO_2 + 2NaOH \rightarrow Na_2CO_3 + H_2O$
2. $Na_2CO_3 + Ca(OH)_2 \rightarrow CaCO_3 + 2NaOH$

The calcium carbonate ($CaCO_3$) precipitates out on the soda lime granules, and the water humidifies the gas in the circuit. The soda lime also contains an indicator dye (e.g., ethyl violet) which changes color (e.g., colorless to purple) as the absorptive capacity of the soda lime is reached. The pressure gauge measures the pressures in the circuit; and the pressure relief valve rids the system of excess gas. The gas leaving the circle through the relief valve is scavenged into an exhaust system for evacuation outside the hospital.

While the anesthesia circle works well with adults and larger children, it is often unsatisfactory for infants since it is cumbersome and presents significant resistance to respiration. Thus, a low-resistance, valveless, non-rebreathing system with low dead space is needed. Such features are provided by the *Jackson-Rees system* (Figure 4-8.) This system consists of a reservoir bag connected by a short corrugated hose to a T-piece having connectors for a gas input hose and for a face mask or endotracheal tube. Fresh gas enters close to the child's face and is exhausted through the reservoir bag.

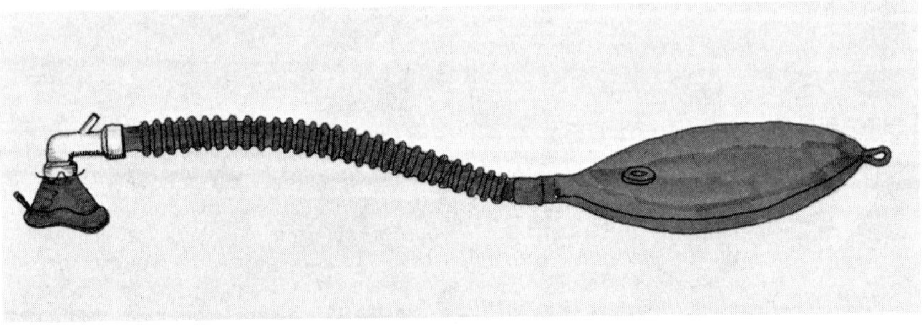

**Figure 4-8.** Diagram of the Jackson-Rees modification of the Ayre's T-piece. Fresh gas enters at the port near the face mask and is exhausted through the hole in the breathing bag. A high rate of fresh gas flow (about 2.5–3.0 times the minute ventilation) minimizes rebreathing of $CO_2$.

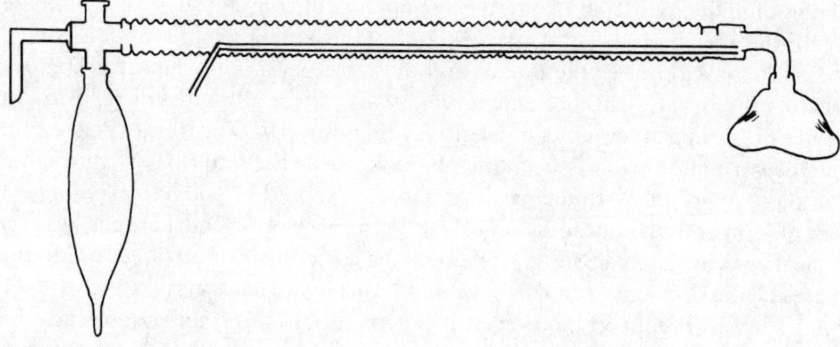

**Figure 4-9.** Diagram of the Bain system.

Since there is no soda lime canister here for absorbing carbon dioxide, rebreathing must be minimized. A fresh gas flow of 2.5–3 times the normal minute ventilation flushes out the exhaled carbon dioxide. Assuming a dead space of 2 mL/kg body weight and a tidal volume of three times dead space, minute ventilation equals tidal volume times respiratory rate. For example, assuming a tidal volume of 6 mL/kg, a 5 kg patient breathing 20 times per minute has a minute ventilation of 600 mL (2 mL/kg x 3 x 5 kg x 20 breaths/min). Therefore, a fresh gas flow of 1.5–1.8 L (2.5–3.0 x 600 mL/min) will prevent rebreathing and carbon dioxide accumulation.

The relatively high gas flows result in some waste of anesthetic gases, but the waste is offset by the system's safety, convenience, simplicity, small dead space, and low resistance. The system does not provide humidification, and tends to lower the child's body temperature. Lack of humidification can cause drying of the respiratory mucosa, with subsequent airway damage and thickening of secretions. To avoid these problems, the anesthetic gases are passed through a heated humidifier before delivery to the infant. Heated humidifiers are commercially available to fulfill this purpose.

Surgical procedures about the head and neck require an anesthetic system that is light in weight, does not create facial distortion, and does not cause excessive drag on the endotracheal tube. In children, the Jackson-Rees system works well, but for adults, the circle absorber system creates bulk and weight about the face, and the one-way valves cannot be located at too great a distance from the patient. To circumvent these problems, Bain and Spoerel (1972) described a system called the *Bain system* (Figure 4-9) in which fresh gas flows through a narrow tube within a corrugated expiratory hose. Its use does not require either valves or a carbon dioxide absorber. The system is particularly useful when the anesthesiologist, for surgical access, must be located at a considerable distance from the patient's head. Data demonstrate that, using this system, patients can be adequately oxygenated and maintain near normal $CO_2$ levels during controlled ventilation at fresh gas flows of 70 mL/kg/min (Chu et al., 1977).

## Apparatus For Intubation

Following the induction of anesthesia with loss of consciousness, it is often necessary for the anesthesiologist to assist or control the patient's ventilation. During the period of unconsciousness, the tongue and the soft tissues of the mouth relax, often obstructing the airway. This obstruction can frequently be alleviated by repositioning the head or inserting an oral or a nasal airway (Figure 4-10). The former displaces the tongue forward and upwards from the pharynx, while the latter passes through the nose into the pharynx. With the nasal airway, care should be taken to avoid injuring the vascular mucous membranes of the nose, because hemorrhage there can be severe. If a nasal airway is to be used, it should be generously lubricated. With these maneuvers, most patients can easily ventilate through a face mask attached to the anesthesia hoses. Frequently, however, it is necessary to insert an endotracheal tube into the trachea. The process of placing this tube into the mouth, between the vocal cords, and into the trachea is referred to as *endotracheal intubation.* The indications for endotracheal intubation are summarized in Table 4-1, and the equipment that should be available is listed in Table 4-2.

To perform endotracheal intubation, the anesthesiologist uses a *laryngoscope,* so that he can see the vocal cords and thus insert the tube under direct vision. A laryngoscope (Figure 4-11) consists of a blade and a metal handle, the latter containing batteries that power a light bulb in the blade. Laryngoscope blades are either straight or curved, with each type available in a variety of styles and sizes. All blades should fit any of the handles.

**TABLE 4-1**
**Some Indications for Endotracheal Intubation**

Patients to have intraabdominal surgeries
Patient with full stomach or intestinal obstruction
Patients whose proper anesthetic management includes the use of muscle relaxants
Patients with an intraabdominal mass
Patients requiring prolonged positive pressure ventilation
Patients requiring tracheal suctioning
Patients in adverse position
- Prone
- Lateral decubitus
- Sitting
- Trendelenburg

Patients who cannot be well fitted with a face mask
Surgeries with intraoral bleeding
Patients with head, neck, or upper airway disease or obstruction
Surgery about the head, neck, or airway
Surgery entailing poor access of the anesthesiologist to the patient's head
Intrathoracic surgery
Situations requiring that the anesthesiologist be free to perform duties other than maintaining mask ventilation

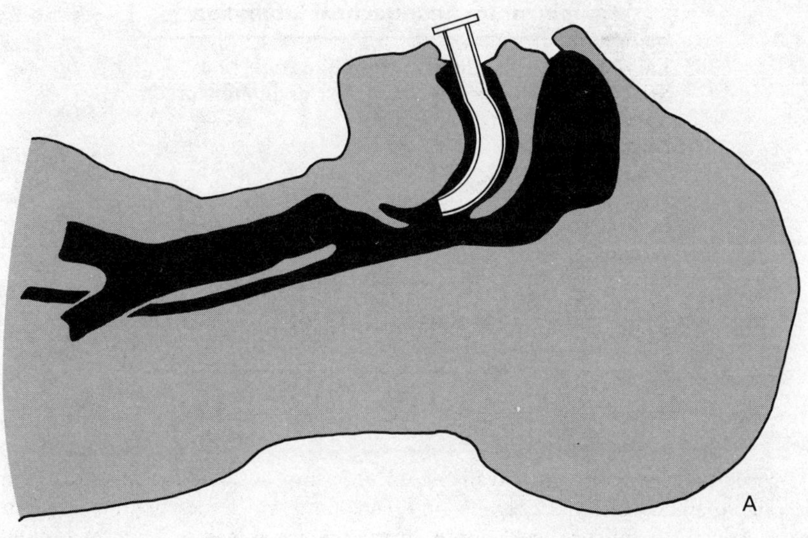


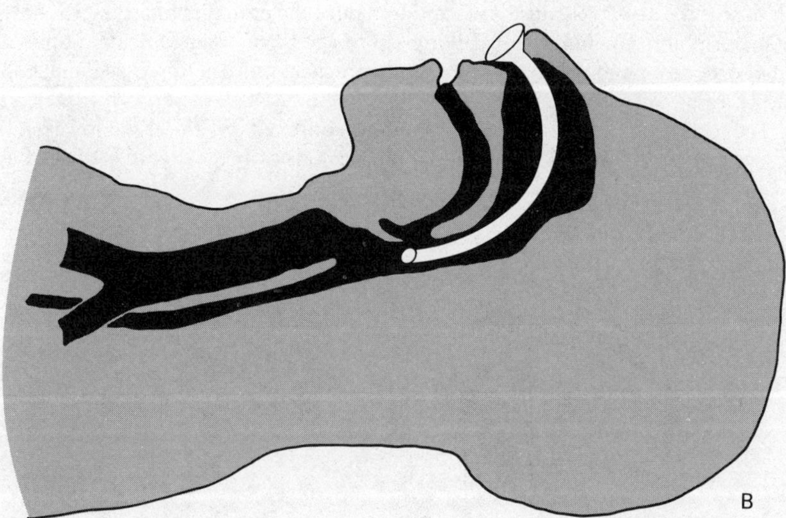


**Figure 4-10.** Oral (A) and nasal (B) airways correctly located to relieve upper airway obstruction.

**TABLE 4-2**
**Equipment for Endotracheal Intubation**

| |
|---|
| Laryngoscope handle with fresh batteries |
| Selection of laryngoscope blades, straight and curved |
| Selection of endotracheal tubes |
| Malleable stylet |
| Magill forceps |
| Lubricant jelly |
| Syringe to inflate cuff of endotracheal tube |
| Tongue blade |
| Selection of oral and nasal airways |
| Suction device |
| Apparatus for positive pressure ventilation |

Endotracheal tubes are available in 0.5 mm inside-diameter increments, although they may also be designated in French units which measure three times the external diameter, a figure which approximates the circumference. Endotracheal tube dimensions and pertinent anatomic measurements are listed in Table 4-3.

Endotracheal tubes are of two types: those with an air-inflatable cuff near the tip, and those without a cuff. Cuffed tubes are used for adults, with the cuff serving both to seal the airway against leaks and to reduce the potential of aspiration of foreign material into the lungs. For children up to age 6 or 7 years, uncuffed tubes are used in order to avoid undue pressure on the tracheal mucosa (discussed in detail in Chapter 13).

The technique of endotracheal intubation is outlined in Table 4-4. However, before attempting to intubate a patient, an intravenous catheter should be placed and

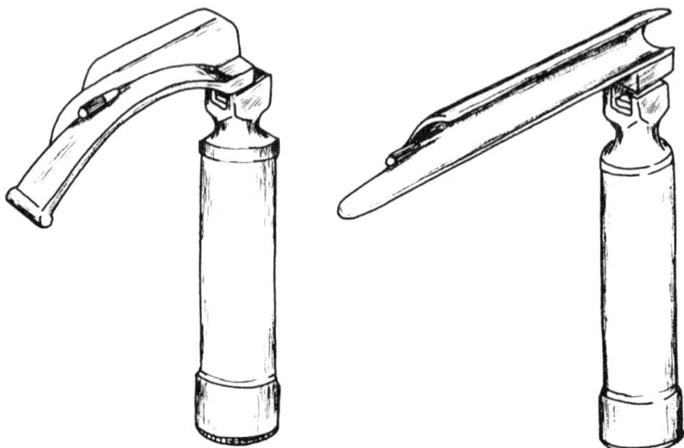

**Figure 4-11.** Curved (MacIntosh-type) and straight (Miller-type) laryngoscope blades for endotracheal intubation.

**TABLE 4-3**
**Endotracheal Tube Dimensions and Patient Anatomy**

| | Anatomic Distance (cm) | | | Tube Sizes* | | |
|---|---|---|---|---|---|---|
| *Age* | *Teeth to Cords* | *Teeth to Carina* | *Lips to Midtrachea* | *Trachea Diameter (mm)* | *Internal Diameter (mm)* | *French* |
| Premature | 6–7 | 10–11 | 10 | 3–3.5 | 2.5 | 10–12 |
| Term newborn | 7–8 | 11–12 | 11 | 4 | 3.0 | 12–14 |
| 1–6 mo | 8–8.5 | 11–12 | 11 | 5–6 | 3.5 | 16 |
| 6–12 mo | 8.5 | 12–13 | 12 | 6–7 | 4.0 | 18 |
| 1–2 yr | 9 | 13–14 | 13 | 7–8 | 4.5 | 20 |
| 2–4 yr | 9–9.5 | 14–15 | 14 | 8 | 5.0 | 22 |
| 4–6 yr | 9.5 | 15–15.5 | 15 | 8.5 | 5.5 | 24 |
| 6–8 yr | 10 | 15.5–16 | 16 | 9 | 6–6.5 | 26 |
| 8–10 yr | 10 | 16–16.5 | 17 | 9.5 | 6.5–7 | 28 |
| 10–12 yr | 11–12 | 16.5–17 | 18 | 10 | 7–7.5 | 30 |
| 12–16 yr | 12–13 | 17–20 | 20 | 11 | 7.5 | 32 |
| Over 16 yr | >13 | >20 | 22–24 | >12 | 8–9 | 32–36 |

*At least one size larger and smaller than stated should also be available.

**TABLE 4-4**
**Technique of Endotracheal Intubation**

1. Preoxygenation (see text).
2. Raise table to comfortable height.
3. Place patient's head 4″ above table on a support (e.g., pillow, towels, folded sheet). This is the "sniffing position."
4. Grasp laryngoscope with left hand.
5. Open patient's mouth with fingers of right hand.
6. Insert laryngoscope blade into right side of mouth.
7. Deflect tongue to the left and locate epiglottis in midline.
8. Avoid pressure on teeth and lips.
9. (a) If using a curved blade: advance blade into the vallecula.* Forward and upward movement (Figure 4-11) of the laryngoscope elevates the epiglottis and exposes the vocal cords.
   (b) If using a straight blade, pass the tip of the blade under the epiglottis. Forward and upward movement (Figure 4-11) of the laryngoscope elevates the epiglottis and exposes the vocal cords.
10. Under direct vision, slip the tip of the endotracheal tube through the vocal cords and advance the tube until the tip lies in the midtrachea.
11. If a cuffed tube was used, inflate the cuff with just enough air to create a seal with the tracheal mucosa. Avoid overinflation.
12. Observe chest motion to positive pressure ventilation.
13. Auscultate both lungs for equality of breath sounds.
14. Reposition tube if necessary.
15. Firmly tape tube in place.
16. Repeat steps 13 and 14.

*The space between the base of the tongue and the pharyngeal surface of the epiglottis.

connected to a free-running bottle of intravenous fluid. The patient should be monitored in a manner consistent with his/her physical condition (Chapter 5). All patients should be monitored with, at a minimum, a blood pressure cuff, electrocardiogram leads, and a precordial stethoscope.

Following injection of a "defasciculating" dose of nondepolarizing muscle relaxant (e.g., pancuronium 0.01 mg/kg IV) general anesthesia is induced, as described in Chapter 10. The patient is ventilated with an anesthesia mask, muscle relaxation is induced by intravenous injection of succinylcholine (1 mg/kg), and the patient ventilated for at least 30 seconds with 100% oxygen ("preoxygenation").

Figure 4-12A illustrates the correct placement of a straight laryngoscope blade within the mouth of an adult. Note that the tip of the blade is slipped just beneath the tip of the epiglottis, clearly exposing the vocal cords. Viewing with a curved blade is similar except that the tip is advanced into the space (the vallecula) between the base of the tongue and the epiglottis but does not actually slip under the epiglottis (Figure 4-12B). Forward and upward motion (i.e., lifting the mandible forward without prying on the upper teeth) exposes the vocal cords. To achieve this motion, the entire laryngoscope handle is lifted forward, away from the anesthesiologist, as shown by the *arrow* in Figure 4-12.

Figure 4-13 illustrates correct placement of a cuffed endotracheal tube within the trachea of an adult. Note that the cuff is located just below the vocal cords, and the tip of the tube is well above the division of the trachea into the right and left bronchi (i.e., located well above the carina).

In some instances, patients must be intubated through the nose rather than through the mouth. This process is referred to as *nasotracheal intubation*. In such an intubation, the nasal mucosa is topically anesthetized (cocaine works best), and the endotracheal tube is passed through the nose, between the vocal cords and into the trachea. Use of the Magill forceps may facilitate tube placement. Nasotracheal intubation is useful for surgery on the mouth, face, or neck when an orally placed tube would normally interfere with surgery. If the patient's mouth opens normally and the anesthesiologist judges that there should be little difficulty viewing the vocal cords, anesthesia can be induced and the tube then placed under direct vision. However, if the patient has a restricted opening of the mouth, or if the anesthesiologist judges that it will be difficult to see the vocal cords, the tube can be passed through the nose and into the trachea with the patient awake and topically anesthetized. This latter technique allows the patient to maintain vocal cord reflexes during intubation, thus making it less likely that aspiration of gastric contents will occur should the patient vomit during intubation. Topical anesthesia of the trachea, vocal cords, and epiglottis, as well as pharmacologic sedation, may increase the possibility of aspiration.

Endotracheal intubation is not without complications. These are related both to the process of intubating a patient and to the results of locating a tube within the trachea. Table 4-5 summarizes these complications. The reader should note that while such complications are rare, they must carefully be weighed against the benefits to be gained.

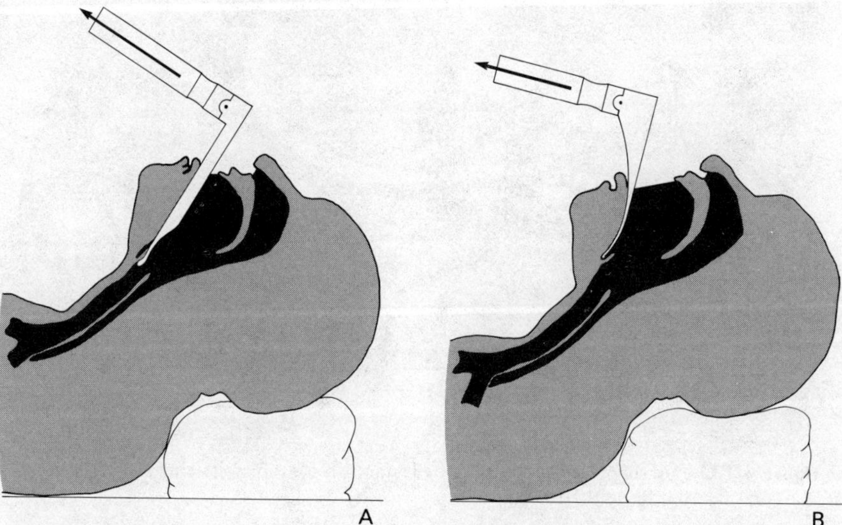


**Figure 4-12.** Technique of visualizing the vocal cords with straight (**A**) and curved (**B**) anesthesia blades. Note the position of the blades in relation to the epiglottis (see text for details).

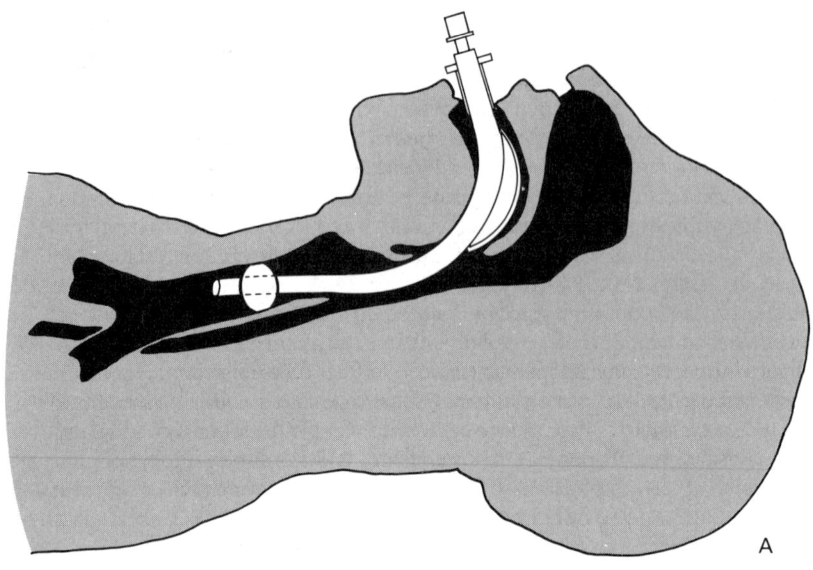


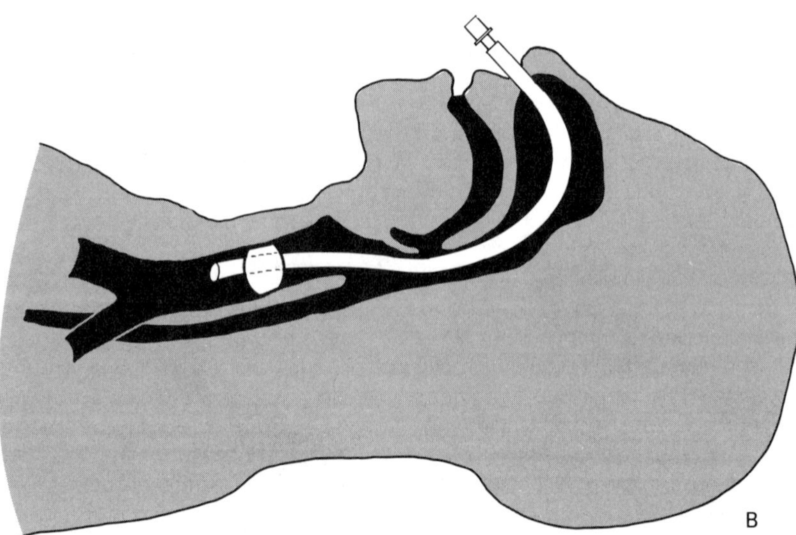


**Figure 4-13.** Correct placement of the cuffed endotracheal tube following oral (**A**) and nasal (**B**) intubation.

**TABLE 4-5**
**Complications of Tracheal Intubation**

Complications at the time of intubation
- Trauma to teeth, lips, and gums
- Hemorrhage
- Hypertension, tachycardia, arrhythmias

Complications while tube is present
- Obstruction of the tube
- Endobronchial intubation
- Esophageal intubation
- Accidental extubation
- Aspiration
- Increased resistance to breathing
- Drying of tracheal mucosa
- Tracheal wall ischemia
- Poor tolerance to tube presence

Complications seen after extubation
- Laryngospasm
- Aspiration
- Laryngeal and tracheal edema
- Subglottic stenosis
- Vocal cord paralysis
- Laryngeal ulceration
- Hoarseness and sore throat

## Apparatus For Intravenous Catheterization

A well-functioning intravenous "line" is a necessity for most anesthetics. Such a line consists of an intravenous catheter connected to a length of tubing that carries sterile fluid by gravity from a bottle located above the patient. The tubing contains one or more injection ports, through which drugs can be injected into the tubing and carried to the patient. Intravenous catheters are used both for patient monitoring and for administering blood and fluids.

Intravenous catheters may be placed in either a peripheral or a central vein. Peripherally placed catheters are most often placed in the subcutaneous veins of the hands or arms. Centrally placed intravenous catheters are those whose tip is located within the chest (i.e., in either the superior vena cava or the right atrium of the heart). Common routes for the placement of central catheters include the internal or the external jugular veins, the subclavian vein, and the brachiocephalic vein. Since these are large veins, relatively large catheters (14 or 16 gauge) can be inserted, and large amounts of blood and fluids can be transfused through them.

While there are several types of venous catheters, the plastic, over-the-needle catheters have proven to be most satisfactory since they cause minimal bleeding at the

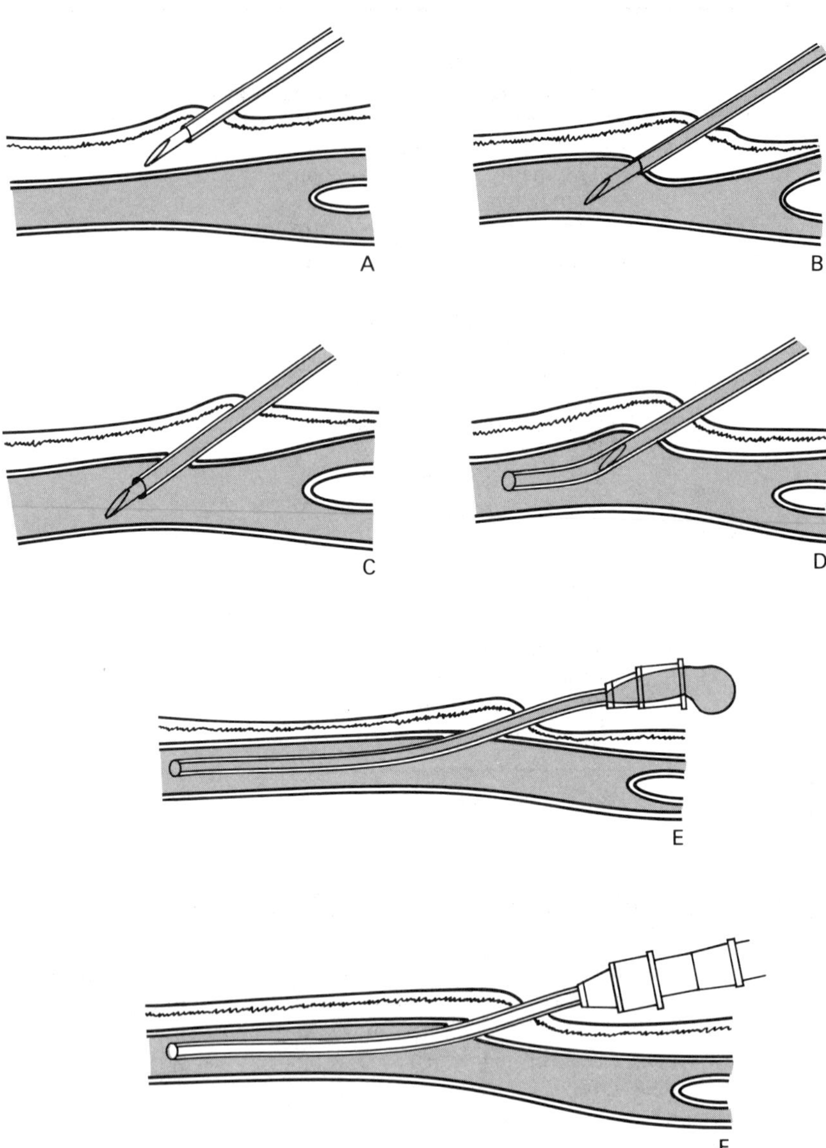


**Figure 4-14.** Technique of intravenous catheterization with an over-the-needle catheter. **A,** Introducer needle and catheter enter the subcutaneous tissue. **B,** Introducer needle enters the vein but the plastic catheter remains outside the vessel. Note the flash of blood backup in the needle. **C,** With further advancement, both the needle and the catheter have entered the lumen of the vessel. The catheter may now be advanced off the needle. **D,** The catheter is being advanced off the needle. **E,** The catheter has been advanced and the introducer needle has been removed. Note free flow of blood from the hub. **F,** The catheter is connected to plastic tubing from the bottle of intravenous fluid.

site of insertion, and their internal diameters are large, relative to the size of venapuncture. The site most often used for placing intravenous catheters is the dorsum of the hand or forearm. Antecubital veins are less frequently used. The distal portions of the saphenous veins are seldom used in adults but are convenient to use in infants and in some adults where placement of a catheter in a hand vein might be difficult.

To increase the chances of successfully cannulating a vein, one should be selected that is easily seen and that has a straight course for the length of the catheter. The tourniquet should be placed well above the site of insertion of the catheter. The hand should be kept below the level of the heart, and several minutes should lapse between placement of the tourniquet and the venapuncture. This allows sufficient time for the vein to become engourged with blood. The skin overlying the vein should be cleaned with alcohol or iodine, then infiltrated with local anesthetic, using a 25- or 27-gauge needle. Gently tapping the skin may assist in causing venous engourgement. The catheter is then passed through the skin and enters the vein at a narrow angle. Venapuncture is indicated by a flash of blood back through the metal needle. At this point, attempts should not be made to advance the plastic catheter into the vein as it my still lie outside the vein (Figure 4-14). The entire unit should be advanced an additional few millimeters into the lumen of the vein before advancing the plastic catheter off the needle. Following successful placement of the catheter, the intravenous tubing is attached and the catheter firmly taped in place.

Details of the placement of *central venous catheters* may be found in Chapter 5.

## Anesthesia Checklist

Before inducing anesthesia, the anesthesia machine, monitors, and anesthesia apparatus must be checked. Obviously, the machine must be in good working order and all pieces of necessary equipment must be available and functional. Table 4-6 has been prepared to be used daily by anyone administering anesthesia. Its use would ensure the presence and proper functioning of important items of equipment, and would provide proper end-of-day procedures that would leave the equipment ready for subsequent use. It is suggested that this table be reproduced and individual boxes be checked following completion of each inspection.

### *Readings and References*

Aldrete, J.A.; Lowe, H.J.; and Virtue, R.W. 1979. *Low flow and closed system anesthesia*. New York: Grune & Stratton.

Bain, J.A., and Spoerel, W.E.: A streamlined anesthetic system., *Can. Anaesth. Soc. J.* 19:426–435, 1972.

Chu, Y.K.; Rah, K.H.; and Boyan, C.P. 1977. Is the Bain circuit the future anesthesia system? An evaluation. *Anesth. Analg.* 56:84–87.

Dorsch, J.A., and Dorsch, S.E. 1984. *Understanding anesthesia equipment*. 2nd ed. Baltimore: Williams & Wilkins.

Dripps, R.D.; Eckenhoff, J.E.; and Vandam, L.D. 1982. *Introduction to anesthesia*. 6th ed. Philadelphia: W.B. Saunders.

**TABLE 4-6**
**Anesthesia Checklist**

**A. Anesthesia apparatus**

1. Two laryngoscope handles with fresh batteries ☐
2. Laryngoscope blades with functioning bulbs ☐
3. Endotracheal tubes with cuff integrity verified ☐
4. Cuff inflator syringe ☐
5. Flexible stylet ☐
6. Oral and nasal airways ☐
7. Tonsil-tip and catheter suction devices ☐
8. Hoses, headstrap, masks, and bag ☐
9. Blood pressure cuffs of appropriate sizes ☐
10. Stethoscopes, blood pressure, precordial, and esophageal ☐
11. Temperature probes and monitor ☐
12. Adhesive tape, benzoin, lubricant, alcohol swabs ☐
13. Electrocardiograph connectors and pads ☐
14. Doppler device and probes (if desired) ☐
15. Nerve stimulator and probes (if desired) ☐
16. Initial drugs (thiopental, atropine, succinylcholine) ☐
17. Check drug drawer for emergency drugs ☐

**B. Anesthesia machine**

1. Wall supply of oxygen and nitrous oxide connected ☐
2. Spare oxygen tanks reading above 500 psi ☐
3. Spare nitrous oxide tanks reading above 700 psi ☐
4. Tank wrench present ☐
5. Oxygen flowmeter works smoothly ☐
6. Nitrous oxide flowmeter works smoothly and oxygen flows also if machine equipped with low oxygen fail-safe device ☐
7. Oxygen analyzer calibrates in room air and in 100% oxygen ☐
8. Oxygen analyzer alarm functions ☐
9. Flush valve works ☐
10. Vaporizers filled, caps and drains closed tightly ☐
11. Circle system free of leaks ☐
12. Suction connected and working ☐
13. Electrocardiograph functional ☐
14. Breath through circle system to assure that:
    a. Inhalation and exhalation valves function ☐
    b. Resistance is not high ☐
    c. Irritant gas is not present ☐
15. Soda lime not exhausted ☐

**C. Ventilator**

1. Operates when turned on ☐
2. Hose present for connection to breathing system ☐
3. Disconnect alarm functions ☐
4. Tidal volume set to patient's estimated requirement. ☐

**D. Pollution control**

1. Circle system pop-off connected to scavenger system ☐
2. Ventilator exhaust connected to scavenger system ☐
3. No observable nitrous oxide leaks from hoses, wall supply or spare tank connections ☐

**E. End-of-day procedures**

1. Turn off spare tanks ☐
2. Turn off all flow meters ☐
3. Turn off oxygen analyzer ☐
4. Turn off electrocardiograph ☐
5. Turn off temperature monitor ☐
6. Turn off Doppler device and recharge ☐
7. Change oxygen tank if <500 psi, change nitrous oxide tank if <700 psi ☐
8. Change soda lime if half-exhausted ☐
9. Place clean hoses, bag, and mask on circle system ☐
10. Check for leaks in circle system ☐
11. Place tape or towel across hoses to indicate that system is ready for use ☐

Hill, D.W. 1980. *Physics applied to anesthesia.* 4th ed. Woburn, Mass.: Butterworth.

Lowe, H.J., and Ernst, E.A. 1981. *The Quantitative practice of anesthesia: use of closed circuit.* Baltimore: Williams & Wilkins.

Orkin, F.K. 1981. Anesthetic systems. In: *Anesthesia,* Miller, R.D., editor. New York: Churchill Livingstone, pp. 117–156.

Stoelting, R.K. 1981. Endotracheal intubation. In: *Anesthesia,* Miller, R.D., editor. New York: Churchill Livingstone, pp. 233–255.

# 5. Patient Monitoring

Patients under general anesthesia are unable to communicate with the medical staff. Constant vigilance on the part of the anesthesiologist is an absolute necessity. The anesthesiologist closely observes certain physical signs indicative of adequate blood pressure, cardiac output, tissue oxygenation, and skin perfusion. The anesthesiologist, in addition, can use a number of mechanical and electronic monitoring techniques that further increase the safety of the patient. These monitoring methods are listed in Table 5-1.

## Physical Signs

The physical examination is the first monitoring technique the anesthesiologist employs, relying on the senses of sight and touch. It has been said that a patient under anesthesia should remain "warm, pink, and dry;" that is, that anesthetic should blunt excessive activity of the sympathetic nervous system.

Peripheral blood flow can be monitored by evaluating the fingernails: they should be pink, and their capillaries should refill rapidly following the release of pressure applied to them. Pupil size or changes in pupil size are useful monitors of anesthetic depth if the patient has not received narcotics. A patient with small pupils is presumed to be in a moderate stage of anesthesia, during which there is amnesia and analgesia. Dilated pupils either indicate very light anesthesia, in which pain is felt and sympathetic discharge is prominent; or they indicate an anesthetic state much deeper than is required for surgery. These two states can be distinguished from each other by evaluating other signs, such as heart rate, blood pressure, and the presence or absence of sweating, as well as knowledge of the inspired concentration of the anesthetic being administered.

**TABLE 5-1**
**Patient Monitoring Methods**

***Physical signs***

Skin: warm, pink, and dry

Pupils: midposition, reactive to light

Nail beds: good capillary filling, pink in color

Pulses: strong carotid or radial artery pulse, regular rhythm

***Mechanical and electronic monitoring***

| *Noninvasive* | *Invasive* |
|---|---|
| Blood pressure cuff | Urine output: Foley catheter |
| Doppler flowmeter | Arterial catheter |
| a. Arterial blood pressure | Central venous catheter |
| b. Precordial: right atrium | Pulmonary artery catheter (Swan-Ganz catheter) |
| Electrocardiograph (ECG) | Intracranial pressure transducer |
| Temperature monitors | |
| a. Thermometer: oral, axilla | |
| b. Temperature probe: nasal, esophageal, rectal, tympanic membrane | |
| Anesthesia stethoscopes | |
| a. Esophageal | |
| b. Precordial | |
| Neurophysiological monitors | |
| a. Electroencephalograph | |
| b. Evoked potential computer | |
| c. Peripheral nerve stimulator | |
| Respiratory monitors | |
| a. Reservoir bag | |
| b. Respiratory spirometer | |
| c. Oxygen analyzer | |
| d. Carbon dioxide analyzer | |
| e. Anesthetic vapor analyzer | |
| f. Transcutaneous oxygen and carbon dioxide analyzer | |
| g. Pulse oximeter | |

If the patient is breathing spotaneously, examination of the movements of the chest wall, abdomen, and suprasternal notch may help in assessing the adequacy of respiratory exchange. But although respiratory rate may easily be counted, the volume of air in each breath is difficult to estimate by merely observing the chest. Instrumental monitoring of tidal volume is discussed in the next section.

Finally, palpation of the arterial pulses (any of the carotid, superficial temporal, or radial pulses are usually accessible) indicates the cardiac rhythm and allows rough estimation of the adequacy of cardiac output.

# Noninvasive Mechanical and Electronic Monitoring

## Blood Pressure

During anesthesia, blood pressure and heart rate are taken at least every 5 minutes and entered on the anesthesia record. Periods of cardiovascular instability demand more frequent measurements. A blood pressure cuff is placed on every patient prior to induction of anesthesia. In addition, a stethoscope is taped in place over a major artery under or distal to the cuff.

The cuff chosen must be appropriate for the particular patient. The width of the cuff should exceed the diameter of the limb by approximately 20%, and the cuff should cover approximately two-thirds of the upper arm. If the cuff is too narrow, a relatively high pressure must be applied to occlude the artery, resulting in an artificially high blood pressure reading. If the patient is obese and has a large upper arm, a very wide blood pressure cuff, such as a thigh cuff, may be necessary. Either arm may be used for pressure measurements because the pressures obtained from both arms are usually equal.

In infants, blood pressure may be difficult to hear with a stethoscope, and in such circumstances a *Doppler flowmeter* (Figure 5-1) is useful. The Doppler device transmits a high-frequency signal towards the artery from a small crystal placed on the skin over the artery. The frequency of the reflected signal changes in relation to changes in blood flow in the artery. As the blood pressure cuff is deflated and blood flow returns to the arm, this frequency change is detected, amplified, and played through a speaker. On the arm, the Doppler flowmeter may be placed over the brachial, radial, or ulnar artery. On the leg, it is usually placed over the dorsalis pedis artery.

Newer automated blood pressure monitors detect the oscillations of the arterial wall, rather than the flow of blood through the artery. They thus are capable of measuring diastolic as well as systolic pressures; they convert the two pressures to a digital display. These devices also calculate and display mean arterial pressure and heart rate (Figure 5-2).

Another alternative to the stethoscope for the measurement of blood pressure is the pulse monitor. This device is a photoelectric detector that senses alterations in the flow of blood in the capillary beds under the fingernail. It functions fairly well in most patients, but may become unreliable when peripheral vasoconstriction occurs, giving only an approximation of systolic blood pressure. It should not be used as a substitute monitor for either blood pressure or electrocardiography.

## The Electrocardiograph

The electrocardiogram (ECG) should be monitored in all surgical patients (Figure 5-3). Information that can be obtained from the ECG monitor are: (a) pulse rate, (b) cardiac rhythm, (c) signs of cardiac ischemia, and (4) signs of electrolyte changes. All electrodes should be placed on the patient where they can easily be checked during surgery and replaced if they become loosened. Note that the ECG displays only the electrical activity of the heart and does not indicate cardiac output or either systemic or central pressures.

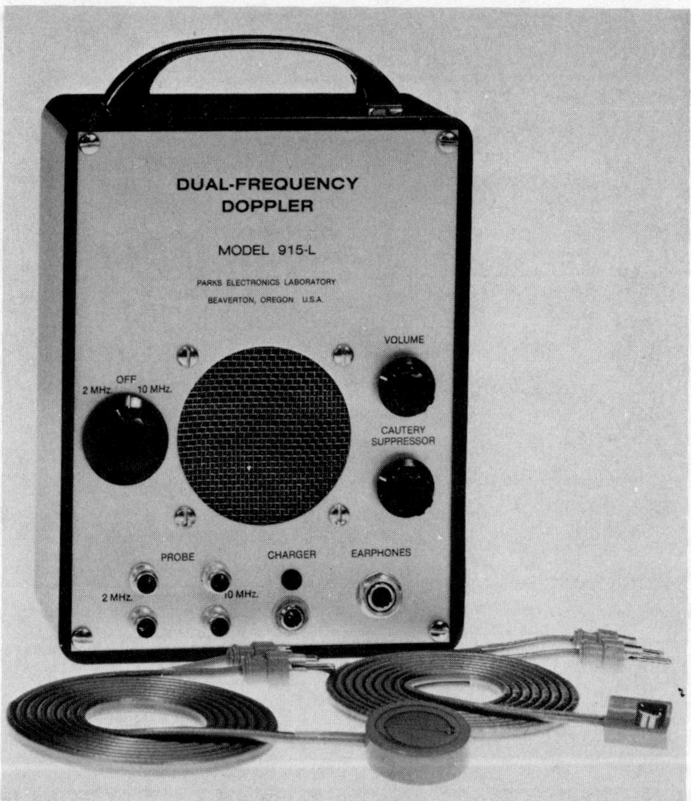


**Figure 5-1.** Doppler flowmeter. Model illustrated is capable of transducing both peripheral pulses and cardiac blood flow (precordial placement). (Photograph courtesy of Parks Electronics Laboratory.)

In a three-wire system, standard limb lead II is the most widely used lead for monitoring, since its electrical axis parallels the electrical axis of the heart, and the complete ECG waveform is easily seen. Lead II allows for diagnosis of inferior wall myocardial ischemia, as well as diagnosis of rate and rhythm disturbances. In a four- or five-wire system, an electrode is placed on the left lateral chest wall, approximately in the V-5 position of a 12-lead ECG tracing. This V-5 lead is used for the diagnosis of myocardial ischemia, as noted by changes in the S-T segment and T wave of the ECG.

Electrolyte alternations also affect the ECG. For example, increased potassium levels produce tall, peaked T waves while decreased potassium results in a decreased amplitude, or even a disappearance of, the T waves.

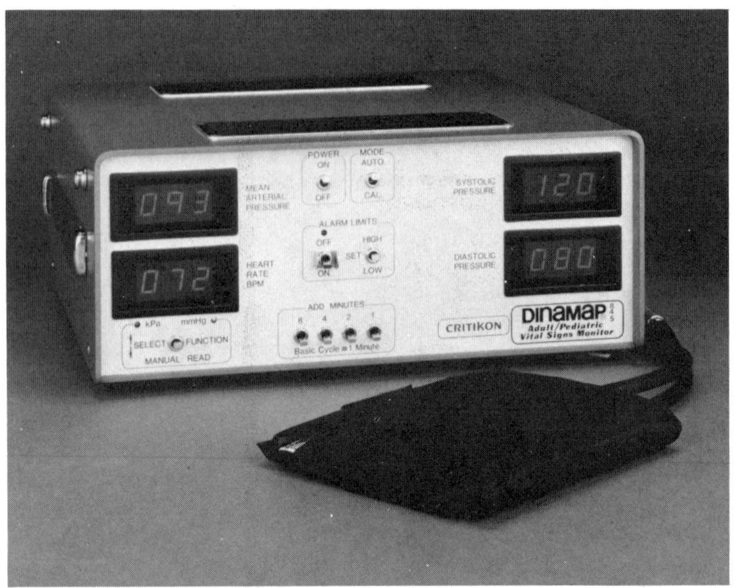


**Figure 5-2.** Dinamap ™ adult/pediatric vital signs monitor. (Photograph courtesy of Criticon, Inc.)

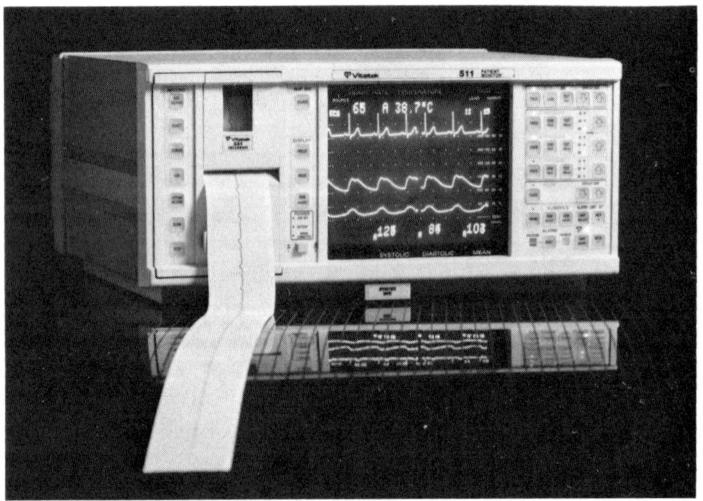


**Figure 5-3.** Vitatek 511 electrocardiograph monitor. (Photograph courtesy of Vitatek, Inc.)

## Body Temperature

The normal thermoregulatory ability of the body is altered by most anesthetics so that body temperature tends to drift towards room temperature. Body temperature should be monitored routinely in all patients undergoing general anesthesia. This is especially important in children, in whom the ratio of body surface area to body weight is large and who may therefore lose body heat rapidly. Body temperature may fall drastically, especially during prolonged surgery, if large amounts of blood and fluids are infused, and if the chest or the abdomen is open. Increases in body temperature are unusual unless: (a) the room is extremely warm, (b) it becomes extremely warm under the surgical drapes, or (c) the serious, very rare, but potentially fatal complication termed *malignant hyperpyrexia* occurs (see Chapter 6).

The usual method for monitoring temperature is to use a temperature probe and a meter, although a simple thermometer placed under the tongue or in the armpit will suffice. Temperature probes have been developed for continuously measuring rectal, esophageal, nasopharyngeal, and tympanic membrane temperatures. If possible, the probe should be accessible to the anesthesiologist so that it can be respositioned if necessary. If a rectal probe is used, care should be taken to tape it firmly in place so that it does not slip out during surgery.

Patients who are allowed to become cold during surgery are prone to cardiac arrhythmias, acidosis, prolonged actions of drugs, profound shivering, and increases in oxygen consumption upon awakening. Hypothermia may be blunted by maintaining warm operating rooms and by using thermal pads, radiant heat lamps, surgical drapes, hot-water circulation blankets, warmed intravenous and irrigation solutions, and humidified and warmed anesthetic gases.

## Anesthesia Stethoscopes

While an ordinary stethoscope is used to monitor blood pressure, there are other stethoscopes especially designed for use in anesthesia. These are of two types: the *esophageal stethoscope* and the *precordial stethoscope* (Figure 5-4). The esophageal stethoscope is a flexible plastic tube inserted through the mouth into the midesophagus. When connected to an earpiece, this tube allows continuous monitoring of heart sounds, of the adequacy of the airway, and of the quality of breath sounds. The precordial stethoscope is a hollow, metal weight connected by tubing to an earpiece. For use, the stethoscope is placed on the patient's chest or in the suprasternal notch.

The Doppler flowmeter can also be used as a precordial monitor in certain neurosurgical procedures where the patient is in the sitting position. Using a special low-impedence pickup (Figure 5-1, left side of photo) placed over the right atrium of the heart, sounds of blood flowing through the right atrium can be monitored. Alteration in these sounds indicate absorption of air through open venous sinuses into the heart. If such absorption is detected, immediate measures should be taken to prevent further air emboli. The surgeon should attempt to prevent the absorption of additional air while the anesthesiologist attempts to aspirate the air already in the right atrium through a previously placed central venous catheter.

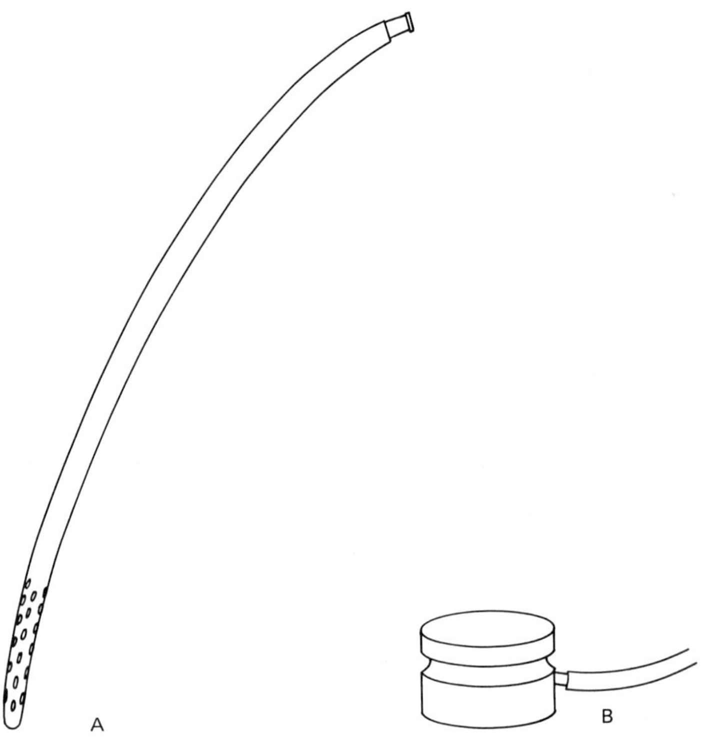


**Figure 5-4.** Illustrations of esophageal (**A**) and precordial (**B**) anesthesia stethoscopes.

## Neuromuscular Function

While muscle tone is often judged by observing the surgical field or by moving the patient's head or jaw, more accurate assessment of neuromuscular function is necessary when neuromuscular blocking agents (Chapter 6) are administered. This is necessitated by the variability in a patient's response to these drugs and by their prolonged respiratory depressant effects. A peripheral nerve stimulator is used for such assessment, with the anesthesiologist visually observing the intensity of the contraction of the fingers (adductor pollicis and flexor digitorum). Most commonly, two needle electrodes are placed subcutaneously over the ulnar nerve as it travels down the forearm, or two pad electrodes are placed over the nerve. Stimuli are delivered to the electrodes from a battery-powered stimulator (Figure 5-5). The type of stimuli commonly used include single twitches, five-second tetanic (high frequency) stimuli, or "train of four" stimuli using four stimuli 0.5 seconds apart.

Figure 5-6 illustrates the use of a nerve stimulator to monitor neuromuscular function. At the beginning of the trace, single stimuli produced a thumb twitch which was virtually abolished by *d*-tubocurarine, a nondepolarizing neuromuscular blocking agent (Chapter 6). Over time, there is a small amount of recovery; however, neuromuscular function is still well below control. Following neostigmine and atropine,

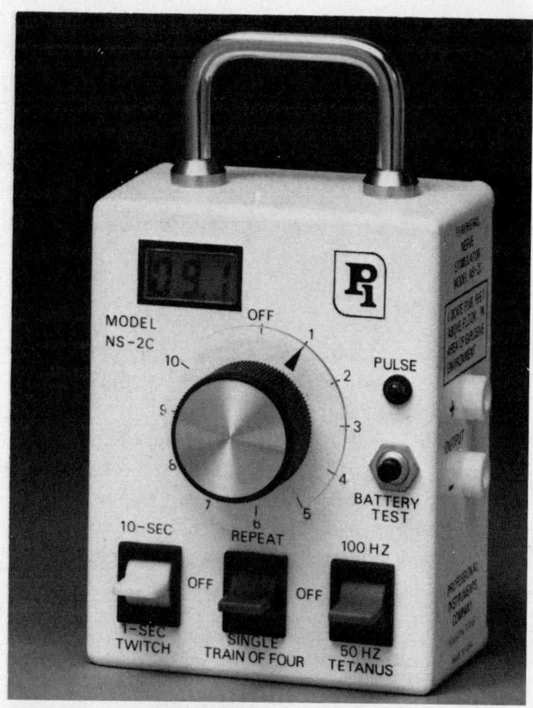


**Figure 5-5.** Peripheral nerve stimulator for monitoring neuromuscular function. (Photograph courtesy of Professional Instruments Co.)

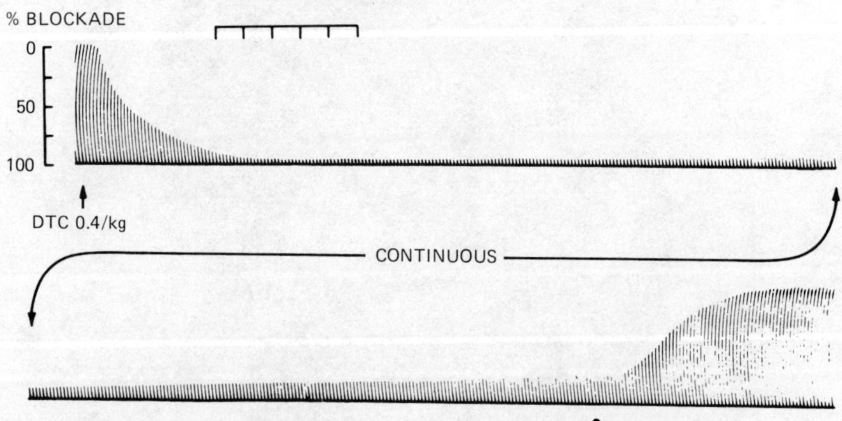


**Figure 5-6.** Nondepolarizing neuromuscular block. Maximal thumb twitches at a stimulus rate of 0.15 Hz. The time scale is in minutes. d-Tubocurarine (DTC) 0.4 mg/kg was administered at the **arrow,** producing gradual neuromuscular block. At the **dot,** neostigmine 0.06 mg/kg was administered, completely reversing the block within 5 min. (Data courtesy of Antonio, R. P., and Basta, S. J. 1982. Nondepolarizing neuromuscular block. In: *Clinical anesthesia procedures of the Massachusetts Hospital.* 2nd ed. Lebowitz, P. W., editor. Boston: Little, Brown and Co.)

normal neuromuscular function is restored (i.e., neuromuscular blockade has been "reversed"). This reversal will be discussed at length in Chapter 11.

In general, when the elicited contraction after a neuromuscular blocking agent has recovered to at least 20% of the control response, a patient can be safely reversed without encountering postoperative respiratory problems.

## Respiratory Measurements

There are several ways to monitor the respiratory system of a patient under general anesthesia. First, the excursions of the reservoir bag may be observed to estimate tidal volume. Second, for more accuracy, tidal volume may be quantitated by a spirometer (Figure 5-7) which measures gas flow through the gauge.

Third, the precordial and esophageal stethoscopes (discussed earlier) allow the anesthesiologist to monitor breath sounds, but such monitoring is only qualitative. Fourth, several relatively inexpensive devices are available for monitoring oxygen concentrations within the anesthesia circle (Figure 5-8). These devices are equipped with alarms that indicate when the inspired oxygen concentration falls below a preset

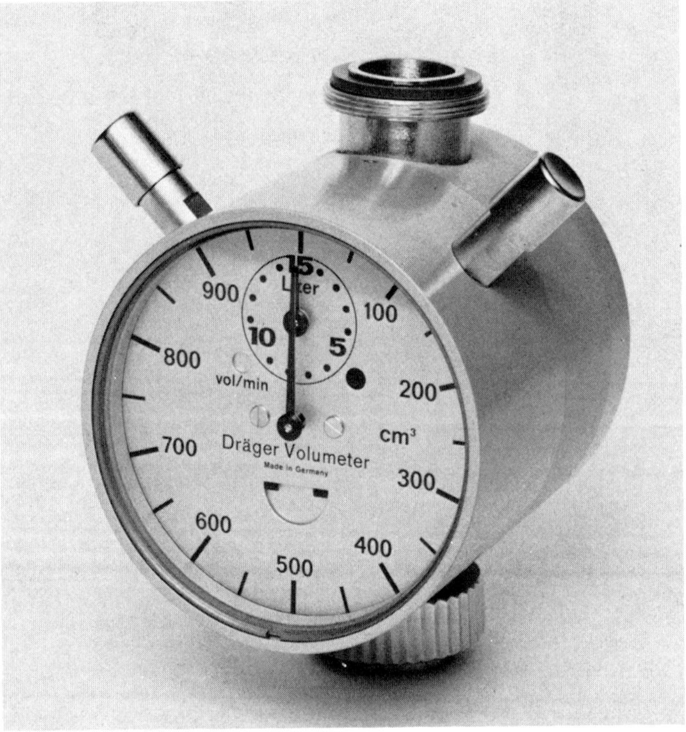


**Figure 5-7.** An anesthesia spirometer (Drager volumeter 3000). (Photograph courtesy of Dragerwerk AG and North American Drager.)

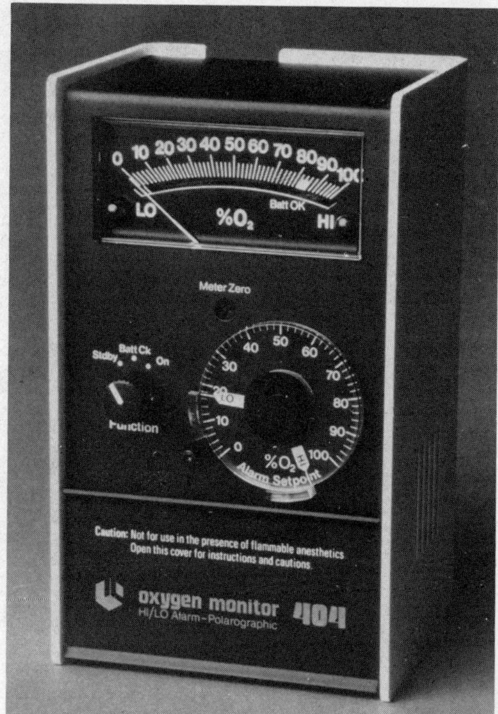


**Figure 5-8.** A polarographic oxygen monitor. (Photograph courtesy of Instrumentation Laboratory, Inc.)

minimum. To compensate for any anesthetic-induced decreases in lung function, most anesthesiologists supply a minimum of 30% oxygen in the inhaled gas mixture.

Fifth, electronically monitoring the amount of carbon dioxide in the expired gas mixture is becoming increasingly important (Figure 5-9). The amount of carbon dioxide in exhaled gas at the end of expiration ("end-tidal" $CO_2$) correlates closely with the level of carbon dioxide in arterial blood, thus providing information on the acid-base balance of the patient, on the adequacy of ventilation, and allowing diagnosis of acute intrapulmonary shunts, such as one that might follow a pulmonary embolus. It can also monitor for a disconnected or obstructed airway.

Sixth, anesthetic vapor analyzers which measure the concentrations of the halothane, enflurance, or isoflurane in the anesthesia circle have become available (Figure 5-10). These devices monitor the amounts of these vapors in the anesthesia breathing circuit, values which correlate with their concentrations in blood.

Finally, transcutaneous oxygen and carbon dioxide electrodes and analyzers are electronic devices that measure and continuously display the oxygen and carbon dioxide tensions of blood perfusing the skin. These electrodes are especially useful for anesthesia in infants in whom high concentrations of oxygen might be detrimental

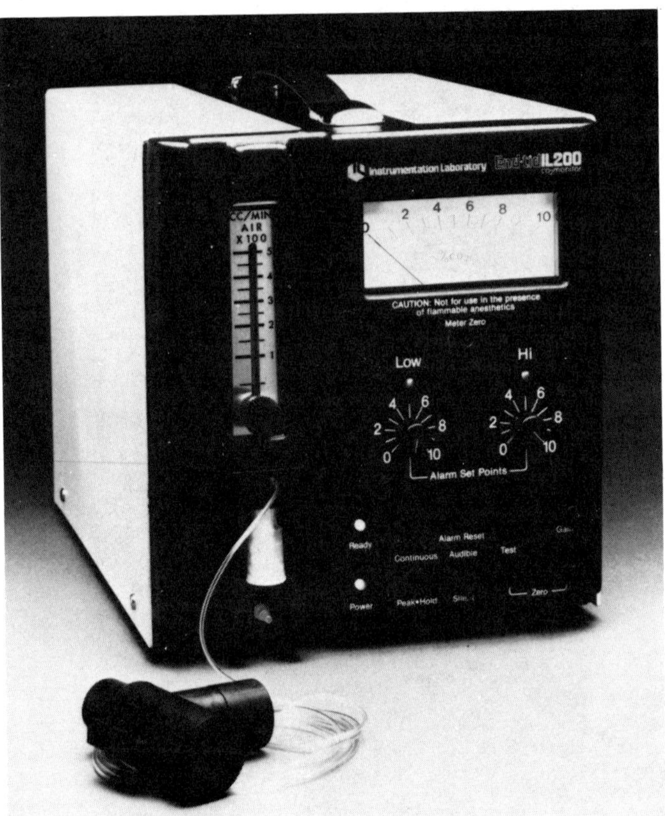


**Figure 5-9.** An on-line device for monitoring expired $CO_2$. (Photograph courtesy of Instrumentation Laboratory, Inc.)

(Chapter 13), and in whom the adequacy of ventilation might be otherwise difficult to assess.

## The Electroencephalograph

Although infrequently used during anesthesia, the electrical activity of the brain can be monitored during surgery by an electroencephalograph (EEG). This machine is occasionally used during neurovascular surgeries and during removal of arteriosclerotic plaques in the carotid arteries.

As an alternative, evoked potential computers are occasionally used. These devices generate pulses that are applied to a nerve; the resulting waveform is transmitted to the brain, where it is measured and analyzed by the recording portion of the computer. Anesthetic drugs usually depress the late-occuring, nonspecific components of the evoked potential, but have less effect on the short-latency, specific response. This

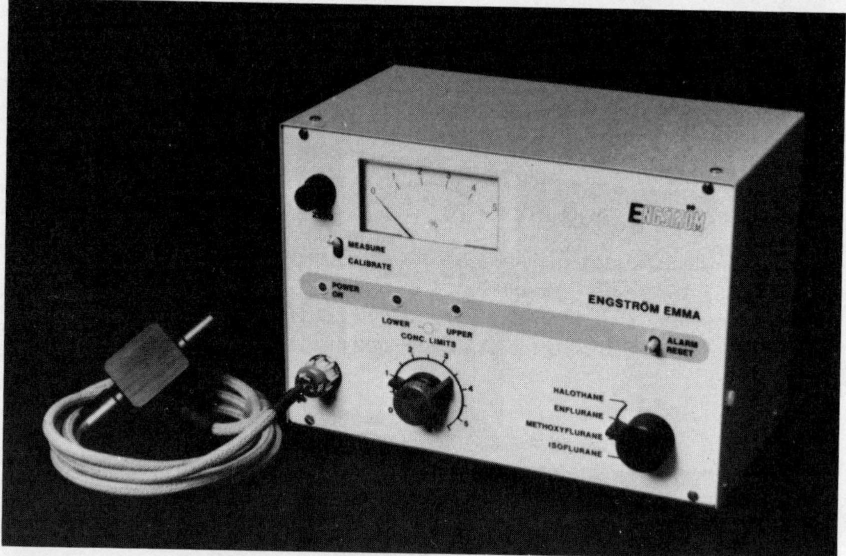


**Figure 5-10.** A multigas monitor for measuring the concentration of anesthetic vapors. (Photograph courtesy of Engstrom Emma, CKB Medical, Inc.)

allows the evoked potential computer to be used to monitor the nervous system for hypoxia, especially that resulting from compression of blood vessels during neurosurgical procedures.

## Invasive Mechanical and Electronic Monitoring

### Urine Output

Measurement of urine output is one of the most important monitors of adequate organ perfusion, and thus is invaluable in determining the adequacy of cardiac output and of blood and fluid replacement. A urine output of 0.5–1.0 mL/kg/hr is consistent with acceptable fluid balance (Chapter 12). Decreased urine output is a cause for concern; it may necessitate giving more fluids, administering diuretics, or increasing cardiac function through the use of such drugs as dopamine (Chapter 9). If decreased urine output persists despite fluid replacement, central venous pressure (CVP) should be measured (see next section) and additional fluids, diuretic therapy, or cardiac stimulants chosen as appropriate. For example, a low CVP with low urine output may indicate need for even more fluid. An increasing CVP in the face of persistently low urine output may indicate need for dopamine. If auscultation of the lungs with a stethoscope reveals rales (a sign of pulmonary edema), a diuretic such as furosemide (Lasix) may be needed, along with the dopamine. Such a situation also calls for the use of more definitive cardiac monitoring, such as can be achieved with a radial artery catheter and a flow-directed pulmonary artery catheter (discussed later).

Monitoring urine output also allows early detection both of hemoglobinuria, a sign of an incompatible blood transfusion, and of glucose excretion in patients with diabetes mellitus.

## Direct Arterial Blood Pressure Measurement

In seriously ill surgical patients, continuous, direct, "beat-to-beat" measurement of arterial blood pressure is frequently desirable. The indications for arterial catheterization are summarized in Table 5-2. Such measurement is made through a catheter placed into a peripheral artery and connected by a fluid-filled line to a transducer,

**TABLE 5-2**
**Indications for Arterial Catheterization**

*Direct measurement of arterial pressure*
- Cardiac surgery, especially with cardiopulmonary bypass
- Deliberate hypothermia
- Deliberate hypotension
- Intracranial operations
- Major vascular surgery: aorta, carotid, iliac, femoral arteries, vena cava
- Extensive surgery with prospect of sudden blood loss or marked shifts of body fluids
- Extensive trauma, especially with uncontrolled hemorrhage
- Thoracic or abdominal surgery with compression of the great vessels
- Noncardiac surgery in patients with significant cardiovascular disease and hemodynamic instability
- Cardiopulmonary resuscitation
- Inability to measure blood pressure indirectly (obesity, burns of the extremities)

*Arterial blood sampling (repetitive)*
- Blood gas analysis
    - Pulmonary disease
    - Lung surgery (one-lung ventilation)
    - Airway surgery (apneic oxygenation)
    - Major surgery (neuro-, cardiac, vascular, thoracic, abdominal)
- Severe metabolic derangements
    - Acid-base evaluation
    - Electrolyte determinations
    - Glucose analysis
    - Serum osmolarity measurement
- Heparin anticoagulation and protamine antagonism
    - Cardiopulmonary bypass
    - Arterial shunts (Gott shunt)

From Hug, Carl C., Jr., 1981. Monitoring. In: *Anesthesia*. Miller, R.D., editor, New York: Churchill Livingstone.

which converts the pressure pulse to an electronic impulse that is displayed on an oscilloscope. This technique allows: (a) continuous measurement of arterial blood pressure, and (b) convenient access for intermittent sampling of arterial blood, so that arterial blood gases and blood chemistries can be measured.

The radial artery is most frequently chosen for insertion of the arterial catheter, provided that the corresponding ulnar artery is intact. The extent of ulnar blood flow to the hand can be judged by the *Allen test,* in which both the radial and ulnar arteries are occluded by manual pressure. When the ulnar pressure is released, perfusion to the hand is visually assessed. Adequate perfusion of the hand through the ulnar artery implies that the radial artery can be catheterized, with possible loss of radial blood flow distal to the catheter, without impairing blood flow to the hand.

Figure 5-11A illustrates the correct positioning of the patient's hand and the technique of inserting the catheter into the radial artery. Following surgical preparation of the skin over the radial artery, the skin is locally anesthetized with 1% lidocaine. The skin is broken with an 18 gauge needle to facilitate passage of the catheter. A 20-gauge (22-gauge in children) over-the-needle catheter is then passed into the artery at an angle of about 30° to the skin surface. Following penetration of the artery, the needle introducer is removed and the catheter is passed full-length into the vessel. Blood should freely pulsate out the catheter. The hub of the catheter is then connected to tubing, as shown in Figure 5-11B. The tubing is filled with heparinized saline under continuous flush (about 4 mL/hr). This is connected to a transducer, attached electrically to an oscilloscope (Figure 5-3), where the pressure tracing is displayed.

Problems associated with this system include distortion of the waveform by distensible tubing, loose connections, air bubbles, poorly positioned catheter, blood clots, and failure to accurately calibrate the transducer.

Complications of arterial catheterization include: pain, trauma to the artery, hematomas, vascular thrombosis, sepsis, and air embolus if the air is flushed through the catheter.

## Central Venous Pressure

A catheter inserted into the superior vena cava or the right atrium allows not only for fluid administration, but for CVP measurement. Such measurement is useful if the factors determining it are understood and its limitations appreciated. Normally, CVP is determined by circulating blood volume, by the capacitance of the venous system, and by the state of myocardial function. Decreased cardiac function, decreased venous capacitance, increased venous tone, and increased intravascular blood volume elevate CVP. Increased cardiac function, increased venous capacitance, decreased venous tone, and decreased blood volume tend to lower CVP. Indications for central venous catheterization are listed in Table 5-3.

The catheter can be introduced through any of the following veins: basilic, subclavian, external jugular, or internal jugular, the last of which has the highest success rate in correctly placing the catheter tip.

The right internal jugular (IJ) vein follows an almost straight path down the neck

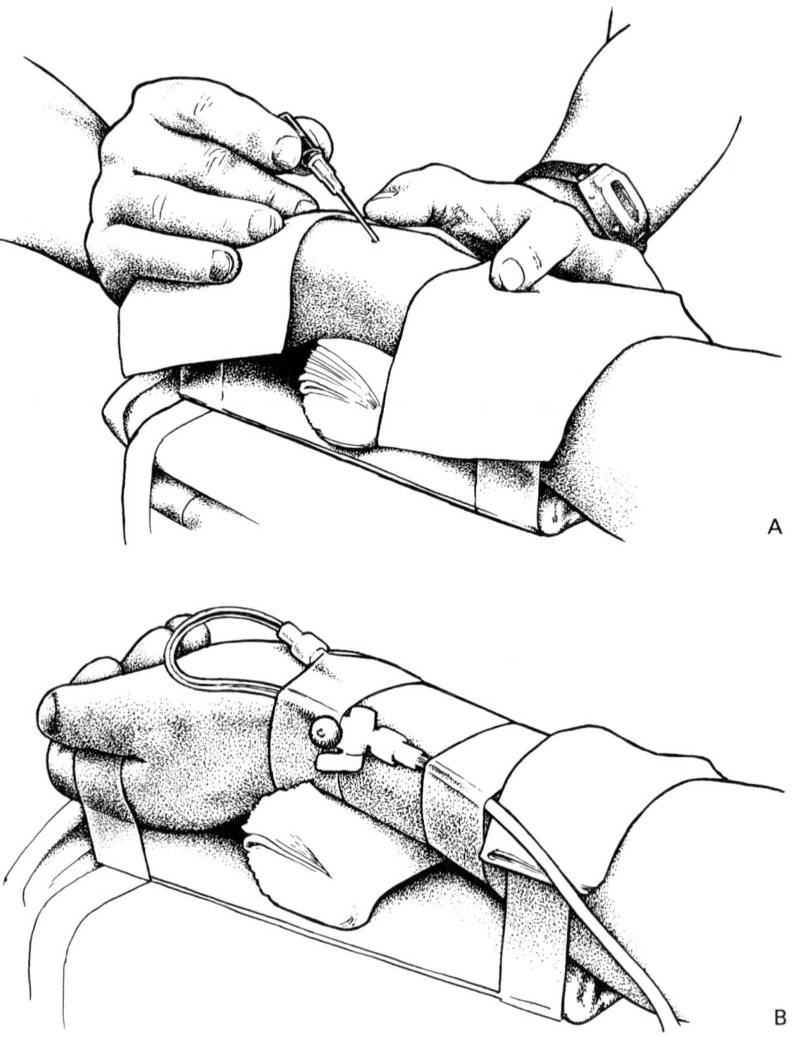


**Figure 5-11.** A, Placement of a percutaneous 20 gauge radial artery catheter. The artery has been entered and the catheter-needle unit is being gently threaded up the vessel. Note the position of the hand. The back wall of the artery has not been punctured. **B**, The radial artery catheter is connected to a short, 4 inch extension tubing, not directly to a stopcock; thus, manipulation of the stopcock will not cause movement of the catheter in the vessel.

**TABLE 5-3**
**Indications for Central Venous Catheterization**

Central venous pressure monitoring
Lack of peripheral veins for cannulation
Intravenous administration of vasopressors, potassium, and other drugs likely to injure peripheral veins and tissues
Rapid infusion of blood and fluids
Removal of autologous blood
Frequent blood sampling
Aspiration of air emboli
Hyperalimentation
Transvenous insertion of temporary pacing leads
Right heart catheterization studies
Insertion of a pulmonary artery catheter (Swan-Ganz)
- Pressure measurements
- Cardiac output determinations by thermodilution
- Pulmonary angiography
- Reduction of pulmonary vascular and left atrial pressures by removal of blood during cardiopulmonary bypass

From Hug, Carl C., Jr., 1981. Monitoring. In: *Anesthesia*. Miller, R.D., editor, New York: Churchill Livingstone.

to the right side of the heart (Figure 5-12). To cannulate the right IJ, the patient is placed in moderate Trendelenburg position with the patient's head turned to the left. The triangle outlined by the clavicle and the two heads (sternal and clavicular) of the sternocleidomastoid muscle is palpated. The skin is prepared with iodine and draped with towels. Under sterile conditions, 1%lidocaine is injected subcutaneously over the right IJ at a point near the apex of the triangle and the vein located with a short (1.0–1.5-inch) 22- or 23-gauge needle attached to a 5 mL syringe (Figure 5-13). The needle is removed and the vessel entered with a 14- or 16-gauge, 5.25-in catheter. Once the catheter tip is within the vessel, it is advanced off its needle introducer until it is located in the right atrium. The catheter is secured in place and connected to a free running intravenous line. Lowering the IV bottle below heart level should be followed by return of blood into the tubing. Pressure monitoring can be either by a water-filled manometer or by connection to a transducer electrically coupled to a pressure input of an ECG monitor.

Depending on the route of insertion of the catheter, complications include puncture of the carotid artery (with the IJ technique), hematoma, infection, local tissue trauma, air embolism, and thrombophlebitis.

In patients with normal cardiovascular function, central venous pressure is used as a guide for fluid and blood replacement during extensive surgical procedures or in hypovolemic, traumatized, or hemorrhaging patients. When combined with values for arterial blood pressure and urine output, clinical judgments can be made, as discussed previously.

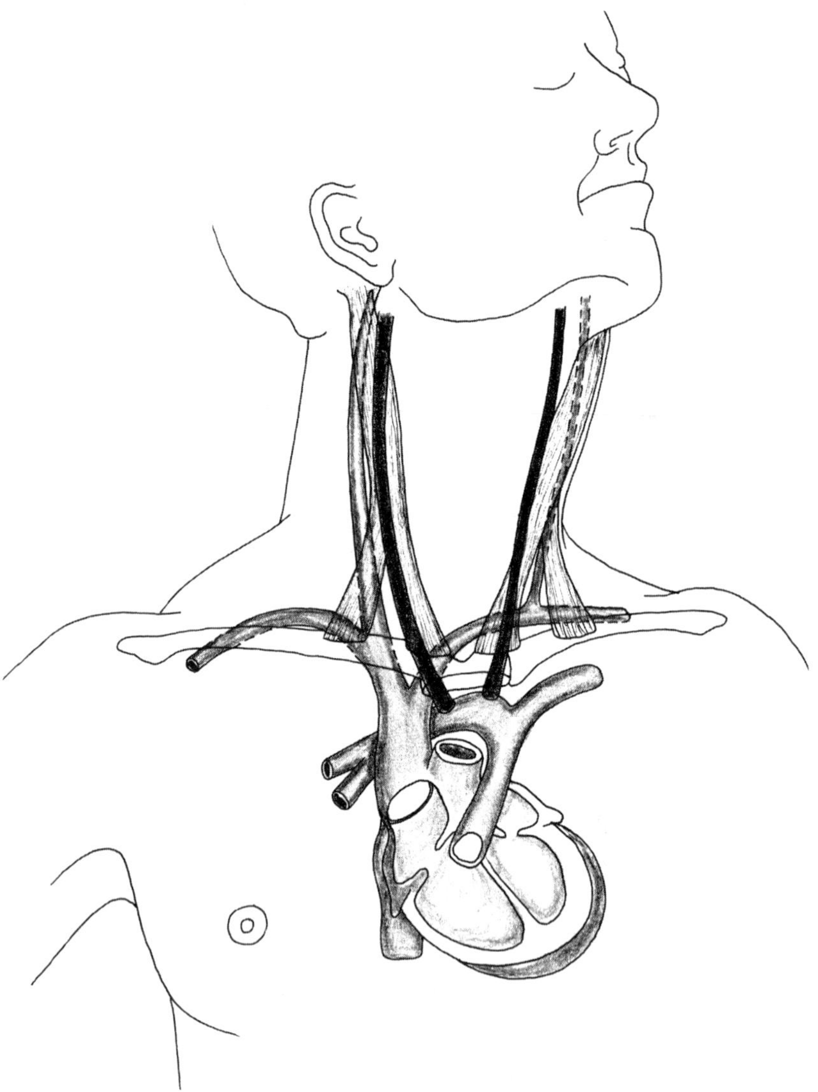

**Figure 5-12.** Anatomy of the internal jugular vein in relation to the carotid artery and the sternocleidomastoid muscles.

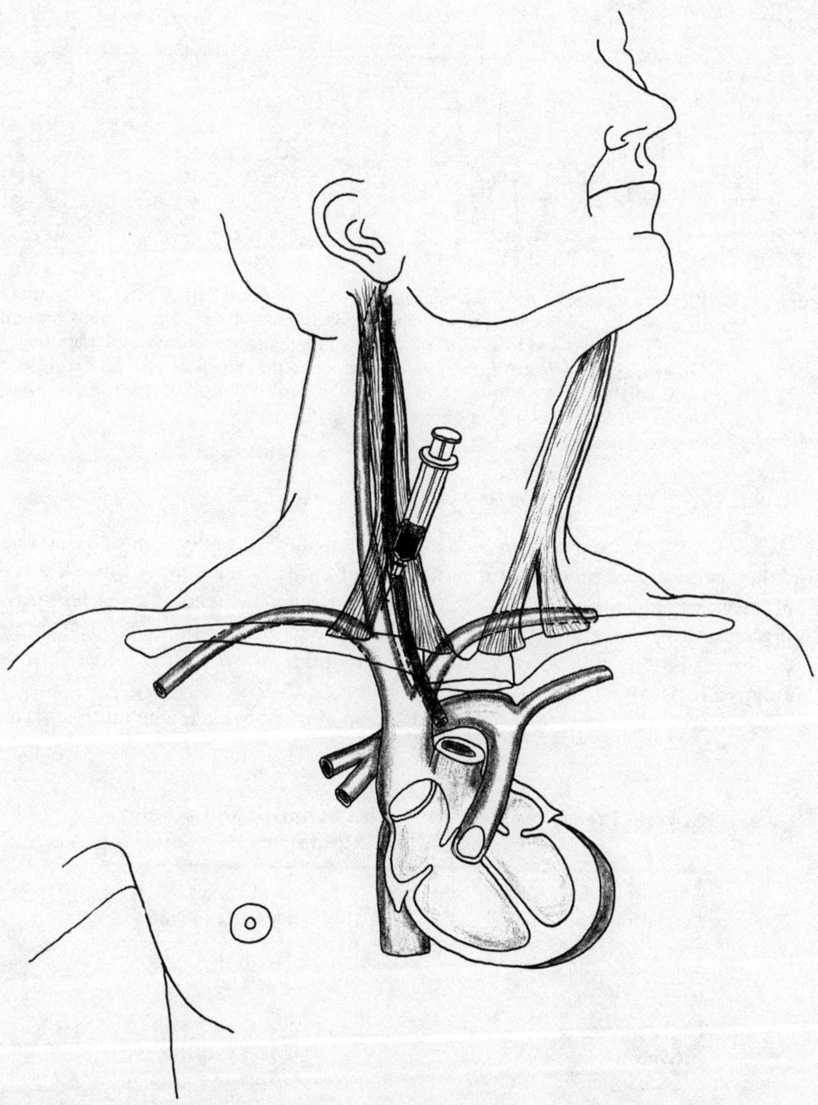

**Figure 5-13.** Locating the right internal jugular vein with a short "seeker" needle attached to a 5 mL syringe. To avoid puncturing the carotid artery, the needle enters the skin at the medial border of the clavicular head of the sternocleidomastoid muscle and is directed towards the ipsilateral nipple.

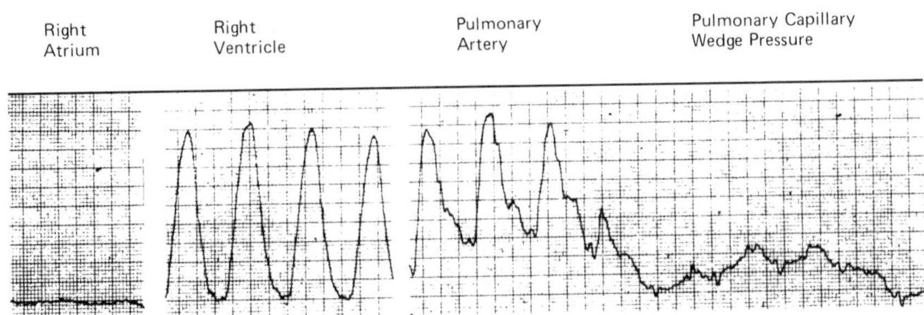


**Figure 5-14.** Pressure tracings recorded from the tip of a Swan-Ganz catheter as it is "floated" through the right atrium, right ventricle, pulmonary artery, and is finally located in the "wedge" position. With deflation of the balloon, return of the pulmonary artery tracing indicates correct placement. (Tracings reproduced with permission from Kaplan, J. A., editor. 1979. Hemodynamic monitoring. In: *Cardiac anesthesia.* New York: Grune & Stratton.)

## Pulmonary Artery Catheters

While CVP measurements provide information about the adequacy of blood volume, they do not give precise information about cardiac function. A flow-directed pulmonary catheter, the Swan-Ganz catheter, has been developed to assess left heart filling pressure (by measuring the pulmonary capillary wedge pressure), to sample mixed venous blood, to measure cardiac output, and to allow calculation of various hemodynamic parameters.

The Swan-Ganz catheter has a small balloon at its tip which, when inflated, can

**TABLE 5-4**
**Normal Pressures Recorded with Swan-Ganz Catheter in Recumbent Adults**

| Recording Location | Pressure (mm Hg) Mean and Range of Normal |
|---|---|
| Superior vena cava | 6 (1–10) |
| Right atrium | 4 (0–8) |
| Right ventricle | |
| Systolic | 25 (15–30) |
| Diastolic | 5 (0–8) |
| Pulmonary artery | |
| Systolic | 24 (15–30) |
| Diastolic | 10 (5–15) |
| Pulmonary artery | |
| Wedge pressure* | 9 (5–15) |

*Correlated closely with left atrial pressure and left ventricular end diastolic pressure.

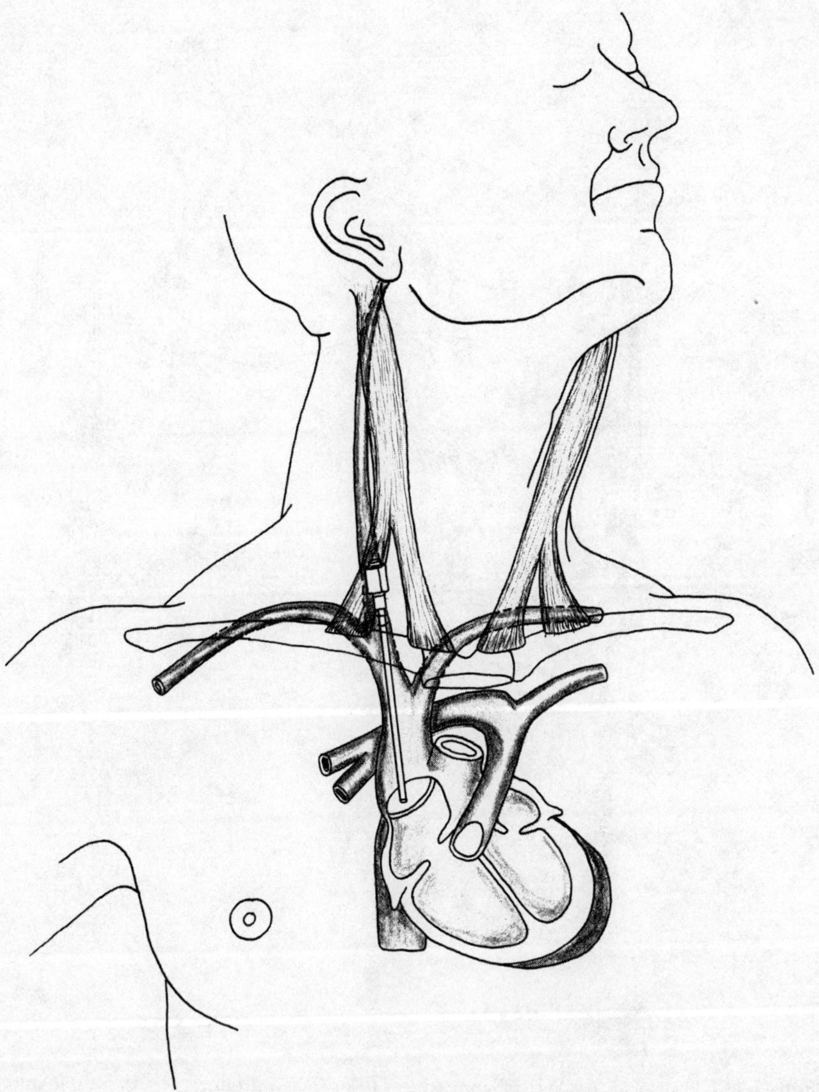

**Figure 5-15.** Location of a Swan-Ganz introducer sheath placed through the right internal jugular vein into the right atrium. A diaphragm in the proximal end prevents backflow of blood.

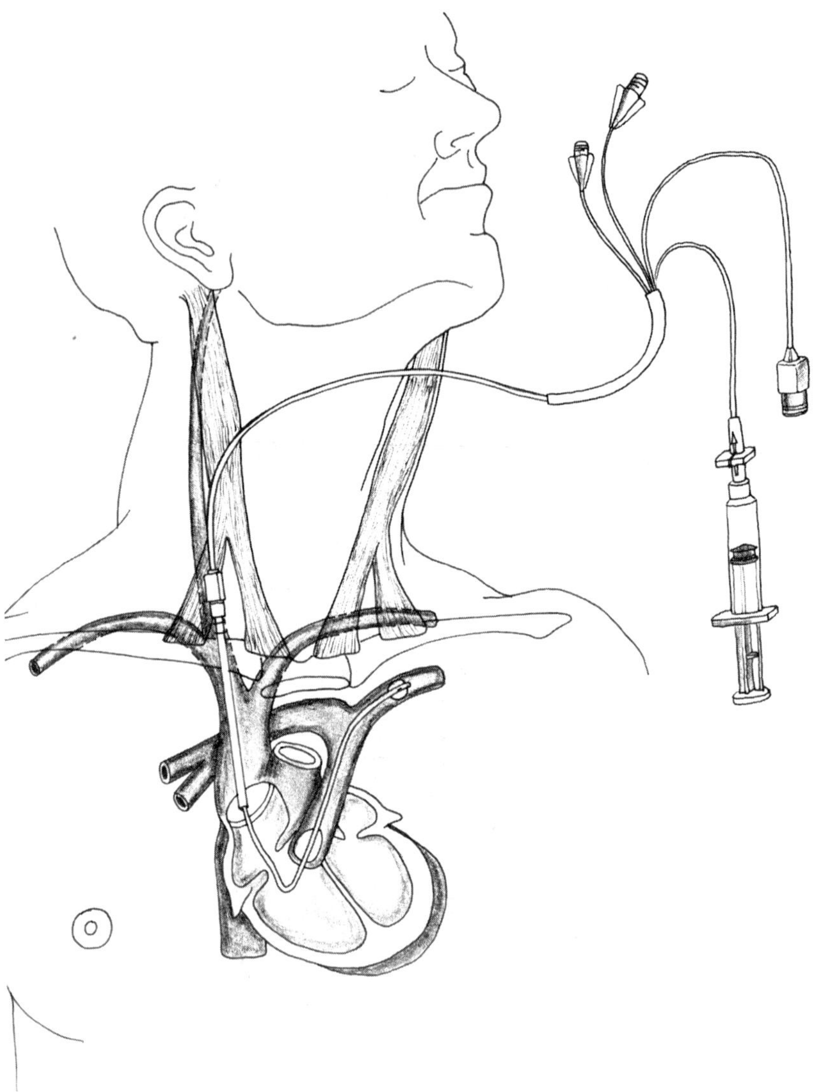

**Figure 5-16.** Placement of a Swan-Ganz catheter through an introducer sheath located in the right internal jugular vein. Illustrated at the proximal end of the catheter are intravenous connectors for injection ports located in the right atrium (proximal port) and the pulmonary artery (distal port), a syringe for balloon inflation, and an electrical connection for calculation of cardiac output measurements by an external computer.

be "floated" through the right atrium and the right ventricle and into the branch of the pulmonary artery. The pressure recordings obtained during advancement of the catheter and during occlusion of the pulmonary artery by the inflated balloon (i.e., the capillary "wedge" pressure) are illustrated in Figure 5-14, with the wedge pressure correlating with left atrial pressure. Normal pressures recorded from the Swan-Ganz catheter are listed in Table 5-4.

Some Swan-Ganz catheters also contain a thermistor probe located near the tip. Injection of ice water through a proximal injection port located in the right atrium results in a mixing of the ice water with the blood in the right atrium and the right ventricle. This cools the blood, which then is ejected by the heart into the pulmonary artery, flowing past the thermistor at the tip of the catheter. This temperature change is fed into a small computer, which calculates the cardiac output by thermodilution. Normal cardiac output in a 70-kg male is 5–6 L/min (3–3.5 L/min/$m^2$ of body surface area). Other Swan-Ganz catheters contain bipolar electrode wires for cardiac pacing when the leads are connected to an external pacemaker.

While pressure data directly obtained from the Swan-Ganz catheter is important, it also enables mathematic calculation of stroke volume, peripheral vascular resistance, pulmonary vascular resistance, and the left ventricle stroke work index. Such values are important in the management of anesthesia in patients with severe cardiac disease.

The placement of the Swan-Ganz catheter is similar to that of the CVP catheter. The right IJ vein is located with a 22- or 23-gauge, 1.0–1.5-inch needle, and 5 mL syringe (Figure 5-13). A short (2.0–2.5-inch) 16- or 18-gauge intravenous catheter is placed in the vessel (instead of the 5.25-inch CVP catheter). A guide wire is then placed through the catheter and the latter removed, leaving the guide wire in the vessel. A # 11 scalpel needle is used to enlarge the skin opening, and a Swan-Ganz dilator and introducer is passed over the wire guide into the vessel. The wire guide and dilator are removed, leaving the introducer in place (Figure 5-15). The Swan-Ganz catheter is then passed through the introducer about 20 cm into the superior vena cava. The balloon is then inflated with about 1.5 mL of air, and the catheter "floated" into the pulmonary artery (Figure 5-16) under constant viewing of the pressure trace on the monitor (Figure 5-14) until the "wedge" tracing is observed. The balloon is then deflated. The proximal and distal injection ports are then connected to constant infusion IV lines. If cardiac output measurements are desired, the thermistor lead is electronically connected to the cardiac output computer.

## *Readings and References*


Gerson, G.R., ed. 1981. Monitoring during anesthesia. In: *International anesthesia clinics*. Boston: Little, Brown and Co., vol. 19, no. 1.

Gravenstein, J.S., and Paulus, D.A. 1982. *Monitoring practice in clinical anesthesia*. Philadelphia: J.B. Lippincott.

Gravenstein, J.S.; Newbower, R.S.; Ream, A.K., et al. 1980. *Essential noninvasive monitoring in anesthesia*. New York: Grune & Stratton.

Gravenstein, J.S.; Newbower, R.S.; Ream, A.K., et al. 1983. *An integrated approach to monitoring*. Woburn, Mass.: Butterworths.

Grundy, B.L. 1983. Intraoperative monitoring of sensory-evoked potentials. *Anesthesiology* 58:72–87.

Hug, C.C., Jr. 1981. Monitoring. In: *Anesthesia.* Miller, R.D., editor. New York: Churchill Livingstone, pp. 157–201.

Kaplan, J.A. 1981. The electrocardiogram and anesthesia. In: *Anesthesia.* Miller, R.D., editor. New York: Churchill Livingstone, pp. 203–32.

——— 1982. Hemodynamic monitoring. In: *Cardiac anesthesia.* 2nd ed. Kaplan, J.A. editor. New York: Grune & Stratton.

Saidman, L.J., and Smith, N.T., editors. 1983. *Monitoring in anesthesia,* 2nd ed. New York: John Wiley & Sons.

Shapiro, B.A.; Harrison, R.A.; and Walton, J.R. 1982. *Clinical application of blood gases.* 3rd ed. Chicago: Year Book Medical Publishers.

Slogoff, S.; Keats, A.S.; and Arlund, C. 1983. On the safety of radial artery cannulation. *Anesthesiology* 59:42–47.

# III

# The Pharmacology of Anesthesia

# 6. Drugs Used for General Anesthesia

## Introduction

Before 1846, surgery was uncommon and usually reserved for emergencies. An understanding of disease processes and aseptic practices was almost unknown. Time-consuming surgical techniques could not be followed because of the lack of satisfactory methods for relieving pain.

Although nitrous oxide had been synthesized by Joseph Priestley in 1776, its anesthetic properties for the most part went unappreciated until the mid-nineteenth century. In 1845, a dentist named Horace Wells attempted to demonstrate the analgesic effect of Priestley's drug at the Massachusetts General Hospital, but the attempt failed when the patient cried out during the procedure. In 1846, another Boston dentist, William T. G. Morton, gave the first public demonstration of surgical anesthesia using inhaled diethyl ether vapors. The success of this demonstration led to the rapid introduction of ether anesthesia throughout the United States and Great Britain.

Ether is a potent anesthetic agent that is readily vaporized and relatively nontoxic. It can be mixed with room air and administered without undue concern that hypoxia will occur. The stimulation of both respiration and circulation was an important consideration during those early days because neither the apparatus for assisting respiration nor the chemicals for supporting circulation were available. But ether is explosive, and this fact, to a great extent, has eliminated the drug from clinical use today.

In 1847, James Simpson, a Scottish obstetrician, introduced chloroform anesthesia, and it became popular throughout Europe. Although chloroform is nonflammable, it is toxic to the liver, severely depresses cardiovascular function, and has a high incidence of producing cardiac arrhythmias. Despite its limitations, however, chloroform, like ether, was widely used for nearly 100 years.

In 1929, the anesthetic properties of cycloproprane were discovered, and this agent was widely used over the next 30 years. But it also is highly explosive, and has been largely abandoned in favor of newer, nonflammable agents.

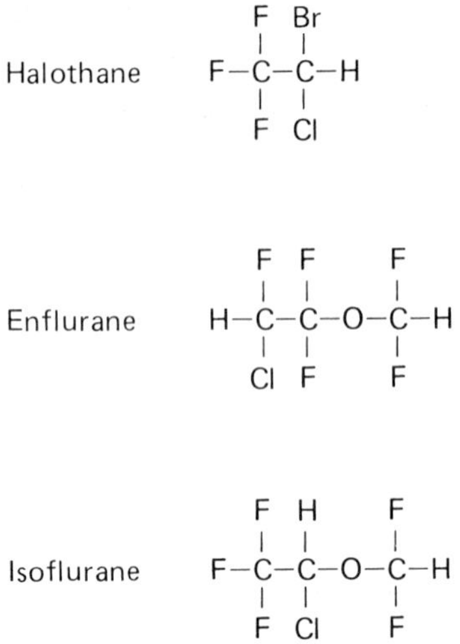

```
              F  Br
              |  |
Halothane   F—C—C—H
              |  |
              F  Cl


              F  F     F
              |  |     |
Enflurane   H—C—C—O—C—H
              |  |     |
              Cl F     F


              F  H     F
              |  |     |
Isoflurane  F—C—C—O—C—H
              |  |     |
              F  Cl    F
```

**Figure 6-1.** Chemical structures of three volatile liquid anesthetics.

A significant advance in 1946 was the demonstration that *d*-tubocurarine, the active product in the naturally occurring substance curare, produces skeletal muscle relaxation by blocking neuromuscular transmission. Muscle relaxation is necessary for certain operative procedures, and using *d*-tubocurarine allowed the anesthesiologist to use less ether than had previously been necessary for obtaining skeletal muscle relaxation. This change reduced the levels of ether vapors in the operating room and decreased the likelihood of explosions.

Another neuromuscular blocking agent, succinylcholine, was introduced in 1951. This drug, which takes effect more quickly (in 1 minute) and has a shorter duration of action (3–5 minutes) than *d*-tubocurarine, simplified endotracheal intubation and allowed its wide acceptance. Thus, by the early 1950s, anesthesia was being induced with thiopental and succinylcholine, and maintained with nitrous oxide, *d*-tubocurarine, and low levels of ether vapors. This technique produced only minimal cardiovascular depression and enabled rapid awakening after surgery.

The ongoing search for a potent inhalation agent that was neither explosive nor highly toxic led to the development of halothane, a halogenated hydrocarbon (Figure 6-1), by the British Research Council and the Imperial Chemical Industries. Introduced into clinical practice in 1956, halothane was one of the most significant advances in general anesthesia since the introduction of ether 110 years earlier. It largely replaced ether and cyclopropane. More recently, two halogenated ethers have been introduced; enflurane, in 1972, and isoflurane, an isomer of enflurane, in 1981 (Figure 6-1).

Although the replacement of ether by the halogenated agents reduced the possibility of explosions, *d*-tubocurarine remains useful for providing relaxation, since it allows use of lighter levels of general anesthesia, thus reducing cardiac and circulatory depression.

Extensive research has provided other drugs that have increased the safety of anesthesia. These drugs, including the narcotics, benzodiazepines, major tranquilizers, and ketamine, are frequently used in various combinations to further minimize the depressant effects on the cardiovascular system. (See Chapter 10 for details on their use in combinations.)

In sum, the years since 1846 have seen an evolution from deep ether-oxygen anesthesia to less profound general anesthesia using a combination of a volatile agent, nitrous oxide, and oxygen, supplemented by drug-induced neuromuscular relaxation. In addition, the development of new drugs for inducing anesthesia, more reliable intravenous catheters, and extensive patient monitoring have made possible a safer anesthesia experience.

For reader convenience, Table 6-1 summarizes many of the significant effects of the volatile anesthetics and nitrous oxide on the cardiovascular system, lungs, and brain.

**TABLE 6-1**
**Summary of Organ System Effects of Inhaled Anesthetics**

| | Halothane | Enflurane | Isoflurane | Nitrous Oxide |
|---|---|---|---|---|
| *Cardiac effects* | | | | |
| Mean arterial pressure | ↓ | ↓ | ↓ | ←→ |
| Heart rate | ↓ | ←→, ↑ | ↑ | ←→ |
| Stroke volume | ↓ | ←→, ↓ | ←→ | ←→ |
| Cardiac output | ↓↓ | ↓ | ←→ | ←→, ↓ |
| Contractility | ↓↓ | ↓↓ | ←→ | ↓ |
| $O_2$ consumption | ↓ | ↓ | ↓ | ←→, ↑ |
| Right atrial pressure | ↑↓ | ↑↓ | ↑↓ | ↑ |
| Systemic vascular resistance | ↓ | ↓↓ | ↓↓↓ | ↑ |
| *Pulmonary effects* | | | | |
| Airway resistance | ↓ | ↓ | ↓ | ←→ |
| Pulmonary vascular resistance | ↓ | ↓ | ↓ | ↑ |
| *CNS effects* | | | | |
| Cerebral blood flow | ↑↑ | ↑↑ | ↑↑ | ↑ |
| Cerebral metabolic rate | ↓ | ↓ | ↓ | ←→, ↑ |
| *Miscellaneous* | | | | |
| Anesthetic potency (MAC*) | 0.75% | 1.68% | 1.15% | 105% |
| % metabolized | 20%–25% | 2%–5% | 0.3%–0.5% | 0% |

*MAC is a useful concept for measuring and comparing the potency of inhaled anesthetics. MAC is defined as the minimum alveolar concentration of an anesthetic (at 1 ATM) that abolishes reflex movement in 50% of subjects given a painful stimulus (e.g., skin incision). MAC is reduced in hypothermia, pregnancy, old age, and by the addition of other anesthetics or narcotics.

Significance: ↑ or ↓ = mild increase or decrease; ↑↑ or ↓↓ = moderate increase or decrease; ↓↓↓ = marked decrease; ←→ = little or no change.

# The Volatile Anesthetics

## Halothane

Halothane (Fluothane) is a potent agent for general anesthesia. A concentration of less than 1% halothane vapor in a mixture of nitrous oxide and oxygen provides general anesthesia for virtually all patients. The relationship between the inspired concentration of halothane and its pharmacologic effects is complex and is discussed at length in the readings listed at the end of the chapter. The texts by Eger (1974) and Wood and Wood (1982) are especially useful.

Some advantges of halothane include rapid onset and rapid termination of effect, qualities that allow for relative ease in controlling anesthesia depth and for rapid awakening when the drug is discontinued. Halothane is nonexplosive and relatively nontoxic when properly used.

*Effects on the Central Nervous System.* Halothane is a general depressant of the central nervous system (CNS), decreasing neuronal activity and cerebral metabolic rate. Halothane also relaxes the smooth muscle of cerebral blood vessels, causing them to dilate, increasing cerebral blood flow, and secondarily increasing intracranial pressure. Halothane is thus contraindicated in patients with increased intracranial pressure, such as might accompany intracranial hemorrhage or tumor. These effects contrast markedly with the reduction in both cerebral blood flow and intracranial pressure that accompanies the intravenous administration of barbiturates.

*Cardiovascular Effects.* At surgical concentrations, halothane decreases both myocardial contractility and stroke volume, reducing cardiac output by 20%–50%. This reduced cardiac output, together with a dilatation of peripheral blood vessels, results in a dose-dependent decrease in arterial blood pressure to 50%–75% of preoperative levels at anesthetic concentrations. But halothane also slightly depresses the responsiveness of the pressure receptors in the aorta and carotid sinus, so that the normal reflex increase in heart rate that follows the induced hypotension is reduced. More importantly, halothane reduces the rate of sinoatrial node depolarization, resulting in a decrease in both heart rate and blood pressure. The cardiac depression does not result in myocardial injury because the volatile anesthetics reduce myocardial oxygen consumption, an effect accompanied by decreased coronary blood flow.

Halothane sensitizes the heart to exogenous catecholamines. Sensitization means that the dose of drugs that stimulate the adrenergic nervous system needed to produce cardiac arrhythmias (especially premature ventricular contractions) is lower in halothane-anesthetized patients than in awake patients. Drugs whose arrhythmogenic doses are lowered by halothane include epinephrine, many antiasthmatic drugs (e.g., aminophylline, isoproterenol), the tricyclic antidepressants (e.g., imipramine), and cocaine. Halothane should be used with great care in patients taking these drugs.

Frequently surgeons inject epinephrine-containing anesthetic solutions locally into anesthetized patients to achieve hemostasis. The dose of epinephrine injected is limited by the inhaled anesthetic used. Patients anesthetized with halothane should receive no more than 1.5 μg/kg body weight of epinephrine, while those anesthetized with isoflurane or enflurane can receive up to 3.0 μg/kg. Thus, a halothane-anesthetized 70 kg adult could be given 14 mL of local anesthetic containing 1:100,000 epinephrine (10 μg/mL), while a 7 kg child could only be given a maximum of 1.4 mL of the same solution. Solutions can be reinjected about every 20 minutes if needed (see Johnson et al. (1976) for discussion of this interaction between epinephrine and inhaled anesthetics).

*Effects on Smooth Muscle.* Halothane relaxes smooth muscle, decreasing both systemic and pulmonary vascular resistance, resulting in hypotension.

Because it affects the smooth muscle of the uterus, it inhibits uterine contractions during parturition and prolongs delivery. After delivery, this uterine relaxation negates the uterine-stimulant effect of oxytocin and increases blood loss. Therefore, halothane is used in low doses in obstetrics. The specific indications for the use of halothane in obstetrics are discussed in Chapter 14.

Halothane also relaxes the smooth muscle of the airways, producing bronchial dilatation. The mechanisms involved appear to be related both to a direct action on the smooth muscle and an indirect action, probably through cyclic adenosine monophosphate, a substance which causes smooth muscle relaxation by activating a cascade of enzymatically catalyzed reactions. Because of this bronchial-relaxant effect, halothane is useful in asthmatic patients, although its use is limited by the drugs the asthmatic may be taking, as discussed above, in order to avoid potentially serious cardiac arrhythmias. Enflurane and isoflurane (discussed later) produce bronchial relaxation similar to halothane's but with less myocardial sensitization, and they are preferable for some asthmatics receiving antiasthmatic drugs.

*Effects on Respiration.* Halothane produces rapid and shallow respirations, and the patient may appear to be panting. Such breathing may result in hypoventilation, decreased minute ventilation, and an increased amount of carbon dioxide in arterial blood.

*Effects on Skeletal Muscle.* Halothane causes only minimal relaxation of skeletal muscle. Thus, when skeletal muscle relaxation is required, neuromuscular blocking agents are used.

Rarely, halothane may induce an uncontrolled hypermetabolic reaction in skeletal muscle, resulting in the syndrome termed "malignant hyperpyrexia." Other drugs associated with this syndrome include other volatile anesthetics and succinylcholine. This syndrome usually occurs in genetically predisposed individuals and is precipitated by drug-induced increases in the calcium permeability of the sarcoplasmic reticulum of muscle cells. The increased permeability leads to cell destruction, acidosis, increased body temperature, increased oxygen consumption, and death. The drug dantrolene (Dantrium) prevents halothane-induced increases in calcium permeability and blunts the manifestations of the syndrome.

*Effects on the Kidney.* Soon after the introduction of halothane, it was noted that, in concentrations used in surgery, it decreased urine output by 40%–50%. This decrease follows the drug-induced reduction in cardiac output, which decreases renal blood flow and glomerular filtration. These effects may be avoided by giving intravenous fluids. Halothane does not appear to have any significant long-term effect on renal function.

*Effects on the Liver.* Halothane was originally thought to be completely eliminated from the body through the lungs. It is now known that, while approximately 80% of the drug is eliminated by that route, 20%–25% undergoes oxidative metabolism in the liver. The end products of its metabolism include trifluoroacetic acid, bromide ions, and chloride ions, all thought to be nontoxic.

In retrospective analysis of approximately one million halothane anesthesia cases, a small number of postanesthetic hepatitis cases were found that could not be explained by blood transfusions, known liver disease, or known liver toxins. The incidence of such cases is approximately one per 10,000 patients receiving a general anesthetic; the cause most often implicated is halothane. Obesity and middle age appear to be contributing factors. (Halothane hepatitis has not been described in children or the elderly.) While a cause-and-effect relationship between halothane exposure and hepatitis remains to be demonstrated, animal models of human "halothane hepatitis" predict that altered biotransformation of halothane may occur in some humans. An altered metabolism could produce reactive intermediates capable of producing liver damage (Dykes, 1983).

## Enflurane

Enflurane (Ethrane) is a fluorinated methylethyl ether (Figure 6-1), approximately half as potent as halothane. Depth of anesthesia is easily regulated with enflurane, and recovery from anesthesia is rapid. Although similar to halothane in many respects, enflurane differs in many others (Table 6-1).

*Effects on the Central Nervous System.* Anesthesia with either enflurane or halothane is characterized by unconsciousness and insensitivity to painful stimuli. But enflurane anesthesia, unlike that with halothane, is accompanied by electroencephalogram (EEG) patterns resembling those seen in epileptics. Initial clinical reports noted occasional tonic-clonic muscle activity, with twitching of the muscles of the face and limbs. It was therefore thought that enflurane might be a convulsant. Indeed, the drug has been used to activate epileptic foci during neurosurgical ablations of such areas of the brain.

Like halothane, enflurane reduces cerebral metabolic rate and oxygen consumption, while dilating cerebral blood vessels and increasing cerebral blood flow. Because intracranial pressure is then increased, enflurane should be avoided in patients with elevated intracranial pressures.

*Effects on the Cardiovascular System.* The cardiovascular effects of enflurane differ significantly from those of halothane. While both drugs decrease arterial blood pressure, the reduction due to enflurane results from a decrease in systemic vascular resistance, rather than from a large decrease in cardiac output. Thus, although enflurane decreases myocardial contractility, it maintains a better stroke volume and cardiac output than does halothane. In addition, enflurane sensitizes the heart less to catecholamines. It is therefore preferred to halothane for patients in whom increased catecholamine levels are expected.

*Effects on Skeletal and Smooth Muscle.* Enflurane relaxes skeletal muscle more than does halothane, but the level of relaxation still is seldom sufficient for abdominal surgery and must frequently be augmented by neuromuscular blocking drugs. The use of enflurane, however, does allow the use of lower doses of muscle relaxants than do halothane- or narcotic-based anesthetics (Chapter 10).

The smooth muscle of the uterus is relaxed by enflurane in the same manner as halothane, and the same restrictions apply to its use in the pregnant patient at term. The smooth muscle of the blood vessels is likewise relaxed. This results in a decrease in vascular resistance, producing hypotension, increased cerebral blood flow, and increased intracranial pressure.

*Effects on Respiration.* Enflurane is also a respiratory depressant and causes increased partial pressures of arterial carbon dioxide during spontaneous breathing. For this reason, ventilation during its use is often controlled by the anesthesiologist. Enflurane, as described above, relaxes bronchial smooth muscle and is often used for anesthesia in asthmatics.

*Effects on the Liver and Kidney.* Like halothane, enflurane decreases urine output secondary to a reduction in cardiac output. Intravenous fluids usually restore normal urine output.

There is little evidence of liver damage as a result of enflurane anesthesia. About 2%–5% of administered enflurane is metabolized in the liver, contrasted with 20% for halothane. Unlike halothane, metabolism of enflurane results in the production of small quantities of fluoride ions. In patients with normal kidney function, fluoride levels remain well below those that would cause renal toxicity. Even in anephric patients, fluoride ion concentrations fall rapidly after termination of anesthesia, presumably due to uptake of the ion by bone. It therefore appears unlikely that enflurane will produce renal toxicity, even in the presence of poor renal function.

## Isoflurane

Isoflurane (Forane), an isomer of enflurane (Figure 6-1), was developed in the early 1970s, but was not released for clinical use until 1981. Since it is less soluble in blood than halothane or enflurane, recovery from anesthesia with isoflurane is more rapid than with either of the other agents. Isoflurane causes little depression of myocardial contractility, in comparison with the other two volatile anesthetics (Table 6-1). However, it may decrease blood pressure, primarily by a decrease in peripheral vascular resistance. Cardiac arrhythmias with isoflurane are uncommon, and it only minimally sensitizes the heart to catecholamines.

The effects of isoflurane on skeletal muscle are similar to those of enflurane; both agents reducing the dosage of neuromuscular blocking drugs required for intraabdominal surgery. The effects of isoflurane on the central nervous system are similar to those produced by halothane. Isoflurane depresses neuronal activity, decreases cerebral metabolic rate, dilates cerebral blood vessels, increases cerebral blood flow, and thus increases intracranial pressure, although somewhat less than does either halothane or enflurane.

Approximately 99% of the inhaled dose of isoflurane is eliminated unchanged through the lungs, and only about 0.3%–0.5% is metabolized in the liver. Not suprisingly, therefore, no toxic effects of isoflurane on the liver or kidney have been reported.

## Gases Used in Anesthesia

### Nitrous Oxide

Nitrous oxide is the most widely used anesthetic in clinical practice, despite the fact that, when used alone, it cannot predictably produce general anesthesia. But its mild analgesic and amnesic properties make it a useful supplement to other, more potent anesthetics.

*Effects on the Nervous System.* In concentrations of 20%–30%, the analgesic properties of nitrous oxide are demonstrable and equivalent to those of low doses of morphine. Concentrations of 70%–75% produce unconsciousness in most patients, but provide inadequate anesthesia for surgery unless narcotics or volatile anesthetics are added. Since a minimum of 21% oxygen (30% during anesthesia) must be inhaled to avoid hypoxia, concentrations of nitrous oxide in excess of 70% should not be administered. Most commonly, the inhaled anesthetic mixture contains 65%–70% of nitrous oxide, plus 30%–35% of oxygen, together with 0.5%–2% of halothane, enflurane, or isoflurane, depending on the MAC, the patient's age, and the presence of narcotics (Table 6-1).

Nitrous oxide increases cerebral blood flow and may increase intracranial pressure, although such increases can be reduced by diazepam or thiopental. Therefore, when nitrous oxide is used for anesthesia for patients with increased intracranial pressure, precautions should be taken to protect the brain from further increases in pressure (i.e., through the use of hyperventilation, glucocorticoids, mannitol, diazepam, or thiopental).

*Effects on the Cardiovascular System.* Nitrous oxide directly depresses myocardial contractility, although such depression is much less than that produced by the volatile anesthetics. Clinically, this results in an increase in right atrial pressure, while little change is seen in cardiac output, stroke volume, heart rate, or blood pressure. The increased right atrial pressure results, not only from myocardial depression, but from an increase in pulmonary vascular resistance, probably occurring secondary to stimulation of the sympathetic nervous system.

When used in combination, nitrous oxide decreases the anesthetic requirement of the volatile anesthetics, allowing lower concentrations of the volatile agent to be given, thus reducing the cardiovascular depression caused by these latter compounds. When nitrous oxide is combined with narcotics, however, especially in critically ill patients, it may produce clinically significant cardiac depression. It must therefore be used with great care in patients in shock or with serious hemodynamic imbalances.

Nitrous oxide produces little relaxation of skeletal muscle, and neuromuscular blocking agents must be administered with it if required for a particular procedure. It does not relax the smooth muscle of the uterus, and can therefore be used safely in obstetrics.

The liver and the kidneys are not significantly affected by nitrous oxide, and nitrous oxide is eliminated through the lungs with little or none of it undergoing metabolic degradation in the body.

*Toxicity from Chronic Exposure.* There is increasing concern over long-term effects on health from occupational exposure to trace amounts of anesthetic gases and vapors. Operating room personnel (anesthesiologists, nurse anesthetists, technicians, and nurses) and many surgeons, dentists, and dental assistants are at risk of significant exposure to those agents. There have been reports of mutagenic, carcinogenic, teratogenic, and systemic alterations associated with chronic exposure.

To summarize this controversial topic is difficult. Much of the data are conflicting and methods of data collection and analysis are often open to criticism. However, a reasonable judgment is that, based on current evidence, the inhaled anesthetics are neither mutagenic or carcinogenic.

Their teratogenic potential is much less clear. Several large-scale, retrospective studies report increased rates of spontaneous abortions in female operating room and dental personnel, and occasionally in wives of male personnel. A cause-and-effect relationship remains to be demonstrated. The possibility of skeletal malformation in newborns of exposed workers has also been investigated, but the data are quite inconsistent. Probably such malformations are not a major hazard of exposure.

Nitrous oxide has been associated with bone marrow abnormalities and neurologic signs of vitamin $B_{12}$ deficiency (polyneuropathy and spinal cord lesions) in chronic abusers of nitrous oxide. It decreases the activity of methionine synthetase, an enzyme that synthesizes methionine and tetrahydrofolate from homocysteine and methyltetrahydrofolate in the liver (Koblin et al., 1982). The reduced levels of tetrahydrofolate after enzyme inhibition by nitrous oxide may decrease DNA synthesis. The monograph by Eger (1984) reviews these and other potential hazards of nitrous oxide.

Further research is needed to evaluate the potential toxicity resulting from long-term occupational exposure to inhaled anesthetics. For the present, anesthesiologists should minimize the levels of waste gases in the operating room by carefully evaluating the integrity of scavenging systems, gas connectors, and the anesthesia circle.

## Oxygen

The administration of oxygen during general anesthesia is taken for granted; thus, discussion of it is often neglected. But the damage that may result from either too much or too little oxygen should be discussed briefly.

*Hypoxia.* The clinical signs of oxygen deficiency in body tissues, or hypoxia, include cyanosis, increased depth and rate of respiration, increased heart rate, and increased cardiac output. Early recognition and reversal of hypoxia are essential for avoiding damage to the brain and the heart.

There are five general causes of hypoxia:

1. Inadequate oxygen content of inspired gas
2. Inadequate delivery of inspired gas to the lungs
3. Inadequate oxygenation of blood because of abnormal pulmonary gas exchange
4. Inadequate transport of oxygen by the circulatory system
5. Excessive oxygen utilization by tissues

Inadequate oxygen content (less than 21%) of the inspired gas at sea level should never occur in clinical anesthesia. Nevertheless, it may occur, usually with grave consequences. Oxygen flows may cease unexpectedly, as when an oxygen cylinder empties during anesthesia. To prevent such disasters, "fail-safe" devices have been incorporated into newer anesthetic machines, and oxygen analyzers with low oxygen alarms should be used to monitor oxygen concentrations in the anesthesia circle (Chapter 5).

Inadequate delivery of inspired gas to the lungs results from inadequate ventilation. This can be avoided by monitoring the patient's breath sounds with a precordial or esophageal stethoscope, and by observing both the pressure in the anesthesia circle and the movement of the reservoir bag. Passing an endotracheal tube below the level of the carina, into the right mainstem bronchus, is a common cause of decreased oxygen delivery during anesthesia as the left lung is not ventilated in such an instance. This situation can be avoided by auscultation of both lungs after carefully inserting the endotracheal tube, and then periodically during the course of surgery.

Inadequate oxygenation of blood due to abnormal pulmonary gas exchange results from thickening of the alveolar-capillary membrane, abnormal shunts of blood through the lungs, bronchial secretions, water in the lungs (e.g., as in cases of near-drowning), or pulmonary edema. Such defects are often present before surgery and should be sought by the anesthesiologist in the preoperative visit.

Intraoperative management of altered gas exchange processes consists of administering higher concentrations of oxygen, along with monitoring blood gases with an indwelling arterial catheter. Positive end-expiratory pressure (PEEP) may be added to further aid oxygenation. Pulmonary edema, should it occur intraoperatively, can be treated by administering diuretics and cardiac stimulants (see Chapter 8), by restricting fluids (see Chapter 12), or by adding PEEP.

Inadequate oxygen transport by the circulatory system usually occurs in patients whose blood has a low oxygen-carrying capacity due to hemorrhage, anemia, or abnormal hemoglobin. In an otherwise healthy patient, inadequate oxygen transport usually follows anesthetic-induced cardiac depression.

Finally, tissues occasionally extract excessive amounts of oxygen from the blood because of their abnormally high metabolic requirements, as might occur in some diseases (e.g., thyroid disease and malignant hyperpyrexia).

*Oxygen Toxicity.* In adults, oxygen toxicity usually occurs after several days' exposure to high concentrations of the gas. Such exposure produces pulmonary irritation, alveolar and interstitial changes, and pulmonary edema, which can result in reduced arterial oxygenation despite increases in inspired oxygen.

In newborns and premature infants, on the other hand, even limited exposure to high concentrations of oxygen can produce retrolental fibroplasia, retinal detachments, and blindness. Infants should not be exposed to oxygen concentrations in excess of about 30%–35% unless absolutely necessary. If possible, arterial oxygen should be monitored with a transcutaneous oxygen analyzer (Chapter 5), and the anesthesiologist should adjust the inspired oxygen concentration to maintain arterial oxygen near or slightly above levels in normal infants breathing room air.

## Sedative-Hypnotic Drugs

The sedative-hypnotic drugs are compounds of diverse chemical structures, all capable of inducing varying degrees of CNS depression. The sedative-hypnotics commonly used in anesthesia are barbiturates (e.g., thiopental and methohexital) and benzodiazepines (e.g., diazepam, lorazepam, and midazolam). In addition, a newer agent, etomidate (Amidate), has become available. All of these produce amnesia and unconsciousness without either analgesia or neuromuscular blockade.

### Barbiturates

The numerous barbiturates available may be conveniently classified as ultrashort, short, intermediate, and long-acting. The ultrashort-acting compounds are of most interest to anesthesiologists. Of these, methohexital (Brevital) and sodium thiopental (Pentothal) are most widely used, primarily for the induction of general anesthesia. Their brief duration of action is primarily determined by redistribution of the drug from highly perfused tissues, such as brain tissue, to less well-perfused tissues, such as muscle, fat, or bone tissue (discussed later). Table 6-2 summarizes their effects on the CNS, the cardiovascular system, and respiration.

*Effects on the Central Nervous System.* All barbiturates produce a dose-dependent depression of the activity of all neurons within the CNS. They are anticonvulsants and they decrease cerebral metabolic rate. Unlike the volatile anesthetics, the barbiturates reduce cerebral blood flow concomitant with their reduction in cerebral metabolic rate. They therefore reduce intracranial pressure. The neuronal depression and reduced intracranial pressure may be of clinical benefit in protecting injured brain in patients with acute increases in intracranial pressure (e.g., after head injury).

Barbiturates are not analgesics and, in low doses, they may actually increase the sensation of pain. Indeed, if pain is present, the lack of analgesia combined with drug-induced intoxication can result in agitation and disorientation instead of sedation.

*Effects on the Cardiovascular System.* In normal patients, low doses of barbiturates exert little effect on the heart or the vasculature. In anesthetic doses, however, they produce myocardial depression and decrease both cardiac output and stroke volume, all of which can lead to precipitous decreases in blood pressure, especially in patients with a poorly functioning circulatory system. While 3–5 mg/kg of sodium thiopental might be tolerated well by a healthy patient, this dose could produce profound hy-

**TABLE 6-2**
**Summary of Organ System Effects of Intravenous Anesthetics**

| | Barbiturates | Benzodiazepines | Narcotics | Ketamine | Etomidate |
|---|---|---|---|---|---|
| *Cardiovascular effects* | | | | | |
| Myocardial contractility | ↓ | 0, ↓ | 0 | ↑ | 0, ↓ |
| Cardiac output | ↓ | 0, ↓ | 0 | ↑ | 0, ↓ |
| Mean arterial pressure | ↓ | 0, ↓ | 0 | ↑ | 0, ↓ |
| Systemic vascular resistance | ↓ | 0, ↓ | 0 | ↑ | 0, ↓ |
| Venous capacitance | ↑↑ | 0, ↑ | 0, ↑ | ↓ | ? |
| *Pulmonary effects* | | | | | |
| Minute ventilation | ↓↓ | ↓ | ↓↓ | 0, ↓ | 0, ↓ |
| $CO_2$ sensitivity | ↓ | 0, ↓ | ↓↓ | 0, ↓ | 0, ↓ |
| Respiratory rate | 0, ↓ | 0, ↓ | ↓↓ | 0, ↑ | 0, ↑ |
| Tidal volume | ↓↓ | ↓ | ↓ | 0, ↓ | 0, ↓ |
| *CNS effects* | | | | | |
| Cerebral blood flow | ↓↓ | ↓ | 0, ↓ | ↑↑ | ↓ |
| Cerebral metabolic rate | ↓↓ | ↓ | 0, ↓ | ↑ | ↓ |
| Analgesia | 0 | 0 | ↑↑ | ↑↑ | 0 |
| Intracranial pressure | ↓↓ | 0, ↓ | 0, ↓ | ↑↑ | ↓ |

Significance: 0 = no change; 0, ↑ or 0, ↓ = little or no increase or decrease; ↑ or ↓ = moderate increase or decrease; ↑↑ or ↓↓ = marked increase or decrease.

potension, even cardiovascular collapse, in patients with cardiac or vascular disease, in hypovolemic patients, or in the elderly.

*Effects on Respiration.* In doses used for anesthesia induction, thiopental (3–5 mg/kg IV) markedly depresses respiration, commonly inducing apnea. However, the degree of muscle relaxation produced by thiopental is inadequate for endotracheal intubation. Succinylcholine (1 mg/kg) is frequently given to produce the 1–3 minutes of skeletal muscle relaxation needed for intubation (discussed later).

The intravenous administration of barbiturates to allergic or asthmatic patients has been reported to induce bronchospasm, although barbiturates do not appear to alter airway resistance (Stoelting, 1983). Barbiturates should probably be used with caution when inducing anesthesia in patients with a history of allergy or asthma. In such patients, a combination of diazepam, ketamine, and lidocaine intravenously, together with oxygen and halothane by mask for a few minutes before intubation, might offer a safer alternative to a barbiturate induction and rapid intubation.

*Termination of Action.* Thiopental is rapidly distributed to the brain, where it induces sleep within seconds after a bolus intravenous injection. Over the next 2–5 minutes, it diffuses into other tissues of high vascularity, such as the heart, lungs, liver, and kidneys. Awakening after a single 3–5 mg/kg dose occurs as a result of this rapid redistribution process. Over the next 15–30 minutes, the drug more slowly distributes to body tissues with less perfusion (muscles and, to a lesser degree, fat), further decreasing the concentration of drug in both brain and plasma. Following these redistribution processes, thiopental is cleared from the body by hepatic metabolism and by renal excretion of its metabolites. The elimination half-life of thiopental is about 11 hours, accounting for the long time course for psychomotor recovery after thiopental anesthesia.

*Methohexital.* Methohexital is an ultrashort-acting barbiturate, resembling thiopental in its pharmacologic actions. However, it is about three times more potent than thiopental and has shorter distribution and elimination half-lives in the body. Following a single bolus intravenous injection (1.5 mg/kg), methohexital redistributes to muscle and fat within about 6 minutes. Thereafter, the drug is rapidly removed from plasma by the liver, is metabolized, and the end products of metabolism are excreted by the kidneys. The elimination half-life of methohexital is about 4 hours.

*Complications of Barbiturates.* Clinical complications with ultrashort-acting barbiturates most frequently involve the cardiovascular and respiratory depression noted above. Other less-frequent, but potentially serious, complications include anaphylaxis, venous irritation and thrombosis, inadvertent intraarterial injection, and precipitation of an attack of porphyria.

Venous irritation and thrombosis are caused by high alkalotic pH levels of the thiopental solution. Fortunately, a concentration of 2.5% thiopental, or 1% methohexital, is well tolerated and uncommonly associated with vascular irritation.

Inadvertent intraarterial injection is rare, but may produce intense pain, vascular spasm, loss of distal arterial pulses, cyanosis, gangrene, and loss of limb function.

Obviously, one should attempt to insure that such injection never occurs. Treatment consists of intraarterial injection at the same site of a dilute solution of a local anesthetic and heparin. A sympathetic blockade of the extremity can also be used in an attempt to decrease the vascular spasm and its sequelae.

Acute intermittent porphyria is a rare syndrome associated with abdominal pain and acute neurologic attacks. It is associated with accumulation of normal precursors of heme, a compound which normally combines with globulin to form hemoglobin. Administration of barbiturates may precipitate an attack.

## Benzodiazepines

Two benzodiazepines are available in parenteral formulation and are commonly used in anesthesia: diazepam (Valium) and lorazepam (Ativan). A third agent, midazolam (Versed), will soon become available. These drugs are used for inducing general anesthesia, for providing sedation during regional anesthesia, and for providing amnesia during balanced anesthesia (Chapter 10). The usefulness of diazepam and lorazepam is limited by poor water solubility and long elimination half-lives (24 hours for diazepam and 16 hours for lorazepam). Elderly patients experience a prolonged half-life of diazepam; the elimination half-life increasing to about 90 hours in an 80-year-old patient. Lorazepam's elimination is not as prolonged in the elderly. Diazepam is very poorly absorbed after intramuscular administration and probably should not be given by this route. Lorazepam is quite well absorbed from intramuscular depots.

Midazolam is water-soluble benzodiazepine, with pharmacologic effects similar to those of diazepam and lorazepam. Midazolam differs, however; in that it is rapidly distributed through the body and is metabolized in the liver, with an elimination half-life of about 2–2.5 hours. This short half-life may increase the usefulness of midazolam in anesthesia as an induction agent since it does not have the prolonged action of the other benzodiazepines, and yet it shares their rather benign effects on the cardiovascular system (discussed later). However, when compared to thiopental, onset of unconsciousness is slower and recovery times are longer. It therefore will likely not replace thiopental as a "routine" induction agent for healthy surgical patients.

The effects of benzodiazepines on the central nervous system resemble those of the barbiturates. As sedative-hypnotics, they depress both the activity and the metabolic rate of neurons, and they are anticonvulsant.

The effects of benzodiazepines on the cardiovascular system are relatively minor, being only very mild cardiovascular depressants. Large doses can be administered without significant alteration in cardiac dynamics. They are therefore useful as induction agents and anesthetic supplements in seriously ill patients with cardiovascular disease. The benzodiazepines exert only minimal effects on respiration, unless they are combined with more specific respiratory depressants, such as the opiates. In such an instance, prolonged respiratory depression may occur.

## Etomidate (Amidate)

Etomidate is a new, nonbarbiturate, induction anesthetic. It produces hypnosis within 1 minute of intravenous injection and unconsciousness persists for about 5 minutes. Like the barbiturates, etomidate is devoid of analgesic or muscle-relaxant properties. Pain on injection and myoclonus are frequently reported side effects. If the trachea is to be intubated, succinylcholine (1 mg/kg IV) will provide the needed muscle relaxation.

As shown in Table 6-2, the cardiovascular effects of an induction dose of etomidate (about 0.2–0.3 mg/kg IV) are minimal, making this agent useful for inducing anesthesia in patients with compromised cardiovascular function (e.g., patients in shock, coronary-risk patients) or in whom high cerebral perfusion pressures need to be maintained (e.g., hypertensive patients with stenotic lesions of cerebral blood vessels).

Etomidate produces similar but less pronounced depressant effects on the CNS than do the barbiturates. Myoclonic activity is not accompanied by seizure-like activity on the EEG. Unlike the barbiturates, subcortical structures are little depressed and a cortical site of action is postulated, accounting for the relative lack of analgesic, cardiovascular, or respiratory depressant effects.

The distribution half-life of etomidate is about 2–3 minutes. The drug is hydrolyzed in the liver, with an elimination half-life of about 4 hours. However, due to extensive tissue uptake, clinical effects are minimal after about 1.0–1.5 hours.

## Opiate Narcotics

### Classification

The opiate narcotics are compounds that exert both a sedative and an analgesic action. They act by attaching to opiate receptors in several brain structures where naturally occurring enkephalins normally appear to act. These receptors have been extensively subclassified by their location in the brain and by their interactions with certain agonists and antagonists. The articles by Jaffe and Martin (1980), Freye et al. (1983), Hameroff (1983), and Thorpe (1984) listed at the end of this chapter will introduce the interested reader to discussion of opiate receptors and their relevance to anesthesia.

Table 6-3 classifies opiate narcotics by their activity as narcotic antagonists or agonists at opiate receptors. As shown, some are pure agonists, meaning that they not only have affinity for opiate receptors, but they exert profound analgesic effects and can substitute for other narcotics in narcotic-dependent patients. In contrast, one agent, naloxone (Narcan), is a pure narcotic antagonist, meaning that it has affinity for opiate receptors but exerts no pharmacologic effects. As a result, naloxone is *not* analgesic and will precipitate withdrawal in narcotic-dependent patients by displacing the agonist from the receptor. Intermediate between pure agonists and pure antagonists are opiates classified as mixed agonists-antagonists (pentazocine, nalbuphine, and butorphanol). These agents exert analgesic effects when other, more powerful agonists (such as morphine) are not present in the body, and they reverse the analgesic effects of more powerful agonists when the latter are present, thus precipitating withdrawal in drug-dependent adults.

**TABLE 6-3**
**Agonist-Antagonist Activity of Opiate Narcotics**

| Analgesic (intrinsic) Activity | No Analgesia | Increasing Analgesia | Complete Analgesia |
|---|---|---|---|
| Agonist-antagonist properties | Pure antagonist | Decreasing antagonist with increasing agonist activity (mixed agonist-antagonists) | Pure agonist |
| Pharmacologic agent | Naloxone (Narcan) | Pentazocine (Talwin)<br>Nalbuphine (Nubain)<br>Butorphanol (Stadol) | Morphine<br>Meperidine (Demerol)<br>Fentanyl (Sublimaze)<br>Oxymorphone (Numorphan)<br>Hydromorphone (Dilaudid) |

Examples of pure agonist narcotics used in anesthesia include morphine, meperidine (Demerol), oxymorphone (Numorphan), hydromorphone (Dilaudid), alphaprodine (Nisentil), fentanyl (Sublimaze), sufentanyl (Sufenta), and alfentanyl (Alfenta). The latter two are fentanyl analogues: sufentanyl is 5–10 times more potent than fentanyl, with a similar or slightly shorter duration of action. Alfentanyl has only one-fourth the potency of fentanyl, but has a duration of action that is one-third to one-half that of fentanyl (Borel, 1983). Thus, alfentanyl can be considered as an ultrashort-acting narcotic (about 5–15 minutes), fentanyl and sufentanyl as short-acting (15–30 minutes), alphaprodine intermediate-acting at 1.5–2.0 hours, meperdine slightly longer at 2.5–3.5 hours, and morphine, oxymorphone, and hydromorphone at 4–5 hours.

The mixed agonist-antagonists all have intermediate to long durations of action (i.e., 3–5 hours). Naloxone, the only parenterally available pure narcotic antagonist, has a brief duration of action, in the range of 15–30 minutes.

*Actions on the Central Nervous System.* Opiates produce analgesia, drowsiness, mood changes, respiratory depression, and mental clouding. With the pure agonists, these effects intensify linearly with increasing doses. With the three mixed agonist-antagonist compounds, there appears to be a maximal dose for each beyond which further respiratory depression or analgesia do not occur; this "ceiling" reflecting either limited receptor binding to selected opiate receptors or a lower level of intrinsic activity than is displayed by the pure agonists.

All opiates depress respiration, principally by reducing the responsiveness of the respiratory centers in the brainstem to increasing levels of carbon dioxide in arterial blood. This causes a "right shift" of the carbon dioxide-ventilatory response curve, an effect which can be reversed by a mixed agonist-antagonist or by naloxone (Figure 6-2). Opiate-induced respiratory depression results in a decrease in minute ventilation, with respiratory rate more affected than tidal volume. One should expect respiratory acidosis (i.e., ↑ $Paco_2$) in narcotic-treated patients breathing spontaneously.

Opiates exert depressant effects on cough centers in the brainstem. Such effects may be detrimental, since patients must be able to cough after surgery in order to clear secretions and prevent mucous plugging of the alveoli.

Opiates produce either no change or slight decreases in cerebral blood flow, cerebral metabolic rate, and intracranial pressure (Table 6-2), provided the patient's ventilation is controlled and $Paco_2$ is maintained below 40 mm Hg.

*Effects on the Cardiovascular System.* It is significant that opiates, even in high doses used in narcotic-based anesthesia (i.e., "balanced anesthesia," Chapter 10), have very little effect on the cardiovascular systems in supine patients (Table 6-3). These drugs are widely used, therefore, for the induction and maintenance of anesthesia in patients with myocardial and valvular disease, and with peripheral vascular-, carotid-, or coronary-occulsive arterial disease.

It should be noted that, in these patients, blood pressure may fall secondary to drug-induced peripheral vasodilatation and venous pooling of blood. Maintaining the supine position, preloading the patient with fluid, maintaining an adequate preload, and judiciously using a vasoconstrictor (such as ephedrine, Chapter 8), all help to minimize hypotensive responses to drug-induced vasodilatation.

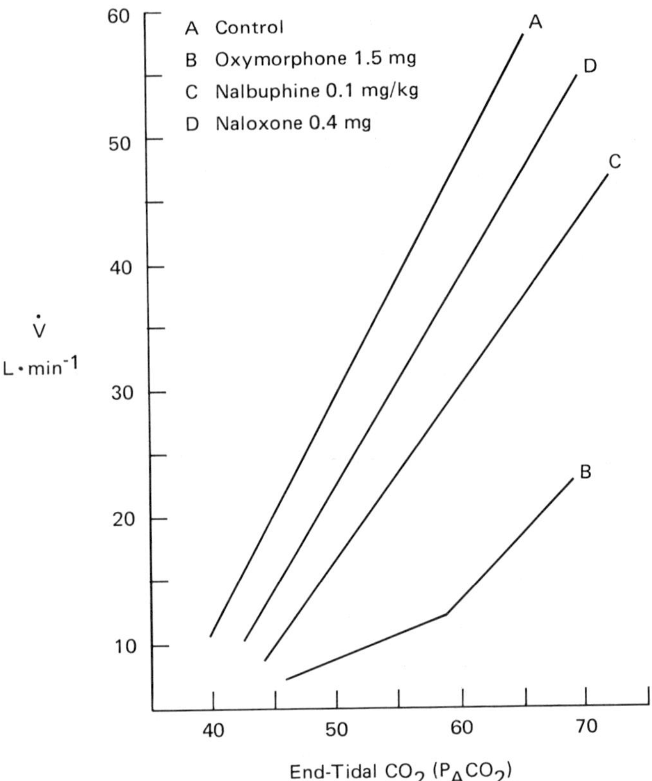


**Figure 6-2.** Ventilatory response to increasing levels of $CO_2$ in nine subjects. (**A**), Control, and after sequential administration of oxymorphone (**B**), nalbuphine (**C**), and naloxone (**D**). Oxymorphone dose equivalent to 10 mg of morphine. Note partial reversal of oxymorphone-induced respiratory depression by nalbuphine and further reversal by naloxone. (Reproduced, with permission, from Julien, R. M. 1982. Effects of nalbuphine on normal and oxymorphone-depressed ventilatory responses to carbon dioxide challenge. *Anesthesiology* 57:A320.)

Narcotics should be used with caution in patients with acute blood loss or with hypovolemia, and in patients dependent on high filling pressures (i.e., cardiac tamponade). In addition, morphine (but not other narcotics) may release histamine from mast cells; thus, it might be advisable to avoid morphine in patients with reactive airway disease.

*Other Clinical Effects of Opiates.* Morphine and the other opiates increase the tone of the smooth muscle of the gastrointestinal tract and its various sphincters. The nausea and vomiting and the constipation produced by opiates result from such increases in smooth muscle tone.

**TABLE 6-4**
**Perioperative Uses of Opiate Narcotics**

| *Use* | Example | | *Discussion* |
|---|---|---|---|
| | *Drug* | *Dose* | |
| Premedication | Morphine | 0.1 mg/kg IM | Chapter 2 |
| | Meperidine | 1.0 mg/kg IM | |
| "Balanced" anesthesia | Morphine | 1.0 mg/kg IV | Chapter 10 |
| | Fentanyl | 25–50 μg/kg IV | |
| Supplement to inhalation anesthesia | Morphine | 0.1–0.2 mg/kg IV | Chapter 10 |
| | Meperidine | 0.5–1.0 mg/kg IV | |
| | Oxymorphone | 0.02–0.03 mg/kg IV | |
| Postoperative, analgesia | Morphine | 0.05–0.15 mg/kg IV or IM | Chapter 11 |
| | Meperidine | 0.25–0.5 mg/kg IV or IM | |
| Supplement to regional anesthesia (conscious sedation) | Nalbuphine | 0.25–0.5 mg/kg IV or IM | |
| | Fentanyl | 0.5–1.0 μg/kg IV | |
| | Meperidine | 0.25–0.75 mg/kg IM | |
| Labor analgesia | Meperidine | 0.5–1.0 mg/kg IM | |
| | Alphaprodine | 0.25–0.75 mg/kg IM | |

The opiates produce miosis of the pupils, probably through an excitatory action on the brainstem.

Like the volatile anesthetics, morphine causes reduced urine flow, secondary to a decrease in glomerular filtration rate.

*Uses of Opiates in Anesthesia.* As might be predicted, the potent analgesic effects of opiates make them useful in a wide variety of situations in the perioperative period. Such uses are discussed throughout this text. However, it may be useful to summarize these uses (Table 6-4). The validity of these uses will not be challenged at this time; such will be discussed at appropriate times elsewhere in this text.

## Naloxone

Naloxone (Narcan) is a pure narcotic antagonist, possessing virtually no agonist activity. Thus, it reverses (antagonizes) the effects of both the pure narcotic agonists and of the mixed agonist-antagonist opiates. While such an effect is clinically useful for reversing narcotic-induced respiratory depression, two important points must be kept in mind.

First, naloxone is lipid-soluble. It therefore penetrates the blood-brain barrier easily, reaching a peak level in the brain almost immediately. It then rapidly redistributes to other tissues of the body, resulting in a very short duration of action. Naloxone is then metabolized, with a half-time of elimination of about 1.0–1.5 hours. Since many agonist opiates, such as morphine, redistribute more slowly and are metabolized at a slower rate, it frequently happens that the naloxone-antagonism dissipates, allowing return of the agonist-induced respiratory depression. Such a return of respiratory depression is termed "renarcotization." Any patient given naloxone to terminate opiate-induced respiratory depression must be carefully monitored for at least two hours as renarcotization can lead to severe respiratory failure, requiring either assisted ventilation or additional doses of naloxone.

Second, naloxone reverses not only opiate-induced respiratory depression but also opiate-induced analgesia. Therefore, the return of spontaneous ventilation may be accompanied by the acute perception of surgical pain with all the cardiovascular sequelae. Catecholamine levels increase and are accompanied by tachycardia, hypertension, increased peripheral vascular resistance, and ventricular arrhythmias. Care must be taken when administering naloxone to patients with cardiovascular disease since myocardial infarction, acute heart failure, pulmonary edema, cardiac arrest, or a cerebrovacular accident may result. Careful titration with naloxone (0.1 mg/70 kg increments) to a suitable respiratory rate is most commonly used in an effort to retain analgesia. To prevent renarcotization, slow intravenous infusion can be tried. Large bolus doses of naloxone (0.4 mg or greater) should be discouraged. It should be remembered that the administration of naloxone is not without potential danger, even in apparently healthy patients.

## Ketamine

Ketamine is an intravenous anesthetic agent chemically related to phencyclidine (PCP or "angel dust"), a psychedelic drug noted for its ability to cause hallucinations. Ketamine induces fewer hallucinations than phencyclidine, and has potent analgesic and amnesic properties. At amnesic and analgesic doses (about 1 mg/kg IV), ketamine induces a behavioral state in which the patient may appear awake but "dissociated" from the environment; hence, its classification as a "dissociative" anesthetic.

Ketamine anesthesia is characterized by active pharyngeal and laryngeal reflexes, increased tone of skeletal muscle, bronchial dilatation, and increased activity of the sympathetic nervous system, resulting in hypertension, tachypnea, increased peripheral vascular resistance, and tachycardia; and intracranial pressure is increased (Table 6-3). Ketamine is contraindicated in patients with increased intracranial pressure. In patients with significant coronary artery disease, the increased sympathetic activity and its accompanying tachycardia and hypertension are undesirable. If ketamine is to be used in such patients, it should be used with caution, minimizing the dose and protecting the cardiovascular system with other agents. Ketamine anesthesia is most useful in patients who are asthmatic, hypovolemic, or hypotensive, since the sympathetic stimulation due to ketamine may be beneficial in such patients in maintaining blood pressure and airway relaxation. Note that it is the indirect effect of ketamine on the cardiovascular system that produces cardiovascular stimulation. If endogenous catecholamines are depleted, a direct cardiovascular depressant effect of ketamine on the myocardium may be observed, resulting in drug-induced hypotension.

The hallucinations or unpleasant dreams that can accompany doses of ketamine above 1.0 mg/kg can be reduced both by restricting it to use as an induction agent whenever possible (0.5–1.0 mg/kg IV) or by giving concurrently a benzodiazepine such as diazepam (0.15 mg/kg IV).

Many of the postoperative psychedelic complications from ketamine reported in the past were probably due to overdosage, since low doses (0.25–0.75 mg/kg IV) produce amnesia and analgesia with only minimal side effects. Nevertheless, ketamine should probably be avoided in patients with psychiatric disorders.

After bolus intravenous administration, ketamine has a distribution half-life of about 10–15 minutes, accounting for the brief period of amnesia and analgesia observed after low doses (0.3–0.5 mg/kg). Ketamine is metabolized and excreted with an elimination half-life of about 2.5–3.0 hours. Continous intravenous infusion (1–2 mg/kg/hr) or intermittant injections (0.25–0.5 mg/kg every 15 minutes) will maintain the state of dissociation, analgesia and amnesia.

Administered intramuscularly, plasma levels of ketamine become maximal in about 20 minutes, delaying the onset of anesthesia when compared to intravenous administration. However, intramuscular ketamine (2–4 mg/kg) may be useful in the otherwise uncontrollable patient who will not allow either awake intravenous catheterization or a mask induction (Chapter 10).

It is important to note that when ketamine is used for analgesia and amnesia, muscle relaxation, if necessary, must be achieved with one of the neuromuscular blocking agents (see next section).

## Neuromuscular Blocking Agents

Neuromuscular blocking agents exert their effects by blocking transmission between motor nerve endings and the postsynaptic receptors on skeletal muscle (Figure 6-3). To understand the action of neuromuscular blocking agents, we must first consider how muscle contractions are initiated. The transmitter at the neuromuscular junction is acetylcholine (ACh), a compound synthesized in the nerve terminals and stored in synaptic vesicles for later release. When an action potential arrives at the nerve terminal, ACh is released from the vesicles into the synaptic cleft. It diffuses across the cleft and attaches to the receptor on the muscle membrane, causing depolarization of the membrane. The depolarization generates an action potential that initiates muscle contraction. The duration of the contraction is brief, since ACh persists at the receptor for only milliseconds, being rapidly metabolized by the enzyme acetylcholinesterase (AChE). After the destruction of the ACh, the membrane potential returns to resting levels, and the membrane again becomes responsive to the ACh from the presynaptic nerve terminal.

Two types of neuromuscular blocking agents are in use: depolarizing and nondepolarizing blockers.

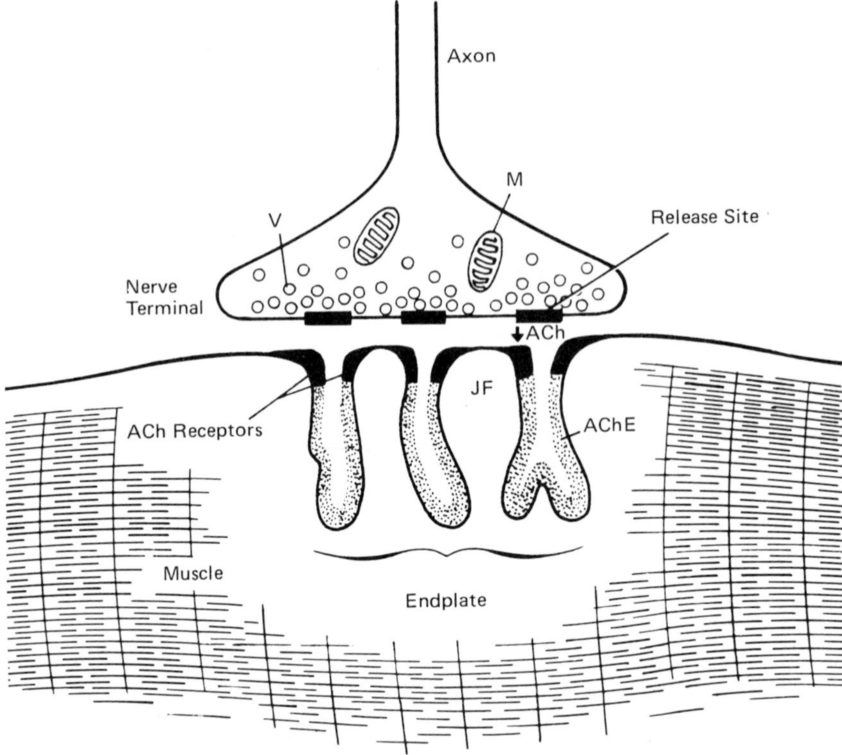


**Figure 6-3.** Schematic representation of the neuromuscular junction. **M**, Mitochondria; **V**, Synaptic vesicles; **JF**, Junctional folds. (Reproduced, with permission, from Drachman, D. B. 1978. Myasthenia gravis. *N. Engl. J. Med.* 298:136.)

## Depolarizing Blocker: Succinylcholine

Succinylcholine (SCh) is the only depolarizing neuromuscular blocker used in anesthesia. As its name suggests, SCh closely resembles the neurotransmitter ACh: the SCh molecule is composed of two molecules of ACh bonded together (Figure 6-4), and produces depolarization at postsynaptic receptors in the same manner as ACh. However, when SCh causes depolarization, it also produces a neuromuscular blockade. This is because SCh persists at the receptors for 3–5 minutes, much longer than ACh does: the more complex structure of SCh requires more time to be metabolized (by an enzyme found in plasma, plasma cholinesterase). During this time, the postsynaptic receptors remain insensitive to ACh released from the nerve terminal.

The intensity and duration of the blockade is determined by the amount of SCh blocking the receptors and by the ability of plasma cholinesterase to metabolize the drug. Some patients produce a structurally modified plasma cholinesterase which metabolizes SCh at a much slower rate than the normal enzyme would metabolize the drug. A normal dose of SCh in such patients may produce complete paralysis of several hours' duration.

In patients with normal acetylcholinesterase, the duration of action of SCh makes it well suited to producing the few minutes of muscle relaxation necessary for tracheal intubation after the induction of anesthesia. Indeed, this is its most common use. The continuous infusion of SCh through an intravenous catheter will provide more prolonged relaxation if necessary.

*Adverse Effects of Succinlycholine.* Side effects of SCh are common. First, as the blockade is established, there is a brief period during which the depolarization produces repeated muscle fasiculations, which have been implicated as a possible cause of postoperative muscle pain. This effect can be much reduced by pretreatment with a low dose of a nondepolarizing neuromuscular blocking agent (see next section).

Second, the depolarization produced by SCh releases potassium ions from the muscle membrane. In most patients, this release is of little clinical significance, since the serum potassium increases only slightly. However, in patients with neuromuscular abnormalities due to burns, trauma, or upper motor neuron lesions (such as spinal cord damage and strokes), the increases in serum potassium can be large, sometimes resulting in cardiac arrhythmias, cardiac arrest, and death. Such a response to SCh begins about 10 days after injury (sooner in some patients), and susceptibility can persist for up to 6 months.

Third, SCh can exert effects on the heart similar to those produced by ACh released by the vagus nerve. Thus, bradycardia can follow SCh administration, particularly in infants. Pretreatment with intravenous atropine will prevent the bradycardia.

Fourth, SCh, along with halothane, is frequently implicated as the causative agent in precipitating malignant hyperpyrexia. Failure of the patient's jaw muscles to relax after SCh is often an early warning sign (Flewellen and Nelson, 1984). When relaxation does not occur, the syndrome should be considered before additional doses of succinylcholine are administered.

Fifth, patients with certain muscle diseases, especially the myotonic syndromes, can experience an abnormally prolonged contracture of muscles following SCh administration. Generalized spasm leads to difficulties in maintaining an airway, intubation, and ventilation.

Sixth, SCh can produce a transient increase in intraoccular pressure which can

```
        H3C           O
           \⊕         ‖
ACh     H3C–N–CH2–CH2–O–C–CH3
           /
        H3C

        H3C                O                 O                 CH3
           \⊕              ‖                 ‖              ⊕ /
SCh     H3C–N–CH2–CH2–O–C–CH2–CH2–C–O–CH2–CH2–N–CH3
           /                                                  \
        H3C                                                    CH3
```

**Figure 6-4.** Structural formulas of acetylcholine (**ACh**) and succinylcholine (**SCh**).

be clinically significant in patients with preexisting states of increased pressure or in patients with open-eye injuries. The mechanism of this increase is not clear but may involve both a direct vascular effect and an indirect effect through spasm of the extraoccular muscles.

Seventh, SCh stimulates secretions normally mediated by ACh (e.g., salivary). This response can be blocked by an anticholinergic (antimuscarinic) agent, such as atropine.

## Nondepolarizing Neuromuscular Blockers: Curare-like Agents

The nondepolarizing, or competitive, neuromuscular blockers are widely used for intraoperative muscle relaxation. Like SCh, nondepolarizing blockers attach to ACh receptors on the membranes of skeletal muscles, but unlike SCh, their attachment is not followed by depolarization and contraction of the muscle. They compete for postsynaptic receptors with ACh and, if present in high enough concentrations, they completely block the access of ACh to the receptor, blocking neuromuscular transmission.

The nondepolarizing agents can be divided into two groups based on their approximate durations of action: (a) intermediate-acting (20–50 minutes), and (b) long-acting (60–150 minutes). Representative of the former are two drugs, atracurium (Tracrium) and vercuronium (Norcuron). Doses of these drugs that are necessary for relaxation sufficient for tracheal intubation within 2–3 minutes of drug injection are 0.4–0.5 mg/kg (atracurium) and 0.1–0.12 mg/kg (vercuronium) (Table 6-5). The duration of clinical relaxation is about 30–45 minutes. Antagonism of residual block at the completion of surgery by anticholinesterase agents (discussed later) is thought to be within about 30 minutes of an intubating dose of either drug.

Representative of the long-acting nondepolarizing neuromuscular blockers are *d*-tubocurarine, pancuronium (Pavulon), gallamine (Flaxedil), and metocurine (Metubine). The intubating doses and durations of action of these agents are listed in Table 6-5. Note from this table that, in the presence of enflurane or isoflurane anesthesia, the required dose of blocking agent is reduced by about one-third to two-thirds over doses necessary during balanced anesthesia, a synergistic action of considerable clinical significance since lower doses of relaxant are easier to "reverse" than are larger doses (discussed later). Note also that four of the drugs in Table 6-5 have relatively long durations of action; durations that limit their usefulness for relatively short procedures. Since their duration of clinical effect is quite long, reversal with anticholinesterase agents probably should not be attempted within about 45 minutes after injection of the neuromuscular blocker.

The duration of the neuromuscular blockade produced by both the intermediate and the long-acting nondepolarizing muscle relaxants is determined by the dose of the particular drug administered and by the rate of its plasma clearance (i.e., by the rate and mode of elimination). Since these drugs are water-soluble (lipid-insoluble), they do not enter the CNS, and their duration of action is not influenced to any great degree by redistribution.

The four long-acting compounds are removed from plasma primarily by excretion of unchanged drug in urine and bile (Table 6-6). Of these four, only pancuronium is metabolized to any significant extent, and that only to about 30%–35% of the

**TABLE 6-5**
**Clinical Doses (mg/kg) and Duration of Action of Nondepolarizing Blockers**
***(suggested dosage in different situations)***

| Drug | Tracheal Intubation | $N_2O$ | Halothane | Enflurane-Isoflurane | Duration of Action (min) |
|---|---|---|---|---|---|
| *d*-Tubocurarine | 0.4–0.6 | 0.3–0.5 | 0.2–0.3 | 0.1–0.15 | 60–150 |
| Pancuronium | 0.06–0.1 | 0.04–0.08 | 0.03–0.06 | 0.02–0.04 | 60–150 |
| Metocurine | 0.25–0.4 | 0.2–0.3 | 0.15–0.25 | 0.06–0.10 | 60–150 |
| Gallamine | 2.0–4.0 | 1.5–2.5 | 1.0–2.0 | 0.8–0.15 | 60–150 |
| Atracurium | 0.4–0.5 | 0.2–0.3 | 0.2 | 0.15–0.2 | 30–45 |
| Vercuronium | 0.10–0.12 | 0.04–0.06 | 0.4 | 0.03 | 40–55 |

*Doses suggested are in the range that usually produced about 95% twitch depression under $N_2O$ (balanced) anesthesia, or at about 1 MAC anesthetic depth with anesthetic vapors in healthy subjects.

Table reproduced, with permission, from Attia, R.R., and Grogono, A.W. 1978. *Practical anesthetic pharmacology*. New York: Appleton-Century-Crofts. Atracurium and vercuronium data from Savarese, J. J. 1983. New muscle relaxants (lecture 304). In: *Annual refresher course lectures*. Park Ridge, Ill.: American Society of Anesthesiologists.

**TABLE 6-6**
**Summary of Disposition of Nondepolarizing Neuromuscular Blockers**

| Drug | Elimination Half-Life (min) | % Metabolized in Liver | % Excreted Unchanged in Bile | % Excreted Unchanged in Urine | Other (%) | Total (%) |
|---|---|---|---|---|---|---|
| *d*-Tubocurarine | 120 | 0 | >50 | <50 | 0 | 100 |
| Pancuronium | 120 | 35 | 5 | 60 | 0 | 100 |
| Gallamine | 120 | 0 | 0 | 100 | 0 | 100 |
| Metocurine | 120 | 0 | 0 | 100 | 0 | 100 |
| Atracurium | 30 | 0 | 0 | 0 | 100* | 100 |
| Vercuronium | 75 | 0 | 40–50 | 5–10 | 50–60† | 100 |

All values are approximate and are intended to give the student a guide to understanding drug disposition and to appropriate selection of an agent for a particular patient.

*Hofmann elimination and ester hydrolysis independent of plasma cholinesterase.

†Spontaneous deacetylation.

total dose of pancuronium administered. In contrast, the intermediate-acting drugs both undergo significant metabolic alteration. Atracurium is almost totally metabolized, although such metabolism does not occur in the liver. The drug undergoes Hofmann elimination (a pH- and temperature-dependent spontaneous breakdown), and a process of plasma ester hydrolysis which is independent of the enzyme plasma pseudocholinesterase. Thus, it is likely that the duration of action of atracurium would be unaffected by either liver or renal failure (or both). Vercuronium is a relatively unstable molecule in the body, and about half of the administered dose undergoes spontaneous breakdown (deacetylation), while the remainder is excreted unchanged, primarily in the bile. Because of this, it is likely that its duration of action will be prolonged in patients with liver disease, as are the durations of action of *d*-tubocurarine and pancuronium in such patients (Savarese, 1983; Fahey and Miller, 1983).

The side effects of nondepolarizing blockers deserve mention. *d*-Tubocurarine produces ganglionic blockade and liberates histamine. It can therefore induce hypotension and precipitate bronchospasm, and should be avoided both in hypotensive patients and in asthmatics. Gallamine and pancuronium both have a vagal-blocking property, causing tachycardia and hypertension. This effect often limits their use in hypertensive patients and in those predisposed to myocardial ischema. Pancuronium also acts to partially block the active reuptake of catecholamines into presynaptic nerve terminals, potentiating catecholamine activity. Thus, pancuronium should be

**TABLE 6-7**
**Situations Requiring Alterations in Dosage of Nondepolarizing Neuromuscular Blockers**

| | |
|---|---|
| Renal disease | Reduced elimination, prolonged durations of action |
| Hepatic and biliary disease | Reduced elimination of pancuronium and *d*-tubocurarine |
| Hypothermia | Prolongation of blockade |
| Age | Reduced elimination with prolonged duration of action in elderly (except atracurium) |
| Myesthenia gravis, myesthenic syndrome and myopathies, muscular dystrophies | Extreme sensitivity to relaxants |
| Lower motor neuron disease | Increased sensitivity to relaxants |
| Hypokalemia | Increased sensitivity to relaxants |
| Hyperkalemia | Reduced sensitivity to relaxants |
| Respiratory acidosis | Potentiation of blockade |
| Metabolic alkalosis | Potentiation of blockade |
| Drug interactions: magnesium, lithium, antibiotics, quinidine, volatile anesthetics | Potentiation of blockade |

used with caution or avoided in halothane-anesthetized patients taking tricyclic antidepressants or other drugs (e.g., aminophylline) which increase their susceptability to cardiac arrhythmias.

It should be noted that, with the exception of gallamine, neither SCh nor the other nondepolarizing blockers cross the placenta in sufficient amounts to produce effects on the fetus. When used for muscle relaxation during Cesarean sections, they do not impair the newborn's breathing (Dailey et al., 1984).

Finally, one should be aware of the numerous factors that alter an individual's response to nondepolarizing neuromuscular blockers (Table 6-7), factors which may necessitate altering doseage. Such factors usually involve either a drug interaction or a physiologic alteration in organ function. Obviously, experience and knowledge should guide the use of these drugs. As a general rule, the lowest dose capable of providing surgical relaxation should be used.

## Acetylcholinesterase Inhibitors

While pharmacologically more appropriate to discuss in a chapter on autonomic drugs (Chapter 8), the inhibitors of acetylcholinesterase will be presented at this time since they are used in anesthesia primarily for their clinical ability to antagonize (or "reverse") the neuromuscular blockade produced by the six nondepolarizing neuromuscular blockers discussed above. Acetylcholinesterase (AChE) inhibitors used in anesthesia include neostigmine (Prostigmin), pyridostigmine (Mestinon, Regonol), and edrophonium (Tensilon). Of these, pyridostigmine has a slower onset (13 minutes) than either neostigmine (6–8 minutes) or edrophonium (3 minutes), but a longer duration of action than either of the latter.

Inhibition of AChE causes acetylcholine to accumulate at cholinergic receptors throughout the body. Thus, cholinergic stimulation of *muscarinic* receptors produces bradycardia, miosis, salivation, sweating, and possible bronchospasm. *Nicotinic* receptor stimulation occurs at the autonomic ganglia and at the neuromuscular junction: the latter being the reason for which the drug was administered. The unavoidable muscarinic stimulation is a side effect which must be prevented as doses of AChE inhibitors necessary to restore neuromuscular transmission produce profound degrees of bradycardia. Thus, one routinely administers a muscarinic blocking agent (atropine or glycopyrrolate) with the AChE inhibitor. Drug combinations used for the reversal of neuromuscular blockade are listed in Table 6-8.

Individual practitioners choose the combination they feel offers the best balance of onsets and durations of action of both the AChE inhibitor and antimuscarinic agent. An ideal antimuscarinic agent should match the onset and duration of the AChE inhibitor, thus avoiding early tachycardia due to vagal blockade and late bradycardia due to loss of antimuscarinic activity in the presence of residual AChE inhibition with AChE accumulation. Popular combinations include neostigmine-atropine (a "traditional" combination despite the wide swings in heart rate), neostigmine-glycopyrrolate, and edrophonium-glycopyrrolate, although edrophonium-atropine has been claimed to have advantages (Cronnelly et al., 1982).

Further discussion of reversal of neuromuscular blockade with AChE inhibitors is presented in Chapter 11.

**TABLE 6-8**
**Drug Combinations for Reversal of Neuromuscular Blockade**

| AChE Inhibitor | | | Antimuscarinic Agent | |
|---|---|---|---|---|
| *Drug* | *Dosage (mg/kg)** | | *Drug* | *Dosage (mg/kg)* |
| Neostigmine | 0.05 | + | Atropine | 0.020 |
| Pyridostigmine | 0.25 | + | Atropine | 0.020 |
| Edrophonium | 0.5 | + | Atropine | 0.01–0.02 |
| Neostigmine | 0.05 | + | Glycopyrrolate | 0.01 |
| Pyridostigmine | 0.25 | + | Glycopyrrolate | 0.01 |
| Edrophonium | 0.5 | + | Glycopyrrolate | 0.01 |

*Doses listed are those used to reverse long-acting nondepolarizing neuromuscular blockers. Lower doses may be adequate to reverse intermediate-acting agents such as atracurium.

From Yang, E.; Lee, C.; and Tran, B. 1984. Optimum dose of edrophonium for reversal of atracurium neuromuscular block. *Anesth. Analg.* 63:283.

## *Readings and References*


Aldrete, J.A., and Britt, B.A. editors. 1977. *Malignant hyperthermia: Proceedings of the Second International Symposium.* New York: Grune & Stratton.

American Society of Anesthesiologists. 1982. *Waste anesthetic gases in operating room air: a suggested program to reduce personnel exposure.* Park Ridge, Ill.: American Society of Anesthesiologists.

Azar, I.; Pham, A.N.; Karambelkar, D.J., et al. 1983. The heart rate following edrophonium-atropine and edrophonium-glycopyrrolate mixtures. *Anesthesiology* 59:139–141.

Borel, J.D. 1983. New narcotics in anesthesia. In: *New pharmacologic vistas in anesthesia.* Brown, B.B., Jr., editor. Philadelphia: F. A. Davis Co.

Bovill, J.G.; Sebel, P.S.; Blackburn, C.L., et al. 1982. The pharmacokinetics of Alfentanil (R39209): a new opioid analgesic. *Anesthesiology* 57:439–43.

Britt, B.A. 1979. Malignant hyperthermia. In: *International anesthesiology clinics.* Boston: Little, Brown and Co., (vol. 17.)

Brown, B.B., editor. 1980. *Anesthesiology and the patient with heart disease.* Philadelphia: F. A. Davis Co.

Brown, B.B., editor. 1983. *New pharmacologic vistas in anesthesia.* Philadelphia: F. A. Davis Co.

Calvey, T.N., and Williams, N.E. 1982. *Principles and practice of pharmacology for anesthetists.* Boston: Blackwell Scientific.

Cohen, E.N. 1980. *Anesthetic exposure in the workplace.* Littleton, Mass.: PSG Publishing Co.

Cronnelly, R.; Morris, R.B.; and Miller, R.D. 1982. Edrophonium: duration of action and atropine requirement in humans during halothane anesthesia. *Anesthesiology* 57:261–66.

Cronnelly, R.; Fisher, D.M.; Miller, R.D., et al. 1983. Pharmacokinetics and pharmacodynamics of Vercuronium (ORG NC45) and pancuronium in anesthetized humans. *Anesthesiology* 58:405–08.

Cullen, B.F., and Miller, M.G. 1979. Drug interactions and anesthesia: a review. *Anesth. Analg.* 58:413–23.

Dailey, P.A.; Fisher, D.M.; Shnider, S.M., et al. 1984. Pharmacokinetics, placental transfer, and neonatal effects of vercuronium and pancuronium administered during cesarean section. *Anesthesiology* 60:569–74.

Dykes, M.H.M. 1983. Hepatic considerations. *Semin. Anesth.* 2:125–34.

Eger, E.I. 1974. *Anesthesia uptake and action.* Baltimore: Williams & Wilkins.

Eger, E.I., editor. 1984. *Nitrous oxide ($N_2O$)*. New York: Elsevier.

Fahey, M.R., and Miller, R.D. 1983. New muscle relaxants. In: *New pharmacologic vistas in anesthesia*. Brown, B.B., Jr., editor. Philadelphia: F.A. Davis Co.

Flewellen, E.H., and Nelson, T.E. 1984. Halothane-succinylcholine-induced masseter spasm: indicative of malignant hyperthermia susceptibility? *Anesth. Analg.* 63:693–7.

Freye, E.; Hartung, E.; and Schenk, G.K. 1983. Bremazocine: an opiate that induces sedation and analgesia without respiratory depression. *Anesth. Analg.* 62:483–88.

Hameroff, S.R., 1983. Opiate receptor pharmacology: mixed agonist/antagonist narcotics. In: *New pharmacologic vistas in anesthesia*. Brown, B.B., Jr., editor. Philadelphia: F.A. Davis Co.

Hilgenberg, J.C. 1983. Comparison of the pharmacology of Vercuronium and Atracurium with that of other currently available muscle relaxants. *Anesth. Analg.* 62:524–31.

Hudson, R.J.; Stanski, D.R.; and Burch, P.G. 1983. Pharmacokinetics of methohexital and thiopental in surgical patients. *Anesthesiology* 59:215–19.

Jaffe, J.H., and Martin, W.R. 1980. Opiod analgesics and antagonists. In: *Goodman and Gilman's The pharmacological basis of therapeutics*. 6th ed. Gilman, A.G., Goodman, L.S., and Gilman, A., editors. New York: Macmillan, pp. 494–534.

Johnson, R.R.; Eger, E.I.; and Wilson, C. 1976. The interaction of epinephrine with enflurane, isoflurane, and halothane in man. *Anesth. Analg.* 55:709–12.

Kaplan, J.A. 1983. Cardiac anesthesia. In: *Cardiovascular pharmacology*. New York: Grune & Stratton, vol. 2.

Koblin, D.D.; Waskell, L.; Watson, J.E., et al. 1982. Nitrous oxide inactivates methionine synthetase in human liver. *Anesth. Analg.* 61:75–78.

Lindeburg, T.; Spotoft, H.; Sorensen, M.B., 1982. Cardiovascular effects of etomidate used for induction and in combination with fentanyl-pancuronium for maintenance of anesthesia in patients with valvular heart disease. *Acta Anaesthesiol. Scand.* 26:205–08.

Miller, R.D., and Cronnelly, R. 1983. A new look at an old drug (editorial). *Anesthesiology* 59:84–85.

Moss, E.; Powell, D.; Gibson, R.M., et al. 1979. Effects of etomidate on intracranial pressure and cerebral perfusion pressure. *Br. J. Anaesth.* 51:347–51.

Prys-Roberts, C., and Hug, C. 1984. *Pharmacokinetics of anesthesia*. (Boston:) Blackwell Scientific.

Renou, A.M.; Vernhiet, J.; Macrez, P., et al. 1978. Cerebral blood flow and metabolism during etomidate anesthesia in man. *Br. J. Aneasth.* 50:1047–50.

Savarese, J.J. 1983. New muscle relaxants (lecture 304). In: *Annual refresher course lectures*. Park Ridge, Ill.: American Society of Anesthesiologists.

Smith, N.T.; Miller, R.D.; and Corbascio, A.N. 1981. *Drug interactions in anesthesia*. Philadelphia: Lea and Febiger.

Sokoll, M.D.; Gergis, S.D., et al. 1983. Safety and efficacy of Atracurium (BW 33A) in surgical patients receiving balanced or isoflurane anesthesia. *Anesthesiology* 58:450–55.

Stanski, D.R., and Watkins, W.D. 1982. *Drug disposition in anesthesia*. New York: Grune & Stratton.

Stoelting, R.K. 1980. Opiate receptors and endorphins: their role in anesthesiology. *Anesth. Analg.* 59:874–80.

Stoelting, R.K. 1983. Allergic reactions during anesthesia. *Anesth. Analg.* 62:341–56.

Symposium on Anesthetic Pharmacology. 1979. *Br. J. Anaesth.* 51:577–710.

Thorpe, D.H. 1984. Opiate structure and activity—a guide to understanding the receptor. *Anesth. Analg.* 63:143–51.

Van Hamme, M.J.; Ghoneim, M.M.; and Ambre, J.J. 1978. Pharmacokinetics of etomidate, a new intravenous anesthetic. *Anesthesiology* 49:274–77.

Ward, S.; Keith, E.A.M.; Weatherley, B.C., et al. 1983. Pharmacokinetics of Atracurium besylate on healthy patients (after a single IV bolus dose). *Br. J. Anaesth.* 55:113–18.

Wood, M., and Wood, A.J.J. 1982. *Drugs and anesthesia: pharmacology for anesthesiologists*. Baltimore: Williams & Wilkins.

# 7. Pharmacology of Local Anesthetics

## Introduction

A local anesthetic is a drug that can temporarily interrupt the conduction of electrical impulses in nerve tissues. An *ideal* local anesthetic should have the following characteristics: it should not irritate any tissue to which it is applied; it should not cause permanent damage to nerve structures; it should not be toxic after absorption into the blood stream; and it should have a predictable duration of action. Reversibility of action is mandatory in local anesthetics, since normal nerve conduction must be regained after the drugs leave the tissues.

Local anesthetics have been used for more than 100 years. Niemann observed in 1860 that cocaine had a peculiar effect on the tongue, making it almost devoid of sensation. In 1884, Koller instilled a solution of cocaine into the conjunctival sac and introduced the drug into ophthalmology as a local anesthetic. In 1905, Einhorn synthesized procaine (Novocaine) which, because it lacked the abuse potential of cocaine, rapidly replaced cocaine for general use. Since 1905, numerous other local anesthetics have been synthesized, tested, and marketed. Agents widely used include bupivacaine (Marcaine), chloroprocaine (Nescaine), etidocaine (Duranest), lidocaine (Xylocaine), mepivacaine (Carbocaine), and tetracaine (Pontocaine).

## Mechanism of Action

Local anesthetics block conduction of nerve impulses by their action on the nerve cell membrane. After a local anesthetic is applied to a peripheral nerve, the loss of neuronal function follows a sequence determined by the diameter of the axons and the concentration of local anesthetic used. In low concentrations, the axons of smaller diameter, primarily sensory and autonomic, are blocked; the large, rapidly conducting axons, primarily motor, are more resistant to blockade. In higher concentrations, all axons within a peripheral nerve are blocked, and complete motor and sensory blockade results.

The neuronal membrane is a semipermeable, lipid-protein structure that separates the potassium-rich axoplasm from the sodium-rich extracellular fluid. In the resting state, the concentration gradient of potassium ions across the membrane produces a resting potential of 75–90 mV, with the interior negatively charged relative to the exterior. While this gradient in potassium ions across the membrane maintains the membrane potential, transient fluctuations in sodium ion permeability are involved in the conduction of electrical impulses.

At rest, sodium ion channels are blocked by calcium ions. To achieve depolarization, membrane permeability to sodium ions is increased, resulting in a large influx of sodium ions across the membrane. This has two results: (a) it generates the action potential, and (b) it causes displacement of calcium ions from adjacent portions of the membrane, which in their turn become depolarized. In this way, the electrical impulse, or action potential, is conducted down the axon. The entire process is extremely rapid, depolarization and repolarization together taking less than 1/1000 sec; some axons conduct more than 500 impulses/sec at conduction velocities greater than 60 meters/sec.

The prevailing theory holds that local anesthetics act by displacing calcium ions from the inner surface of the neuronal membrane, blocking the sodium channels and preventing the movement of sodium ions into the axoplasm. The process of depolarization and the propagation of the nerve impulse are prevented. Evidence in favor of this theory includes the observation that the potency of a local anesthetic can be correlated with drug-induced displacement of calcium ions from the neuronal membrane. For example, tetracaine is 10 times as effective as an equal concentration of procaine in displacing calcium from the membrane, and these results correlate well with the known relative potencies of the two drugs in clinical use (Table 7-1).

## Structure and Classification

The chemical structure of local anesthetics allows the three components of the molecule to be described as an aromatic ring, an intermediate chain, and an amine portion (Figure 7-1). The aromatic ring accounts for the lipid solubility of the anesthetic, and the amine portion accounts for its water solubility. Changes in either the aromatic or amine portions therefore alter the drug's lipid/water distribution, and also alter its ability to bind the membrane proteins. The latter effect is thought responsible for the efficacy and the duration of action of each drug.

The intermediate chain in the anesthetic molecule can be either an ester or an amide. Anesthetics with ester intermediate chains are metabolized in plasma by plasma cholinesterase; those with amide chains are metabolized by enzymes in the liver. The metabolic end-product of the ester-type anesthetics is *p*-aminobenzoic acid (PABA), a compound that contributes to the development of allergic reactions in a small percentage of patients. Allergic reactions to the amide-type of local anesthetic

**TABLE 7-1**
**Classification of Local Anesthetics**

| Generic Name | Trade Name | Class | Onset | Potency | Toxicity | Duration (min) |
|---|---|---|---|---|---|---|
| Low potency, short duration of action | | | | | | |
| Procaine | Novocain | Ester | Moderate | 1 | 1 | 60 |
| Chloroprocaine | Nesacaine | Ester | Fast | 1 | 1 | 45 |
| Intermediate potency and duration of action | | | | | | |
| Lidocaine | Xylocaine | Amide | Fast | 2 | 2 | 120 |
| Mepivacaine | Carbocaine | Amide | Moderate | 2 | 2 | 150 |
| High potency, long duration of action | | | | | | |
| Tetracaine | Pontocaine | Ester | Slow | 10 | 10 | 180 |
| Bupivacaine | Marcaine | Amide | Moderate | 10 | 10 | 200+ |
| Etidocaine | Duranest | Amide | Moderate | 6 | 6 | 200+ |

are exceedingly rare. Multiple dose vials of amide-type anesthetics contain a preservative, methylparapen, which has been postulated as the cause of the allergic reactions alleged to the amide-type compounds.

In addition to their classification as either esters or amides, local anesthetics can be classified by their potencies (i.e., how many milligrams of drug are required to block nerve condition) and by their durations of action (Table 7-1). With the exception of tetracaine, the ester-types of anesthetics are of lesser potency and shorter duration than the amide-types. Note that as potency increases, toxicity (discussed below) also increases.

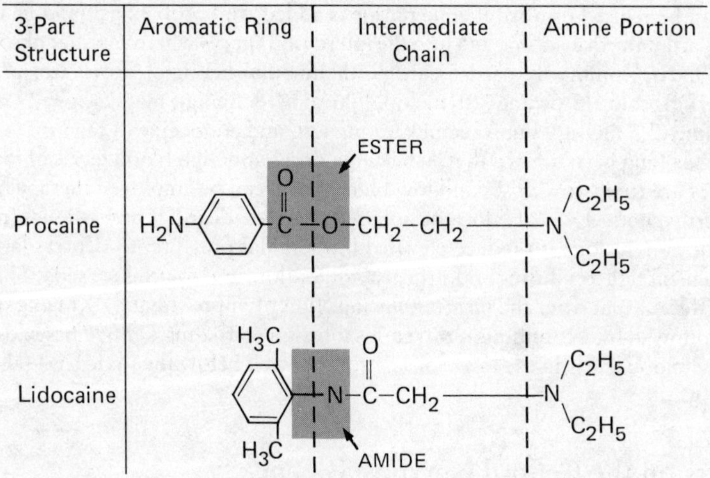

**Figure 7-1.** Structural formulas of procaine and lidocaine illustrating the three-part structure of each.

# Concentrations in Blood and Systemic Effects

## Concentrations in Blood

Since local anesthetics are metabolized only minimally at their sites of injection near nerve membranes, they must be absorbed from those sites into the vascular system in order to be metabolized. Adding a vasoconstrictor such as epinephrine to local anesthetic solution constricts blood vessels in the region of the injection, decreasing the rate of absorption into the circulation and prolonging the duration of the block.

The rate of absorption of local anesthetic (and hence the termination of local anesthetic action) depends not only on the presence of a vasoconstrictor but on the site of injection. Vascular absorption of the drug occurs most rapidly after its injection into the intercostal spaces, followed by injection into the caudal canal, epidural space, brachial plexus, sciatic-femoral nerves and subcutaneous tissues in that order. For example, 400 mg of lidocaine injected into the intercostal space results in an average maximum blood level of the drug of approximately 7μg/ml, while the same dose used for brachial plexus block or injected into the epidural space results in maximum blood levels of about 3.5 and 2.5 μg/mL, respectively.

From the above, it is obvious that the maximal dose of local anesthetic that can be safely administered to a patient is determined not only by the drug involved but by the site at which the drug is injected. In addition, adding epinephrine, 5 μg/mL (1:200,000), to the anesthetic solution decreases the rate of absorption from its site of injection, decreasing the maximal blood level of the local anesthetic and thereby increasing the dose that can be safely administered.

The following values reflect a conservative value for the minimal toxic dose (i.e., maximal safe dose) of local anesthetics without added epinephrine. These doses should be used only as a guide for the maximal dose that should be administered. The dose can be revised upward if epinephrine is added, and probably should be revised downward if the drug is injected into the intercostal spaces where vascular absorption is rapid. For commonly used local anesthetics, the maximal doses are: procaine (20 mg/kg), chloroprocaine (20 mg/kg), lidocaine (6 mg/kg), mepivacaine (9 mg/kg), tetracaine (2.5 mg/kg), bupivacaine (1.5 mg/kg), and etidocaine (3 mg/kg).

It has long been known that, while high doses and high blood levels of local anesthetics are toxic, low doses and low blood levels can be employed therapeutically. Low intravenous doses of lidocaine are used to prevent cardiac arrhythmias, to treat epileptic convulsions, to reduce elevated intracranial pressure, to depress laryngeal and tracheal reflexes during endotracheal intubation, and to produce sedation. All of these effects occur after the intravenous injection of approximately 1 mg/kg of lidocaine followed by a continous intravenous infusion of 1–2 mg/kg/hr. These doses will produce blood levels in the range of 1–4 μg/mL, well below the toxic level (about 8–15 μg/mL).

## Effects on the Central Nervous System

When local anesthetics are absorbed from injection sites into the vascular system, they are distributed throughout the body and readily cross the blood-brain barrier. Their effects on the CNS are related to their concentrations in the plasma. Lidocaine will be discussed as a prototype, since its effects on the CNS have been the most widely studied.

At low doses (1–2 mg/kg) and low concentrations in the blood, (0.5–5 μg/mL), lidocaine produces sedation and depresses brain excitability (i.e., it has an anticonvulsant effect). Patients report light-headedness, dizziness, ringing in the ears, drowsiness, and an altered sensation of taste; voices may seem distant. As blood levels of the drug increase to the range of 5–8 μg/mL, slurred speech, shivering, and muscular twitching may appear. With increases to about 10 μg/mL, muscle twitching increases, convulsions may occur, and the patient may lose consciousness. A further increase in blood levels of the drug may produce respiratory arrest and death, probably from hypoxia.

High-dose toxicities of lidocaine and other local anesthetics may be reduced by benzodiazepines such as diazepam (Valium) or by barbiturates. If high blood levels of a local anesthetic are attained inadvertently and unconsciousness or convulsions are produced, support of respiration is essential: the patient should be given a general anesthetic, intubated, and ventilated with oxygen.

## Effects on the Cardiovascular System

Local anesthetics can produce significant effects on the cardiovascular system. Most local anesthetics dilate arterioles, by directly relaxing their smooth muscle walls after being absorbed into the vascular system. This vasodilation can produce significant hypotension. But cocaine, which has use as a local anesthetic, potentiates the action of catecholamines, and therefore causes vasoconstriction and hypertension.

Local anesthetics can profoundly affect the myocardium, an effect employed clinically in treating cardiac arrhythmias. Lidocaine, for example, decreases the electrical exictability of the myocardium and decreases both the rate of conduction and the force of contraction. These depressant effects, combined with the dilatation noted above, may lead to hypotension and cardiovascular collapse.

The long-acting local anesthetics that bind strongly to protein, bupivacaine and etidocaine, may bind to cardiac tissue, depressing contractility even more strongly than does lidocaine (Tanz et al., 1984). When this effect is recognized early, cardiotonic agents such as dopamine (Chapter 8) may support cardiac contractility until the local anesthetic can be absorbed and metabolized.

When local anesthetics are employed for spinal or epidural anesthesia, the sympathetic nerve fibers are blocked, reducing venous tone to a much greater extent than arterial tone. Venous dilatation results in hypotension unrelated to the direct cardiovascular effects already noted. As the veins dilate, they hold an increased volume of blood, venous return to the heart is reduced, and cardiac output and blood pressure fall. Thus, hypotension during spinal or epidural anesthesia may be produced not only by the sympathetic blockade that occurs in anesthesia, but by the vascular dilatation and the myocardial depression, which can result from direct effects of local anesthetics on the blood vessels and the heart. Treatment consists of positioning the patient head-down, administering intravenous fluids and small doses of vasoconstrictors, and judicious use of atropine if bradycardia is severe.

## Placental Transport

All local anesthetics cross the placenta by passive diffusion, some at a greater rate and degree than others. The amount that diffuses across is inversely related to the binding of the drug by maternal plasma proteins. Highly bound anesthetics are poorly distributed to the fetus, while those of low binding tendency are well distributed. More than 90% of bupivacaine and etidocaine molecules are bound to plasma proteins, and these agents are found in low concentrations in blood from the umbilical vein. Mepivacaine and lidocaine, 65%–70% protein-bound, are found in somewhat higher concentrations in umbilical blood than are the first two. Only 6% of procaine is bound to plasma protein, and procaine can be found in high concentrations in the fetus. These characteristics influence the choice of local anesthetic for labor and delivery.

Chapter 10 discusses the clinical use of local anesthetics in regional anesthesia techniques while Chapter 14 discusses their use in obstetrical anesthesia and analgesia.

## *Readings and References*

Covino, B.G., and Vassalo, H.S. 1976. *Local anesthetics: mechanisms of action and clinical use.* New York: Grune & Stratton.

DeJong, R.H. 1977. *Physiology and pharmacology of local anesthesia.* 2nd ed. Springfield, Ill.: C.C. Thomas.

Ritchie, J.M., and Greene, N.M. 1980. Local anesthetics. In: *Goodman and Gilman's The Pharmacological Basis of Therapeutics.* Gilman, A.G., Goodman, L.S. and Gilman, A., editors. New York: Macmillan, pp. 300–20.

Savarese, J.J., and Covino, B.G. 1981. Pharmacology of local anesthetic drugs. In: *Anesthesia.* Miller, R.D., editor. New York: Churchill Livingstone, pp. 563–91.

Tanz, R.D.; Heskett, T.; Loehning, R.W., et al. 1984. Comparative cardiotoxicity of bupivacaine and lidocaine in the isolated perfused mammalian heart. *Anesth. Analg.* 63:549–56.

Wood, M. 1982. Local anesthetic agents. In: *Drugs and anesthesia: pharmacology for anesthesiologists.* Wood, M., and Wood, A.J.J., editors. Baltimore: Williams & Wilkins, pp. 341–71.

# 8. Pharmacology of the Autonomic Nervous System

## Introduction

The two previous chapters have focused on the pharmacology of both the general and the local anesthetics. The drugs discussed next are those whose primary effects are exerted on the autonomic nervous system (ANS).

While both the general and the local anesthetics alter certain functions of the ANS, such changes are not the primary purposes for which those drugs are used. The general anesthetics are used primarly to produce amnesia, analgesia, unconsciousness, and muscle relaxation; alterations in cardiovascular function are side effects that often result from drug-induced changes in ANS function. The blockade of nerve conduction produced by local anesthetics is, again, the primary purpose for their use. The alteration of ANS function resulting from spinal and epidural blocks and the cardiac depression and arteriolar dilatation that follow the drugs' vascular absorption are side effects of the ANS alterations.

The compounds classified as autonomic drugs either mimic or antagonize the actions of the body's own neurotransmitters at autonomic ganglia or target organs. The anesthesiologist uses autonomic drugs to maintain homeostasis in efforts to compensate for disrupted autonomic regulation. The wise use of these drugs requires an understanding of the physiology of the ANS.

## Components of the Autonomic Nervous System

The autonomic nervous system is frequently called the visceral nervous system, since it regulates the function of the internal organs without the brain's conscious control. In the *afferent,* or sensory, component of the ANS, information is transmitted from the internal organs to the CNS. In the *efferent,* or motor, component, information from the CNS is transmitted to these same internal organs, regulating their function.

The autonomic drugs do not appear to act on the afferent fibers; they seem to act only on the efferent portion of the ANS.

## The Efferent Limb: Sympathetic and Parasympathetic Divisions

The efferent limb of the ANS is divided into two major divisions, the sympathetic and the parasympathetic (Figure 8-1). In each division, nerve fibers (preganglionic fibers) arising from cell bodies in the spinal cord or the brain stem synapse on the postganglionic neurons that group to form the autonomic ganglia. In turn, the neurons that make up the autonomic ganglia (and upon which the preganglionic fibers synapsed) give rise to postganglionic fibers that innervate the internal organs.

The neurotransmitter released by all preganglionic fibers and by the postganglionic parasympathetic fibers is acetylcholine (ACh); the neurotransmitter released by postganglionic sympathetic fibers is norepinephrine (NE [noradrenaline]). The terms *cholinergic* and *adrenergic* describe those neurons that liberate ACh and NE, respectively. Thus, all preganglionic neurons and the postganglionic parasympathetic neurons are cholingergic, while postganglionic sympathetic fibers are adrenergic.

The adrenal medulla is a structure homologous to a sympathetic ganglion. It is innervated by preganglionic (cholinergic) fibers; and the medulla cells themselves secrete both norepinephrine and epinephrine.

## Responses of Internal Organs to Autonomic Impulses

To understand the actions of autonomic drugs that mimic or antagonize cholinergic or adrenergic neurons, it is necessary first to understand the normal response of the various internal organs to autonomic nerve impulses. In general, the parasympathetic and sympathetic systems can be viewed as antagonistic to each other; one system augmenting an autonomic function and the other antagonizing it. For example, in the heart, the adrenergic system produces tachycardia and increases both conduction rate and contractility, while the cholinergic system produces bradycardia and decreases both conduction rate and contractility.

The location and function of other receptors are listed in Table 8-1. Note from the table that the receptors innervated by adrenergic neurons are termed $\alpha$ and $\beta$ with the latter subdivided into $\beta_1$ and $\beta_2$. To avoid confusion, Table 8-1 does not subdivide adrenergic receptors beyond $\alpha$, $\beta_1$, and $\beta_2$. Additional subdivision of $\alpha$-receptor deserves brief mention, as do the dopamine receptors. First, the alpha receptors can be subdivided into $\alpha_1$ and $\alpha_2$ receptors. $\alpha_1$-Receptors are the traditional postsynaptic $\alpha$-receptors which, when stimulated, produce the effects shown in Table 8-1. $\alpha_2$-Receptors are located on presynaptic nerve endings. When these receptors are stimulated, norepinephrine release is inhibited. Of clinical significance are two antihypertensive drugs, methyldopa and clonidine (Table 8-1), which stimulate $\alpha_2$-receptors in the

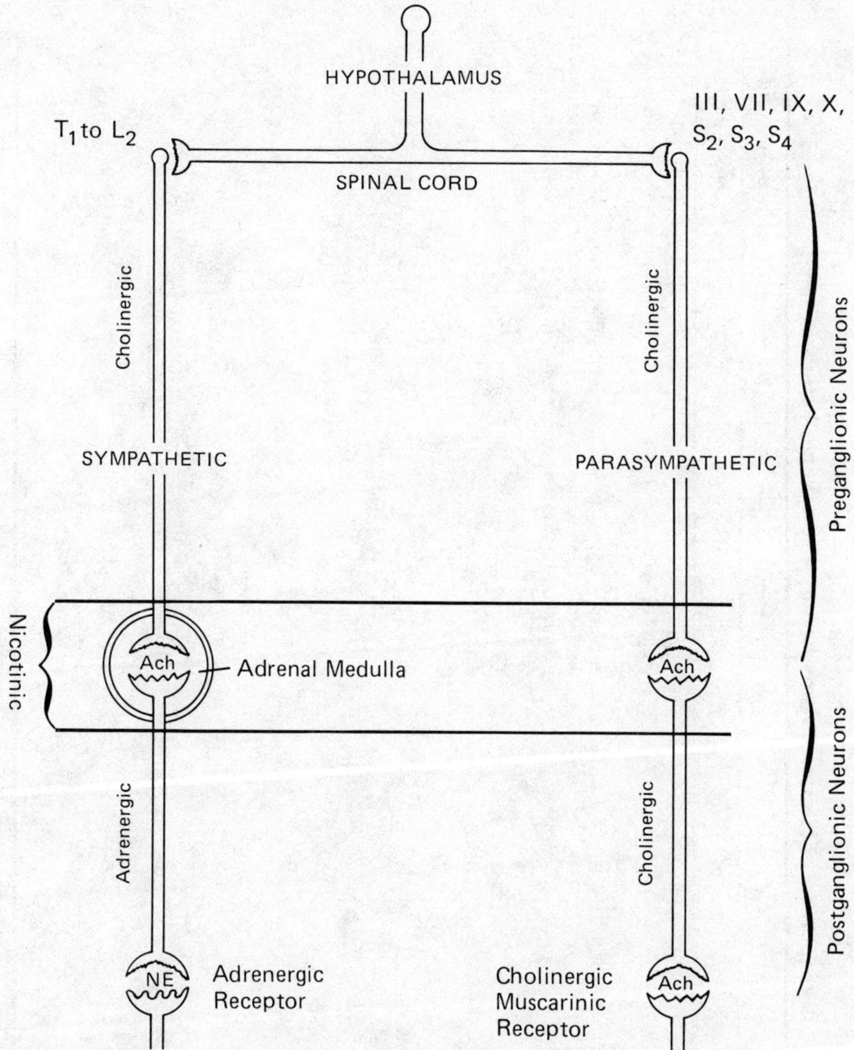


**Figure 8-1.** Sympathetic and parasympathetic divisions of the efferent limb of the autonomic nervous system.

brain, thus reducing sympathetic outflow from the CNS to the peripheral sympathetic nervous system and which, incidentally, potentiate the analgesia of centrally administered opiates (Collins et al., 1984). Second, dopamine is both a precursor of norepinephrine and a transmitter in its own right. Receptors specific for dopamine are located in the brain and on certain blood vessels, especially the renal and mesenteric, and produce vasodilation when stimulated.

**TABLE 8-1**
**Responses of Effector Organs to Autonomic Nerve Impulses**

| Effector Organ | Adrenergic Stimulation | | Cholinergic Stimulation |
|---|---|---|---|
| | *Receptor Type* | *Response* | *Response* |
| Eye: iris, radial muscle, | $\alpha$ | Mydriasis | Miosis |
| ciliary muscle | $\beta$ | Relaxation for far vision | Contraction for near vision |
| Heart | $\beta_1$ | Increased heart rate | Decreased heart rate |
| | | Increased contractility and conduction velocity | Decreased contractility and conduction velocity |
| Blood vessels | | | |
| Skin | $\alpha$ | Constriction | Dilatation |
| Skeletal muscle | $\beta_2$ | Dilatation | |
| Abdominal viscera | $\alpha$ | Constriction | |
| Lung | | | |
| Bronchial muscle | $\beta_2$ | Relaxation | Contraction |
| Gastrointestinal | | | |
| Motility and tone | $\beta_2$ | Decrease | Increase |
| Sphincters | $\alpha$ | Contraction | Relaxation |
| Kidney | $\beta_2$ | Renin secretion | |
| Bladder | | | |
| Muscle | $\beta_2$ | Relaxation | Contraction |
| Sphincter | $\alpha$ | Contraction | Relaxation |
| Uterus | $\beta_2$ | Relaxation | |
| Sex organs, male | $\alpha$ | Ejaculation | Erection |
| Skin (sweat glands) | | | Secretion |
| Liver | $\beta_2$ | Glycogenolysis | |
| Fat cells | $\beta_1$ | Lipolysis | |
| Salivary glands | | | Secretion |

# Drug Action at Adrenergic Nerve Terminals

Adrenergic transmitters are synthesized, released, and act upon receptors on effector organs, all in a series of steps. Available drugs can alter each of these steps, modulating the activity of the sympathetic nervous system. Such drugs include agents that either mimic or prolong the transmitter's effect (adrenergic stimulants) or that antagonize the transmitter's action at the receptor (adrenergic blockers). The effects of the adrenergic stimulants are summarized in Tables 8-2 and 8-3. The former lists six compounds, including the endogenous neurotransmitters called *catecholamines* because of their chemical structure. The noncatecholamines listed in Table 8-3 are of a variety of chemical structures. The effects of adrenergic blocking agents are presented in Table 8-4.

## Adrenergic Stimulants: Catecholamines

*Dopamine.* The substance dopamine is the immediate precursor of the adrenergic transmitter, norepinephrine. Dopamine can be synthetically prepared and is available commercially as a solution for intravenous use. It is also a neurotransmitter in the brain, and its deficiency there is associated with the disease Parkinsonism.

Within the sympathetic nervous system, dopamine exerts dose-dependent effects on adrenergic receptors. As shown in Table 8-2, low doses of dopamine (1–5 μg/kg/min) primarily affect the renal vasculature, producing vasodilation and increased renal blood flow, which result in increased glomular filtration rate and an increase in excretion of both sodium and water. At moderate doses (5–15 μg/kg/min), the increased renal blood flow persists, and is accompanied by an increase in heart rate and cardiac output, and a modest increase in arterial blood pressure. At high doses (above 15–20 μg/kg/min), the $\alpha_1$-receptors, in addition to the $\beta_1$-receptors, are stimulated. $\alpha_1$-Receptor stimulation results in an increase in total peripheral resistance with further increases in blood pressure. But the $\alpha$-receptor activation offsets the dopamine-induced increase in renal blood flow, which now decreases. Indeed, high doses of dopamine used for prolonged periods of time may produce renal failure. At doses below 15–20 μg/kg/min, however, dopamine is used to treat certain types of shock because of its ability to increase both cardiac output and renal blood flow.

Dopamine is available for intravenous use as a 5 mL solutioin containing a total of 200 mg. When diluted to 250 mL, a concentration of 0.8 mg/mL is produced. If a microdrip infusion set (60 drops/mL) is connected to this dilution, each microdrop of dopamine solution yields 13.33 μg of active drug. If a 60 kg patient requires 5 μg/kg/min, a flow rate of 22 drops/min would deliver the desired dosage. Table B-1 is included (see Appendix B) for reader convenience in calculating these flow rates. Table B-2 is similar and presents calculations for a double-strength solution. The latter is useful for patients in whom the total volume of infused liquids must be restricted.

*Norepinephrine.* Norepinephrine, the transmitter released from most adrenergic nerve endings, primarily affects $\alpha$-receptors and mildly affects $\beta_1$-receptors. It in-

**TABLE 8-2**
**Relative Effects of Natural and Synthetic Catecholamines on Mean Arterial Pressure (MAP), Heart Rate (HR), Cardiac Output (CO), Total Peripheral Resistance (TPR), and Renal Blood Flow (RBF).**

| | | Effect | | | | |
|---|---|---|---|---|---|---|
| *Drug* | *Receptor* | *MAP* | *HR* | *CO* | *TPR* | *RBF* |
| Dopamine (DA) | DA (low doses) | 0 | 0 | 0 | 0 | ↑↑ |
| | DA & $\beta_1$ (moderate doses) | ↑ | ↑↑ | ↑↑↑ | 0 | ↑↑↑ |
| | DA, $\beta_1$, $\alpha$ (high doses) | ↑↑ | ↑↑ | ↑↑ | ↑↑ | ↑↓ |
| Norepinephrine | $\alpha$, mild effect on $\beta$ | ↑↑↑ | 0, ↓ | 0, ↓ | ↑↑↑ | ↓↓↓ |
| Epinephrine | $\alpha$, $\beta_1$, $\beta_2$ | ↑↑ | ↑↑ | ↑↑ | ↑↑ | ↓↓ |
| Isoproterenol* | $\beta_1$, $\beta_2$ | ↓ | ↑↑↑ | ↑↑↑ | ↓↓ | ↓ |
| Dobutamine* | $\beta_1$ | ↑, 0 | ↑, 0 | ↑↑↑ | ↑, 0 | ↑, 0 |

*Synthetic catecholamines.

Modified from Kaplan J.A. 1978. The autonomic nervous system: pharmacology. *1978 annual refresher course lectures;* and Stoelting, R.K. 1980. Physiology and pharmacology of the ANS. *1980 annual refresher course lectures.* Park Ridge, Ill.: American Society of Anesthesiologists.

Key: ↑, 0 or ↓, 0 = little or no change.
↑ or ↓ = slight increase or slight decrease.
↑↑ or ↓↓ = moderate increase or moderate decrease.
↑↑↑ or ↓↓↓ = marked increase or marked decrease.

**TABLE 8-3**
**Receptor Targets and Pharmacologic Effects of Noncatecholamine Adrenergic Stimulants**

| | Receptor | | | |
|---|---|---|---|---|
| *Drug* | α | $\beta_1$ | $\beta_2$ | *Action* |
| 1. Ephedrine | + | ++ | ++ | Directly stimulates receptor, releases NE (weak) |
| 2. Mephentermine (Wyamine) | ++ | + | + | Directly stimulates receptor, releases NE |
| 3. Metaraminol (Aramine) | +++ | + | + | Directly stimulates receptor, releases NE |
| 4. Phenylephrine (Neosynephrine) | +++ | 0 | 0 | Directly stimulates receptor |
| 5. Methoxamine (Vasoxyl) | +++ | 0 | 0 | Directly stimulates receptor |
| 6. Amphetamines | +++ | +++ | +++ | Releases NE, directly stimulates receptor (weak) |
| 7. Terbutaline (Brethine) | 0 | 0 | +++ | Directly stimulates receptor |
| 8. Isoetharine (in Bronkosol) | 0 | 0 | +++ | Directly stimulates receptor |
| 9. Metaproterenol (Alupent) | 0 | 0 | +++ | Directly stimulates receptor |
| 10. Imipramine (Tofranil) | ++ | + | + | Blocks NE resorption |
| 11. Cocaine | ++ | + | + | Blocks NE resorption |

creases arterial blood pressure by inducing vasoconstriction, thereby increasing total peripheral resistance and decreasing renal blood flow. The increase in blood pressure can lead to reflex slowing of the heart rate, which reduces cardiac output, despite the increase in myocardial work and oxygen consumption, both of which result from the increase in peripheral resistance.

*Epinephrine.* Epinephrine is a direct stimulant of α-, $\beta_1$-, and $\beta_2$-receptors. It therefore increases heart rate, contractility, cardiac output, and peripheral resistance, all of which increase mean arterial pressure. Renal blood flow falls as a result of the vasoconstriction.

Because it can cause serious ventricular arrhythmias, especially when used with halothane, epinephrine is infrequently used by anesthesiologists. When it is used, it is primarily to relieve acute bronchospasm; to provide local vasoconstriction and reduce bleeding when mixed with local anesthetic solutions; and to produce vigorous ventricular stimulation during cardiopulmonary resuscitation.

**TABLE 8-4**
**Mechanism of Action and Clinical Uses of Adrenergic Blocking Agents**

| Drug | | Mechanism of Action | Clinical Use |
|---|---|---|---|
| *Generic* | *Trade* | | |
| Phentolamine | Regitine | α-Receptor blockade | Control of hypertension, acute and chronic |
| Tolazoline | Priscoline | α-Receptor blockade | Control of hypertension, acute and chronic |
| Phenoxybenzamine | Dibenzyline | α-Receptor blockade | Control of hypertension, acute and chronic |
| Prazosin | Minipress | α-Receptor blockade | Control of hypertension, acute and chronic |
| Propranolol | Inderal | $\beta_1$- and $\beta_2$-receptor blockade | Control of hypertension<br>Control of angina pectoris<br>Control of arrhythmias, acute and chronic |
| Metoprolol | Lopressor | $\beta_1$-, mild $\beta_2$-receptor blockade | Control of hypertension<br>Control of angina pectoris<br>Control of arrhythmias, acute and chronic |

| | | | |
|---|---|---|---|
| Clonidine | Catapres | Reduced central sympathetic outflow | Control of chronic hypertension |
| Methyldopa | Aldomet | Reduced central sympathetic outflow | Control of chronic hypertension |
| Guanethidine | Ismelin | Adrenergic neuron blocker | Control of chronic hypertension |
| Reserpine | Serpasil | Adrenergic transmitter depletion | Control of hypertension<br>Control of psychosis, acute and chronic |
| Methyl-tyrosine | Demser | Inhibition of catecholamine synthesis | Control of hypertension<br>Control of pheochromocytoma |
| Droperidol | Inapsine | Dopamine receptor blockade | Control of psychosis<br>Control of emesis |
| Chlorpromazine | Thorazine | Dopamine receptor blockade | Control of psychosis<br>Control of emesis |
| Trimethaphan | Arfonad | Ganglionic blockade | Control of acute hypertension |

Available as a 1mg/mL solution (i.e., 1:1000), dilution to 250 mL yields a concentration of 4 μg/mL. Each microdrop (60 drops/mL) thus contains 0.066 μg/drop. A dosage of 0.01–0.02 μg/kg/min (12–24 drops/min in an average adult) causes predominately β stimulation. Mixed α and β effects follow doses of 0.02–0.15 μg/kg/min (24–175 drops/min in an average adult). Higher doses cause predominately α effects.

Of more use in anesthesia is a 1:10,000 solution of epinephrine (0.1 mg/mL). Here, 2–5 mL (0.2–0.5mg) intravenously in an adult is useful for cardiac emergencies to provide a rapid but brief stimulation of the heart, often converting ventricular fibrillation to a coarse pattern which is more easily defibrillated.

*Isoproterenol.* The synthetic catecholamine isoproterenol is a direct stimulant of $\beta_1$- and $\beta_2$-receptors, producing an increase in heart rate, automaticity, contractility, and cardiac output; a decrease in peripheral resistance (due to vascular dilatation in skeletal muscle) and bronchodilatation; and a small decrease in renal blood flow. The drug is used in the treatment of acute bronchospasm, but such use is accompanied by tachycardia and hypertension. The latter two effects may reduce coronary blood flow and produce myocardial ischemia.

Isoproterenol is useful as a potent inotropic agent in patients with heart failure who are able to tolerate the drug-induced tachycardia. Such patients include those with valvular disease and infants with heart failure secondary to severe congenital heart defects. The coexistence of pulmonary bronchoconstriction is a further indication for isoproterenol. An intravenous solution of 4 μg/mL can be made by diluting 1 mg of isoproterenol (5 mL of 0.2 mg/mL) to 250 mL. Each microdrop then contains 0.066 μg of isoproterenol. Dosage is titrated to patient response, starting at about 0.01 μg/kg/min. For reader convenience, Table B-3 has been prepared to simplify dosage calculation.

*Dobutamine.* Dobutamine, a synthetic catecholamine, has preferential effects on $\beta_1$-receptors to increase myocardial contractility. As a result, it increases cardiac output with small or no increases in arterial blood pressure, heart rate, peripheral vascular resistence, or renal blood flow. Dobutamine is unique in its ability to increase myocardial contractility with only minimal increases in heart rate and peripheral vascular resistence.

As a continuous infusion, dobutamine is administered in a dose of 2.0–20 μg/kg/min. Available in 250 mg vials, dilution either to 125 or 250 mL yields solutions of either 1 mg/mL or 2 mg/mL, corresponding to 16.66 μg/drop or 33.33 μg/drop. A 70 kg adult receiving 5 μg/kg/min would therefore receive 10 or 21 drops/min, depending upon the solution used. Tables B-4 and B-5 are provided for convenience in calculations.

## Adrenergic Stimulants: Noncatecholamines

Several drugs structurally not classified as catecholamines mimic or potentiate sympathetic activity. Some of these directly stimulate adrenergic receptors; some cause nerve terminals to release norepinephrine, which then stimulates the receptors;

some prolong the action of norepinephrine by blocking its resorption into nerve terminals; and some act through a combination of these mechanisms. Table 8-3 lists a number of such drugs and their effects.

The first five noncatecholamines in the table are used in anesthesia, administered either as an intravenous bolus injection, or by continous intravenous infusion. Ephedrine both releases norepinephrine and directly stimulates $\alpha$-, $\beta_1$-, and $\beta_2$-receptors. Its effects on the cardiovascular system and the lung resemble those of epinephrine but last about 10 times longer. Ephedrine is widely used to treat the hypotension which can follow spinal and epidural anesthesia (Chapter 10). Because it maintains uterine blood flow during labor, ephedrine is also used to treat hypotension in obstetric anesthesia (Chapter 14). Usual doses are in the range of 5–15 mg intravenously and 15–30 mg intramuscularly in adults.

Drugs 2 to 5 in Table 8-3 predominately stimulate $\alpha$-receptors, producing peripheral vasoconstriction. They are therefore used to maintain blood pressure when hypotension is due to loss of sympathetic tone in blood vessels, or when it is necessary to increase blood pressure without increasing heart rate. Drug-induced decreases in renal blood flow can limit the use of drugs 2 to 5; such decreases are less of a problem with ephedrine.

Phenylephrine will be used as an example of an $\alpha$-stimulant used by intravenous infusion. It is available in 1 mL vials containing 10 mg of drug. Dilution to 250 mL yields a concentration of 40 $\mu$g/mL or 0.66 $\mu$g/drop (Table B-6).

Dosage is titrated to patient response, starting at a dose of 0.1–0.2 $\mu$g/kg/min. In seriously ill patients, measurement of left atrial filling pressure may be needed in order to avoid acute cardiac failure secondary to the drug-induced increase in peripheral vascular resistance.

Drugs 6 to 11 in Table 8-3 are not intended for parenteral administration and are infrequently used in anesthesia. They are listed to demonstrate the variety of adrenergic stimulants. The amphetamines exert strong $\alpha$ and $\beta$ effects, primarily by causing the release of norepinephrine from adrenergic nerve terminals. Terbutaline, isoetharine, and metaproterenol are direct stimulants of $\beta$-receptors, with some selectivity for $\beta_2$-receptors at low doses. When the latter three are used to produce bronchodilatation in asthmatics or to reduce premature labor in obstetrical patients, their usefulness is often limited by the tachycardia resulting from $\beta_1$-receptor stimulation. Anesthesiologists would benefit from a more specific $\beta_2$-stimulant, one that could be administered intravenously to produce bronchodilatation or uterine relaxation without the cardiac stimulation.

Imipramine is one of many drugs classified as tricyclic antidepressants. Imipramine prolongs adrenergic neurotransmission by blocking the resorption of norepinephrine into presynaptic nerve terminals. The same effect is caused by cocaine, a local anesthetic with adrenergic stimulant properties. Recall that such stimulation may increase cardiac irritability, especially during halothane anesthesia.

## Adrenergic Blocking Agents

Excessive activity of the sympathetic nervous system can have deleterious effects on cardiovascular function, especially in patients with hypertension or coronary artery disease. A number of agents can reduce such excessive sympathetic activity through a variety of mechanisms (see Table 8-4).

Agents such as phentolamine, tolazoline, phenoxybenzamine, and prazosin are blockers of $\alpha$-receptors. They therefore antagonize the effects of norepinephrine and reduce peripheral vascular resistance. In anesthesia, they are used to control episodes of acute hypertension, although such use has decreased since the advent of newer intravenous agents for this purpose, such as nitroprusside and nitroglycerine (see Chapter 9).

Propranolol and metoprolol affect $\beta$-receptors; propranolol blocking both $\beta_1$- and $\beta_2$-receptors, metoprolol primarily blocking $\beta_1$- but mildly blocking $\beta_2$-receptors. Both drugs are used therapeutically to decrease cardiac output, heart rate, and cardiac contractility, thereby contributing to the control of hypertension, angina pectoris, and certain cardiac arrhythmias. Since stimulation of $\beta_2$-receptors leads to bronchodilatation, inhibition of these same receptors can precipitate bronchoconstriction. An advantage of using metoprolol, the more selective $\beta_1$-blocker, is that drug-induced bronchoconstriction is less likely with it than with propranolol.

Currently, propranolol is the only $\beta$-adrenergic blocker available in parenteral form in the U. S. Intravenously, in the perioperative period, it is indicated for the control of supraventricular tachycardia (although the calcium channel blockers [Chapter 9] may supplant this use) and for the treatment of hypertension, especially that accompanied by tachycardia. In adults, doses of 0.25 mg are administered slowly to a total dose of 1–3 mg. Signs of either bronchoconstriction and excessive myocardial depression should be carefully sought. It should be noted that calcium, glucagon, and digoxin are all effective as positive inotropes in patients taking propranolol or other $\beta$-blockers.

As stated above, clonidine and methyldopa stimulate $\alpha_2$-receptors in the CNS to reduce sympathetic outflow from the brain, decreasing cardiac output and peripheral resistance. The use of clonidine presents a significant problem, since it is not available in parenteral form, and after oral administration it has a relatively short duration of action. Therefore, when it is not administered in the perioperative period, rebound hypertension occurs within hours as the drug is metabolized. Such hypertension can be severe.

Guanethidine and reserpine act on presynaptic adrenergic nerve terminals to deplete them of transmitter, reducing sympathetic activity. Both drugs are used to control hypertension, but have many side effects associated with the generalized reduction in sympathetic activity.

Methyl-tyrosine inhibits the synthesis of adrenergic transmitters, thereby depleting the body of its stores of these substances. The drug is marketed for the preoperative control of hypertension in patients with norepinephrine- or epinephrine-secreting tumors of the adrenal medulla (pheochromocytoma).

Droperidol and chlorpromazine are blockers of dopamine receptors in the brain. Blockade of dopamine receptors in the limbic system appears to be responsible for their efficacy in controlling psychosis. Dopamine receptors are also found in the brainstem emesis centers, and blockade of these brainstem receptors seems to underlie their effectiveness in controlling vomiting. Their weak blockade of $\alpha$-receptors appears to account for their side effects and their modest effects in controlling hypertension.

Trimethaphan blocks receptors in the autonomic ganglia of both the sympathetic and parasympathetic nervous systems. This blockade, which reduces sympathetic activity, was formerly used for treating hypertension, less so today since the advent of the vasodilators discussed in the next chapter.

# Drug Action at Cholinergic Nerve Terminals

## Cholinergic Stimulants

Because acetylcholine is released by sympathetic and parasympathetic preganglionic fibers and by parasympathetic fibers, cholinergic stimulants affect the autonomic ganglia and the effector organs innervated by the parasympathetic nervous system (Table 8-1). (In addition, cholinergic stimulants affect the receptors on skeletal muscle, where acetylcholine is again the neurotransmitter [Chapter 6]).

Like the adrenergic receptors discussed above, cholinergic receptors can be subdivided; with the two subdivisions termed nicotinic and muscarinic because two drugs, nicotine and muscarine, differentially stimulate these receptors. Nicotinic receptors are located on the autonomic ganglia and skeletal muscle while muscarinic receptors are located at postganglionic parasympathetic effector organs.

Nicotinic stimulants are rarely used in anesthesia, so only muscarinic stimulants and drugs which increase ACh at all its receptors are discussed in this section.

Drugs that stimulate muscarinic receptors in the parasympathetic nervous system include pilocarpine (used to lower intraocular pressure in patients with chronic simple glaucoma); bethanechol (used to relieve postoperative gastrointestinal distention, gastrointestinal atony, and urinary retention); and carbachol (used to produce postoperative miosis following intraocular surgery and to treat chronic simple glaucoma).

Drugs that block the enzyme acetylcholinesterase increase the levels of acetylcholine, thereby augmenting cholinergic neurotransmission at both nicotinic and muscarinic receptors. The anticholinesterase inhibitors include neostigmine, physostigmine, pyridostigmine, and edrophonium. Their therapeutic uses include: (a) treatment of atony of the smooth muscle of the gastrointestinal tract and urinary bladder; (b) treatment of glaucoma; (c) increase of muscle strength in patients with myasthenia gravis; and (d) reversal of the skeletal muscle paralysis produced by competitive neuromuscular blocking agents such as pancuronium (Chapter 6).

## Cholinergic Blockers

Cholinergic blockers are effective at either nicotinic or muscarinic receptors. The neuromuscular blocking agents such as pancuronium are examples of nicotinic blockers. Their pharmacology was discussed in Chapter 6, as was the pharmacology of the antimuscarinic drugs atropine and glycopyrrolate. These drugs block acetylcholine receptors on organs innervated by postganglionic parasympathetic neurons. Such blockade produces pupillary dilatation, bronchodilatation, increased conduction velocity of cardiac impulses, tachycardia, reduced bronchial, salivary and sweat gland secretions, and reduced tone of visceral smooth muscle, resulting in gastric atony and urinary retention. They may also inhibit penile erection.

Atropine (and other antimuscarine agents) have several uses in the perioperative period. These include suppressing the muscarine effects of both succinylcholine (Chapter 6) and the inhibitors of acetylcholinesterase. It is also of use during eye surgery to inhibit the occulocardiac reflex that produces bradycardia in response to traction on the extraoccular muscles.

## Note

This chapter, as well as the next, refers to dosage calculation charts for determining the correct infusion rates for several drugs. These charts, while useful, can be confusing to the student because of their apparent complexity and because they do not provide a reasonable "starting dose," which will be therapeutically effective in the majority of patients.

To solve this dilemma, Henry Casson, M.D. (Department of Anesthesiology, Oregon Health Sciences University, Portland, Oregon) has noted a consistency between drugs that allows one to use a simple formula for determining this "starting dose." This formula applies to "single strength" dilutions of dopamine (200 mg in 250 mL), dobutamine (250 mg in 250 mL), isoproterenol (1 mg in 250 mL), epinephrine (1 mg in 250 mL), phenylephrine (10 mg in 250 mL), nitroglycerin (50 mg in 250 mL), and nitroprusside (50 mg in 250 mL). The latter two agents will be discussed in Chapter 9.

Using these dilutions, the starting dose (Table 8-5) is achieved by delivering a number of drops per minute (or milliliter per hour) calculated as 0.3 times the body weight in kilograms. Thus, a reasonable "starting dose" of any of these drugs in a 70

**TABLE 8-5**
**"Starting Dose" Approximations for 70-kilogram Patient***

| Drug | Ampule Contents (mg)† | Drops/Minute‡ | "Starting Dose" (μg/kg/min) |
|---|---|---|---|
| Dopamine | 200 | 21 | 4 |
| Dobutamine | 250 | 21 | 5 |
| Isoproterenol | 1 | 21 | 0.02 |
| Epinephrine | 1 | 21 | 0.02 |
| Phenylephrine | 10 | 21 | 0.2 |
| Nitroprusside | 50 | 21 | 1 |
| Nitroglycerin | 50 | 21 | 1 |

*Number calculated as 0.3 times body weight in kilograms.
†Contents of each ampule diluted to 250 mL.
‡Assuming 60 drops/mL.

kg patient is achieved by multiplying 70 by 0.3, which equals 21 drops/min. Table 8-5 lists the starting dose achieved by this formula for each of the above listed drugs. For doses outside this "starting dose," the dosage calculations charts in Appendix B should be consulted.

## *Readings and References*

Collins, J.G.; Kitahata, L. M.; Matsumota, M., et al. 1984. Spinally administered epinephrine suppresses noxiously evoked activity of WDR neurons in the dorsal horn of the spinal cord. *Anesthesiology* 60:269–75.

Mayer, S.E.; Taylor, P.; and Weiner, N. 1980. Drugs acting at synaptic and neuroeffector junctional sites. In: *Goodman and Gilman's The Pharmacological Basis of Therapeutics*. Gilman, A. G., Goodman, L.S., and Gilman, A. editors. New York: Macmillan, pp. 56–234.

Miller, R. D., and Stoelting, R. K. 1981. Pharmacology of the autonomic nervous system. In: *Anesthesia*. Miller, R. D., editor. New York: Churchill Livingstone, pp. 539–560.

# 9. Vasodilators and Calcium Channel Blockers

## Arteriolar and Venous Dilators

The management of hypertension in the perioperative period has undergone tremendous advancement in recent years. Many of the drugs that are used are those which primarily alter the function of the sympathetic nervous system (Table 9-1). A few of these continue to be used (i.e., β-receptor antagonists and central $\alpha_2$-receptor agonists [see Chapter 8]), while many are now used less frequently (peripheral $\alpha_1$-receptor antagonists, ganglionic blocking agents, and adrenergic neuron blockers).

Since one of the major goals of antihypertensive therapy is a reduction in peripheral vascular resistance (i.e., a reduced "afterload"), much attention is focused on those agents whose primary site of action is vascular smooth muscle and whose primary effect is to reduce arterial or venous tone. This arterial vasodilation produces a reduced afterload (as measured by a reduced mean arterial blood pressure) that results in a decrease in left ventricular work during systole, resulting in a decrease in left ventricular oxygen consumption. In addition, the venous vasodilation produces a reduced preload (decreased return of blood to the heart) that reduces left ventricular filling pressure and further decreases left ventricular oxygen consumption.

Therefore, vasodilators are used in anesthesia to reduce both afterload and preload so that both left ventricular work and myocardial oxygen consumption are reduced (Table 9-2). Such effects are beneficial in patients with either left ventricular failure or myocardial ischemia. The resulting hemodynamic improvement can be measured by an increase in cardiac output, a reduction of left ventricular work, and improvements in cardiac contractility. In addition, combining vasodilator therapy with small doses of a cardiac inotrope such as dopamine or dobutamine results in further hemodynamic improvement, especially in patients with both a high pulmonary capillary wedge pressure and a high systemic vascular resistance, and in patients in cardiogenic shock coming off cardiopulmonary bypass.

Limitations of vasodilator therapy are significant: all vasodilators can produce greater than desired decreases in blood pressure, resulting in decreased coronary and cerebral blood flow (reduced myocardial and cerebral perfusion). The reduced ven-

**TABLE 9-1**
**Classification of Antihypertensive Drugs**

Central $\alpha_2$-receptor agonists
- Clonidine
- $\alpha$-Methyldopa

Peripheral $\beta$-receptor antagonists
- Propranolol
- Metaprolol

Peripheral $\alpha_1$-receptor antagonists
- Phenoxybenzamine
- Phentolamine
- Prazosin

Ganglionic blocking drugs
- Pentolinium
- Trimethaphan

Adrenergic neuron blockers
- Guanethidine
- Reserpine

Dilators of vascular smooth muscle
- Sodium nitroprusside
- Nitroglycerin
- Hydralazine
- Minoxidil
- Diazoxide

ous tone can produce reduction in venous return to the point where cardiac filling, and therefore cardiac output, fall to undesirable levels. Finally, unless $\beta$-blockade is present, the reduction in blood pressure can result in a reflex tachycardia that may increase myocardial oxygen demand in the face of reduced coronary perfusion, resulting in myocardial ischemia. Therefore, vasodilator therapy should be employed only by practitioners skilled in the use of these agents. Patients should, in general, be monitored at least with central venous, arterial, and urinary catheters, and with an ECG with V-5 recording capabilities (Chapter 5). A flow-directed pulmonary artery catheter is also desirable for measurement of pulmonary capillary wedge pressure and cardiac output, and for calculation of improvements in stroke volume, cardiac work, and peripheral vascular resistance.

## Nitroprusside

Sodium nitroprusside (SNP) is a very potent vasodilator, and its effect results from relaxation of vascular smooth muscle in both the arterial and the venous vessels. It has no clinically significant effect on other types of smooth muscle, or on either cardiac or skeletal striated muscle. SNP is widely used for the immediate reduction in peripheral vascular resistance and mean arterial blood pressure in patients with acute

**TABLE 9-2**
**Actions of Vasodilator Drugs**

| Drug | Arteriolar tone | Venous tone | Systemic vascular resistence | Pulmonary vascular resistence | Mean arterial pressure | Cardiac output | Left and right ventricular filling pressure | Heart rate | Myocardial $O_2$ consumption |
|---|---|---|---|---|---|---|---|---|---|
| Sodium nitroprusside | ↓↓↓ | ↓↓ | ↓↓↓ | ↓↓ | ↓↓↓ | ↑ | ↓↓ | ↑ | ↓↓ |
| Nitroglycerin | ←→↓ | ↓↓↓ | ↓ | ↓↓ | ↓ | ←→↑ | ↓↓ | ←→↑ | ↓↓↓ |
| Hydralazine | ↓↓↓ | ←→ | ↓↓↓ | ↓↓ | ↓↓ | ↑↑ | ↑ | ↑↑ | ↑ |

←→ = no change.
←→↑or ←→↓ = minimal change.
↑ or ↓ = small increase or decrease.
↑↑ or ↓↓ = moderate increase or decrease.
↑↑↑ or ↓↓↓ = large increase or decrease.

heart failure, acute hypertensive crises, and in instances where deliberate, drug-induced hypotension may benefit the surgical technique (e.g., clipping of intracranial aneurysm). Advantages include a rapid onset and a brief duration of action, allowing for fine adjustment of blood pressure by titrating the infusion rate. The primary disadvantage is its potential for producing severe hypotension. Other disadvantages and limitations are discussed below.

Because SNP has a balanced vasodilator effect on arterial resistance and venous capacitance vessels, the hemodynamic response to it represents a combination of decreased afterload and reduced preload. Thus, SNP reduces systematic and pulmonary vascular resistance, increases cardiac output (if preload reduction is not excessive), decreases left and right ventricular filling pressures, reduces pulmonary capillary wedge pressures, and reduces myocardial oxygen consumption (Table 9-2). At low doses, blood pressure may be only slightly changed, since the reduction in afterload is counterbalanced by an increase in stroke volume and cardiac output. Higher doses result in the predicted dose-related hypotension.

The chemical structure of SNP ($Na_2Fe(CN)_5NO \cdot 2H_20$) is a ferrous center surrounded by five cyanide groups and a nitrosyl group; the latter is responsible for the pharmacologic effects. Cyanide is released in the body and is combined enzymatically in the liver with thiosulfate to form thiocyanate. Either inadequate levels of thiosulfate or overdose of SNP (due to high infusion rates) can result in cyanide toxicity (accumulation). To minimize this risk, blood gases should be closely monitored for signs of metabolic acidosis and infusion rates should be limited to less than 8 μg/kg/min. The total daily dose should be limited to 1 mg/kg. Cyanide levels in blood can be measured and sodium thiosulfate administered if needed.

Thus, the major complications of SNP are primarily two-fold: (a) excessive and undesirable hypotension, and (b) cyanide toxicity. Thiocyanate levels in blood should be measured if SNP infusions continue for prolonged periods. Levels should not exceed 10 mg/100 mL of blood.

The usual infusion range of SNP during anesthesia is about 0.5–5.0 μg/kg/min, with a "starting dose" of about 0.8 μg/kg/min (see Appendix B, Tables B-7 and B-8). Due to its brief duration of action, SNP infusions should not be abruptly terminated since the rebound increase in systemic vascular resistance may precipitate acute left ventricular failure with a decrease in cardiac output. This is especially likely in patients with congestive heart failure.

## Nitroglycerin

For decades, sublingual nitroglycerin (NTG) has been used for the symptomatic relief of angina pectoris. Originally thought to produce coronary vasodilation, it is now recognized that the primary effect of NTG is to increase the venous capacitance, thus reducing cardiac preload, left atrial filling pressure, left ventricular volume, wall tension, myocardial work, and ultimately, myocardial oxygen demand. In addition, there is recent evidence that NTG may cause redistribution of coronary blood flow to areas of subendocardial ischemia, reducing the size of acute myocardial infarctions.

Intravenous preparations of NTG are available for patients with cardiac failure (especially those with pulmonary capillary wedge pressures in excess of 15 mm Hg), for the management of myocardial ischemia during coronary revascularization surgery, for the control of severe angina pectoris and coronary insufficiency, for inducing deliberate hypotension, and to reduce infarct size following acute myocardial infarction. The drug is titrated by intravenous infusion to the desired effect, using a starting dose of about 0.8 μg/kg/min (see Appendix B, Table B-9). Because NTG is rapidly metabolized in the liver, its duration of action is brief, approaching that of SNP. To date, the only toxicities of NTG that have been reported involve acute hypotension associated with overdosage.

Hypotension with NTG can be treated either by reducing the infusion rate or by administering an α-agonist, such as phenylephrine or methoxamine, to ensure adequate coronary perfusion pressure. NTG is readily absorbed into most plastics. Therefore, it should be diluted in glass bottles rather than plastic bags, and it should be administered through intravenous administration sets specifically manufactured for NTG infusion.

## Arteriolar Vasodilators

Hydralazine, diazoxide, and minoxidil are arteriolar vasodilators: they reduce systemic vascular resistance by a direct action on arterioles, without significantly affecting venous capacitance vessels. These drugs reduce peripheral and pulmonary vascular resistance, thus increasing venous return, right and left ventricular filling pressures, and cardiac output. Renal blood flow may also be improved. Blood pressure will decrease moderately, limited by a barorecepter reflex-induced tachycardia. The increases in heart rate and cardiac output may increase myocardial work and therefore increase myocardial oxygen consumption, effects which may precipitate acute oxygen insufficiency in patients with coronary artery disease. These effects can be minimized by the administration of a β-adrenergic blocker such as propranolol. With all three drugs, sodium retention can occur secondary to increased plasma renin activity. Concomitant use of a diuretic may be necessary.

Administered intravenously, these agents have a slower onset of action than is seen after SNP or NTG (2–5 minutes). Their durations of action are similarly prolonged, in the range of at least 4 hours. Thus, under careful supervision, these agents may be used intravenously in the absence of invasive hemodynamic monitoring. Hydralazine can be titrated intravenously in 5 mg increments; diazoxide can be given by intravenous injection to a dose of 1–3 mg/kg over a 30-second infusion period. Minoxidil is available only for oral administration.

# Calcium Channel Blockers

## Physiologic Roles of Calcium

Calcium ions play important roles in a number of biological systems, including the functions of myocardial and smooth muscle cells. In the heart, calcium is involved in the genesis of the cardiac action potential, in excitation-contraction coupling, and in energy storage and utilization. In the smooth muscle of both the coronary and the peripheral vascular vessels, calcium movement across cellular membranes controls vascular tone.

Extracellular calcium concentration far exceeds intracellular concentration. The entrance of calcium into cells through specific "channels" raises intracellular calcium concentration and initiates events that lead to contraction. Two types of membrane channels are described. "Fast channels" conduct the inward movement of sodium ions, producing cellular depolarization. These channels are selectively blocked by the local anesthetics (Chapter 7); "slow channels" conduct inward calcium movements and are blocked by verapamil, nifedipine, and diltiazem. Indeed, these latter agents reduce the tone of vascular smooth muscle and decrease cardiac excitability and work (Table 9-3). As a result, they are clinically useful in treating angina pectoris and hypertension, and as antiarrhythmics.

Most myocardial cells (atrial and ventricular conductile tissues, intracardiac conducting fibers, and the distal A-V node) depend on both rapid inward sodium currents and slow inward calcium currents for action potential generation, and thus for contraction. However, pacemaker cells of the S-A node and cells in the proximal region of the A-V node differ in that they are much less dependent upon rapid inward sodium currents for excitation and are activated largely by the slow calcium current. Thus, the calcium channel blockers (especially verapamil) depress the rate of S-A node depolarization (a negative chronotropic effect), reduce conduction velocity through the A-V node (a negative dromotropic effect), prolonging the refractory period, and depress myocardial contractility (a negative inotropic effect). These effects appear to underline their usefulness in preventing reentrant tachycardias and controlling supraventricular arrhythmias.

**TABLE 9-3**
**Comparison of Three Calcium Channel Blockers**

| | Verapamil | Nifedipine | Diltiazem |
|---|---|---|---|
| Rate of SA node depolarization (chronotropic effects) | ↓↓ | ←→ | ↓↓ |
| A-V conduction (dromotropic effects) | ↓↓ | ←→ | ↓ |
| Contractility (inotropic effects) | ←→↓ | ↓ (direct)<br>↑ (indirect) | ↓ |
| Vasodilation | ↑ | ↑↑ | ↑↑ |
| Heart rate | ↓ | ←→ (direct)<br>↑ (indirect) | ↓ |
| Cardiac output | ↓ | ↑ (indirect) | ↓ |
| Blood pressure | ↓ | ↓↓ | ↓ |

As stated above, calcium is involved in controlling the tone of smooth muscle of coronary arteries. Calcium channel blockade results in an increase in blood flow through coronary arteries, nifedipine being the most effective of currently available drugs. In addition, the smooth muscle of arterioles is relaxed in a manner similar to that produced by hydralazine.

## Verapamil

Verapamil affects S-A node depolarization, cardiac conduction, myocardial contractility, and vascular smooth muscle tone to varying degrees. Because of its depressant action on the S-A and A-V nodes, it has received wide clinical application as an antiarrhythmic, especially those which are supraventricular in origin (paroxysmal supraventricular tachycardia, atrial fibrillation, atrial flutter). Verapamil has not been particularly useful in treating ventricular tachycardias. It does, however, increase the threshold for catecholamine-induced ventricular arrhythmias during halothane anesthesia. Verapamil has little depressant effect on cardiac contractility and does not affect either the QRS or the QT intervals of the ECG. Verapamil as a vasodilator appears to be less effective than nifedipine, and therefore is not as effective as nifedipine in treating angina pectoris or coronary spasm in Prinzmetal's angina.

Verapamil is well absorbed orally with a peak effect occuring 5 hours after administration (Table 9-4). With intravenous administration, peak action occurs at 10–15 minutes, although the effects on the S-A and A-V nodes can persist for up to 6 hours. Verapamil is rapidly taken up and metabolized by the liver; therefore, oral doses are about 10-fold higher than intravenous doses. Primary side effects are extensions of the pharmacologic effects: hypotensioin and delays in A-V nodal conduction. A reflex tachycardia can also occur.

The negative inotropic, chronotropic, and dromotropic effects are additive with those of β-adrenergic blocking agents; and, thus, verapamil should not be used in combination, especially in patients with preexisting cardiac dysfunction. Verapamil should be avoided in patients with hypotension, left ventricular dysfunction, atrioventricular blockade, and S-A node dysfunction. Oral doses start at 40–60 mg every 8 hours; intravenous doses are 0.15 mg/kg injected over 1–2 minutes with constant electrocardiographic and blood pressure monitoring.

**TABLE 9-4**
**Pharmakokinetics of Calcium Channel Blockers**

| Drug | Dose | Route | Onset | Peak Effect | Duration |
|---|---|---|---|---|---|
| Verapamil | 40–60 mg q 8 h | Oral | 2 hr | 5 hr | 6–10 hr |
| | 0.15 mg/kg | IV | 1–2 min | 10–15 min | 6 hr |
| Nifedipine | 10–20 mg q 8 h | Oral | 20 min | 1–2 hr | 4–5 hr |
| Diltiazem | 40–80 mg q 8 h | Oral | 15 min | 30 min | 4–5 hr |

## Nifedipine

Nifedipine is much more effective than verapamil as a vasodilator (Table 9-3). At clinical doses (10–20 mg every 4–8 hours), nifedipine reduces coronary and peripheral vascular resistance and lowers mean arterial blood pressure. Reflex baroreceptor activation increases heart rate, contractility, and cardiac output, all secondary to increased catecholamine and plasma renin levels. Because of the increased catecholamine levels, the drug has less utility as an antiarrhythmic. Nifedipine is clinically indicated for use in ischemic heart disease, especially for the treatment of coronary vasospasm (Prinzmetal's or variant angina). Its usefulness may be limited by a diastolic hypotension (which limits coronary blood flow) and by the reflex tachycardia.

## Diltiazem

Diltiazem is very rapidly absorbed orally with peak effect occurring at 30 minutes. It appears to be similar to verapamil on heart rate and A-V conduction, and it resembles nifedipine in its vasodilatory action. Because of its cardiac depressant effects, the reflex tachycardia and the catecholamine-induced increases in contractility and cardiac output may not be as much of a therapeutic problem when it is used as a coronary vasodilator. However, A-V nodal conduction disturbances may limit its use.

## Drug Interactions

Calcium channel blockers are effective in treating many diseases that can also be treated with β-adrenergic blockers. Thus, it is not uncommon to see these drugs used together. Since both verapamil and diltiazem exert depressant effects in the heart, combination with a β-adrenergic blocker can worsen A-V conduction and cause complete heart block. Therefore, nifedipine might be a better choice of calcium channel blocker if the patient is already taking a β-adrenergic blocker, such as propranolol.

The vasodilation produced by calcium channel blockers is additive with the vasodilation produced by arteriolar and venous vasodilators discussed earlier in this chapter. Consequently, extreme caution should be exercised when using these drugs in combination, since profound hypotension can result.

Since calcium channel blockers can delay A-V nodal conduction and prolong A-V nodal refractory periods, the addition of a cardiac glycoside such as digoxin may intensify the block. Furthermore, since the calcium channel blockers are highly protein-bound, they can displace glycosides that are also protein-bound, increasing plasma levels of the glycoside. Thus, calcium channel blockers should be used cautiously in patients taking digitalis preparations.

The increased catecholamine activity seen with nifedipine may predispose patients to cardiac arrhythmias, especially during halothane anesthesia. Also, the cardiac depressant effect of calcium channel blockers may intensify the cardiac depressant effects of volatile anesthetic agents. The interactions between calcium channel blockers and anesthetics are now being investigated (Durant et al., 1984; Nugent et al., 1984).

## Readings and References


Antman, E.M.; Stone, P.H.; Muller, J.E., et al. 1980. Calcium channel blocking agents in the treatment of cardiovascular disorders: I. Basic and clinical electrophysiologic events. *Ann. Intern. Med.* 93:875–85.

Durant, N.N.; Nguyen, N.; and Katz, R.L. Potentiation of neuromuscular blockage by verapamil. *Anesthesiology* 60:298–303.

Henry, P.D. 1980. Comparative pharmacology of calcium antagonists: Nifedipine, Verapamil, and Diltiazem. *Am. J. Cardiol.* 46:1047–57.

Johnston, W.E., and Lowenstein, E. 1983. Calcium channel blocking drugs. In: *New Pharmacologic Vistas in Anesthesia.* Brown, B.B., Jr., editor. Philadelphia: F.A. Davis Co., pp. 163–91.

Kraynack, B.J. 1983. Calcium channel blocking agents: side effects and drug interactions (lecture 238). *ASA Annual Refresher Course Lectures.* Park Ridge, Ill.: American Society of Anesthesiologists.

Nugent, M.; Tinker, J.H., and Moyer, T.P. Verapamil worsens rate of development and hemodynamic effects of acute hyperkalemia in halothane-anesthetized dogs: effect of calcium therapy. *Anesthesiology* 60: 435–439.

Reves, J.G.; Kissin, I.; Lell, W.A., et al. 1982. Calcium entry blockers: uses and implications for anesthesiologists. *Anesthesiology* 57:504–18.

Robertson, D., and Robertson, R.M. 1982. Calcium antagonists. In: *Drugs and anesthesia: pharmacology for anesthesiologists.* Wood, M., and Wood, A.J.J., editors. Baltimore: Williams & Wilkins, pp. 565–74.

Stone, P.H.; Antman, E.M.; Muller, J.E., et al. 1980. Calcium channel blocking agents in the treatment of cardiovascular disorders: II. Hemodynamic effects in clinical applications. *Ann. Intern. Med.* 93:886–904.

# IV

# THE PERIOPERATIVE PERIOD

# 10. Choice of Anesthesia Technique

This chapter will discuss the two types of anesthesia techniques: those that provide *general anesthesia* and those that provide *regional anesthesia*. General anesthesia techniques are those that produce unconsciousness and amnesia. Regional anesthesia techniques are those that use local anesthetics to interrupt the sensory pathways between the surgical site and the brain. Regional anesthesia is often supplemented with sedating drugs to decrease the patient's sense of awareness during surgery and to provide additional comfort.

## Techniques for General Anesthesia

### Introduction

The administration of a general anesthetic can be divided into four parts: (a) preparation for anesthesia, (b) induction of anesthesia, (c) maintenance of anesthesia, and, (d) emergence from anesthesia. Preparation for anesthesia (preoperative visit, premedication, equipment, and monitoring) has already been discussed, and should include review of the "Anesthesia Checklist" (Table 4-6). The induction and maintenance of anesthesia are the subjects of this chapter, while emergence, drug "reversal" and postanesthetic recovery will be discussed in Chapter 11.

General anesthesia can be defined as a state of absence of awareness that consists of three components: (a) amnesia with unconsciousness, (b) analgesia, and (c) muscle relaxation. Amnesia is an absence of memory, most often accompanied by unconsciousness. Analgesia is often defined as an insensibility to pain and is assessed by stability of autonomic responses (i.e., blood pressure, pulse rate, pupillary dilation, and sweating). The muscle relaxation that occurs during general anesthesia is a depression of neuromuscular transmission and skeletal muscle tone that ultimately leads to muscular paralysis. The adequacy of muscle relaxation can be determined by use of a peripheral nerve stimulator (Chapter 5).

**TABLE 10-1**
**The Contribution by Pharmacologic Agents to Each of the Three Components of the State of General Anesthesia**

| | Barbiturates | Etomidate | Opiates | Nitrous Oxide | Halothane | Enflurane | Isoflurane | Ketamine | Benzodiazepines | Succinylcholine | Non-depolarizing Neuromuscular Blockers |
|---|---|---|---|---|---|---|---|---|---|---|---|
| Amnesia and unconsciousness | 4 | 4 | 1–2 | 2 | 4 | 4 | 4 | 4 | 2–3 | 0 | 0 |
| Analgesia | 0 | 0 | 3–4 | 2 | 4 | 4 | 4 | 3 | 0 | 0 | 0 |
| Muscle relaxation | 0 | 0 | 0 | 0 | 1–2 | 2–3 | 2–3 | 0 | 0 | 4 | 4 |

The number 0 to 4 in each box refers to the relative intensity of effect induced by each agent, with 0 indicating no effect and 4 the greatest effect.

Before describing specific techniques for induction and maintenance, it might be well to assess the contribution that various drugs make to the state of general anesthesia (Table 10-1). Ultrashort-acting *barbiturates,* widely used as induction agents for general anesthesia, provide amnesia and unconsciousness, but do not provide either analgesia or muscle relaxation. This fact, together with their relatively brief duration of action, implies that they are primarily useful for rendering patients unconscious for short periods of time, during which the patient may be given a muscle relaxant (usually succinylcholine) and intubated. After intubation, anesthesia is maintained with other drugs (discussed later). Barbiturates are rarely used as sole anesthetic agents. When they are, it is for such brief procedures as closed reduction of fractures, electroconvulsive therapy, and cardioversion of patients with abnormal heart rhythms.

Etomidate is similar to the barbiturates in its rapid onset and short duration of action, predictable unconsciousness and amnesia, and its lack of analgesic and muscle relaxant properties (Chapter 6). *Opiate narcotics* and *ketamine* are potent analgesics, with ketamine also providing amnesia. Neither the narcotics nor ketamine provide muscle relaxation. *Nitrous oxide* ($N_2O$) contributes modest amnesic and analgesic properties in concentrations ranging from 40%–70% of the inspired gas mixture. As discussed in Chapter 6, $N_2O$ is not sufficiently potent to be used as a sole anesthetic, but it lowers the dosage requirements of other, more potent anesthetics.

The three *volatile liquid* anesthetics are potent amnesics and analgesics and they contribute mild to moderate muscle relaxation. The *benzodiazepines* can produce sedation and unconsciousness with amnesia, but they do not provide either analgesia or muscle relaxation. Finally, *succinylcholine* and the *nondepolarizing neuromuscular blockers* produce paralysis of skeletal muscle. These drugs are neither analgesics nor anesthetics. They do not produce effects on the CNS; they act only at the neuromuscular joint where they block synaptic transmission.

As will now be described, these drugs can be combined in various ways to produce combinations satisfactory for either inducing anesthesia or maintaining a state of anesthesia.

## Anesthesia Induction

Induction is the process of taking the patient from a waking state to a state in which surgery can be performed. Table 10-2 lists several advantages and disadvantages of the drugs used as induction agents. The anesthesiologist will combine two or more of these in an effort to minimize the disadvantages of each while maximizing the amnesic, analgesic, and muscle-relaxing properties of the combination.

While the *barbiturates* rapidly and reliably produce unconsciousness, they are cardiovascular depressants and do not protect against bronchospasm; they should therefore be used with care in hypovolemic or asthmatic patients and in patients with cardiovascular disease.

*Narcotics* can provide cardiovascular stability during induction, as well as analgesia for the subsequent surgical procedure. But induction with them is slow, and

**TABLE 10-2**
**Drugs Used for Anesthesia Induction**

| Drug Class | Example and Dose | Advantages | Disadvantages |
|---|---|---|---|
| Barbiturates | Thiopental (3–5 mg/kg, IV) | Rapid induction<br>Good patient acceptance<br>Decreased intracranial pressure | No analgesia or muscle relaxation<br>Cardiovascular depression and hypotension<br>Possible bronchospasm |
| Narcotic | Morphine (05.–1.0 mg/kg, IV) | Cardiovascular stability<br>Excellent analgesia | Poor relaxation and amnesia<br>Respiratory depression<br>Slow induction |
| Benzodiazepine | Diazepam (0.25–0.75 mg/kg, IV) | Cardiovascular stability<br>Amnesia | Long duration<br>Poor analgesia and relaxation<br>Pain on injection<br>Phlebitis |
| Ketamine | (0.5–2.0 mg/kg, IV) | Excellent analgesia and amnesia<br>Bronchial relaxation<br>Increased heart rate and blood pressure | Poor relaxation<br>Tachycardia and hypertension<br>Postoperative delirium<br>Increased intracranial pressure<br>Salivation, nystagmus, increased intraoccular pressure |
| Gas | Nitrous oxide (70%) plus halothane | Good controlability<br>Administered through the lungs<br>Bronchial relaxation | Slow induction<br>Prolonged excitement period<br>Increased intracranial pressure<br>Cardiovascular depression and hypotension |
| Etomidate | (0.2–0.3 mg/kg, IV) | Rapid induction<br>Brief duration of unconsciousness<br>Hemodynamic stability | Increased muscle tone with myoclonus<br>Lack of analgesia |

an induction dose may necessitate postoperative assisted ventilation. Use of short-acting narcotics, as well as limiting the total dose, reduces the incidence of this latter problem. The use of narcotics during induction is particularly useful for patients with cardiac disease, in whom it is necessary to maintain cardiac contractility and stability of cardiac output and blood pressure.

*Benzodiazepines* produce amnesia without analgesia or muscle relaxation when used for induction. Their major disadvantages include a slow onset of action, prolonged durations of action, and phlebitis and pain at the site of injection. A new benzodiazepine (midazolam) has a shorter half-life and does not irritate the veins. It may thus be a more useful benzodiazepine for anesthesia induction.

*Ketamine* used as an induction agent provides amnesia, analgesia, bronchial relaxation, tachycardia, and hypertension. Because of these effects, ketamine is most useful as an induction agent in two types of patients: (a) those with reactive airway disease (asthma), and (b) those who are hypovolemic. The drug should be avoided in patients with coronary artery disease, cardiac ischemia, hypertension, or increased intracranial pressure.

Finally, induction can be carried out with the inhalation of nitrous oxide, oxygen, and a volatile anesthetic (a "gas induction"). Thus, the drugs are administered through the lungs rather than through an intravenous catheter. Anesthesia can therefore be induced more easily in patients in whom preoperative intravenous catheterization is difficult. Such patients include young children with significant amounts of subcutaneous fat. Venapuncture for administering fluids, blood products, or other medications can be done after the patient is asleep. The major disadvanatages are that induction is slow and intravenous access has not been made for rapidly administering drugs in case cardiovascular or respiratory problems develop. In addition, an excitement phase, characterized by involuntary movements, hyperventilation, and struggling, frequently occurs. Because of these potential problems, inhalation inductions are seldom used for older children or adults.

Table 10-3 lists seven different techniques widely used for inducing anesthesia. The first, a thiopental (4 mg/kg) and succinylcholine combination (1mg/kg), is mostly used for healthy patients and will be described in detail. The remaining six techniques provide alternatives for special situations and will be elaborated upon later.

## Induction Technique for the "Routine" Patient

In discussing the thiopental-succinylcholine technique for "routine" inductions, a caveat must first be stressed:

> Just as there is no such person as an "average patient," there is no such thing as a "routine anesthetic." Each patient is unique in his or her response to the drugs we administer.

However, despite this caveat, to form a basis for understanding, an anesthetic sequence can be described which will safely and effectively result in anesthesia induction for healthy, fasted patients with normal head and neck anatomy, and without evidence of systemic disease. This sequence is detailed in Table 10-4.

A few comments regarding this sequence are in order. Use of a "defasciculating" dose of nondepolarizing neuromuscular blocking agent, such as pancuronium (0.015

## TABLE 10-3
## Drug Combinations for Anesthesia Induction

| Drugs and Technique | Indications for Use |
|---|---|
| 1. Thiopental (4 mg/kg)<br>Succinylcholine (1 mg/kg)* | Normal, healthy patients |
| 2. Thiopental (1–2 mg/kg) or etomidate (0.2–0.3 mg/kg)<br>Succinylcholine (1 mg/kg)* | Elderly patients<br>Patients with mild-to-moderate systemic illness |
| 3. Combination of narcotics, benzodiazepine, +/− ketamine<br>Succinylcholine (1 mg/kg)* | Patients who will be maintained with a "balanced" technique<br>Patients with moderate-to-severe systemic illness |
| 4. Technique 1, 2, or 3 above; succinylcholine replaced with a nondepolarizing agent* | Patients in whom succinylcholine is to be avoided<br>Patients who will receive a nondepolarizing neuromuscular blocker as part of the anesthesia maintenance technique<br>Patients with open-eye injuries |
| 5. Rapid-sequence induction†<br>(a) Thiopental (4 mg/kg)<br>Succinylcholine (1 mg/kg)<br>(b) Ketamine (1–2 mg/kg)<br>Succinylcholine (1.5 mg/kg)<br>(c) Pancuronium (0.15 mg/kg)<br>Thiopental (4 mg/kg) | Nonfasted patients<br>Patients with intraabdominal mass<br>Patients with intestinal obstruction<br>Pregnant patients<br>Patients with hiatal hernia<br>Nonfasted patients with open-eye injuries |
| 6. Inhalation induction | Patients in whom it is difficult to start a preoperative intravenous line (especially young children) |
| 7. Awake intubation<br>(a) Blind nasal<br>(b) Direct laryngoscopy<br>(c) Fiberoptic<br>Followed by thiopental (4 mg/kg) | Patients in whom a difficult intubation is anticipated<br>Patients with intraoral masses or bleeding<br>Patients who are unable to open their mouth adequately<br>Patients with cervical spine injuries |

*Assuming that proper anesthetic management requires endotracheal intubation.
†Choice of (a) or (b) depends upon the cardiovascular status of the patient.

**TABLE 10-4**
**Anesthesia Induction***

1. Review of anesthesia checklist (Table 4-6).
2. Apply ECG, blood pressure, and precordial monitors.
3. Test face mask for proper fit.
4. Verify integrity and adequacy of intravenous line.
5. Have patient breathe 100% oxygen for 2–3 min.
6. Check vital signs.
7. Administer "defasiculation" dose of a nondepolarizing neuromuscular blocking agent (e.g., pancuronium, 1.0 mg or gallamine, 20 mg).
8. Administer test dose of thiopental (1 mg/kg).
9. Check vital signs.
10. Administer remainder of thiopental (3–4 mg/kg).
11. Following loss of eyelid reflex, verify ability to mask-ventilate patient.
12. Administer succinylcholine (1 mg/kg).
13. Ventilate patient with 100% oxygen for 1–2 min (oral airway may be of assistance).
14. Intubate trachea as described in Chapter 4.
15. Inflate cuff of endotracheal tube.
16. Verify bilateral breath sounds and reposition tubes if necessary.
17. Tape tube firmly in place.
18. Verify bilateral breath sounds.
19. Check vital signs.
20. Administer 60%–70% nitrous oxide, decreasing oxygen to 30%–40%.
21. Administer sufficient amount of volatile anesthetic, narcotic or muscle relaxant to maintain the anesthetic state.
22. Lubricate eyes and tape eyelids closed.
23. Check patient positioning, especially pressure points (Chapter 3).

*Healthy, fasted patient (70 kg) with normal head and neck anatomy and without evidence of systemic disease.

mg/kg, or about 1.0 mg/70 kg patient) or gallamine (about 20 mg/70 kg patient), reduces succinylcholine-induced muscle fasciculations and reduces the postoperative muscle aches and pains that can result from the use of succinycholine without defasciculation. At least 3 min should be allowed between injection of the nondepolarizing agent and injection of the succinylcholine.

The test dose of thiopental is used to determine the effects of the drug on the cardiovascular and nervous systems prior to administering a full "sleep dose". If pain occurs with the test dose, one must rule out an intraarterial or subcutaneous injection of drug before proceeding. After the test dose, one evaluates the drug's effects on vital signs and on the level of consciousness. Assuming that vital signs remain normal and that the patient is sleepy but still responsive, the induction dose (4 mg/kg) can be administered. Either cardiovascular depression or patient unresponsiveness necessitate withholding the sleep dose and reevaluating the planned technique of anesthesia induction.

To help avoid the situation where one might be unable to ventilate an unconscious, paralyzed patient, one should always verify his or her ability to ventilate the patient by mask before the paralyzing dose of succinylcholine is administered (Table 10-4, step 11). This step should be omitted only in patients with a full stomach, abdominal mass, or in any other situation where an awake or a rapid-sequence (or "crash") induction is required, and where the benefits of omitting this step outweigh the risk taken. Consultation with experienced anesthesia faculty is necessary before a paralyzing dose of relaxant or rapid sequence or awake intubations are attempted.

Following step 18 of Table 10-4, anesthesia is maintained with one of the techniques described below, using nitrous oxide and a volatile anesthetic.

## Alternative Techniques of Anesthesia Induction

Several situations necessitate alterations in the induction technique (Table 10-3). Such alterations can be summarized as follows:

1. Intravenous induction using lower doses of thiopental
2. Replacement of thiopental with combinations of etomidate, narcotics, benzodiazepines, and/or ketamine
3. Replacement of succinylcholine with a nondepolarizing blocking agent
4. Replacement of the intravenous induction technique with an inhalation technique
5. "Rapid-sequence" induction
6. Awake intubation followed by intravenous thiopental

Deciding when to choose an alternative technique is a skill learned only by experience and is based on knowledge, judgment, and common sense. In general, should the patient have a systemic disease, especially cardiovascular, and a "normal" sleep dose of thiopental is poorly tolerated, reductions in dose or replacement with drugs that are less of a cardiovascular depressant are indicated. Similarly, succinylcholine should be avoided and replaced with a nondepolarizing agent in patients who are susceptible to the adverse effects of succinylcholine (Chapter 6).

Finally, one must be aware of patients with facial deformity, trauma, or masses, and in patients in whom a difficult intubation (or difficult visualization of the vocal cords) might be anticipated, and those in whom positive pressure ventilation by face mask might be difficult or dangerous. Such patients are candidates for an awake intubation, followed by induction of anesthesia. Identification of such patients can be difficult, especially for the novice, but occasionally even for the most experienced anesthesiologist. Some deformities may present minimal abnormal physical findings, yet may result in major problems with airway management.

## Maintenance of Anesthesia

Following induction, the state of anesthesia is maintained with combinations of the agents listed in Table 10-1. The choice of agents depends upon the patient's physical status, patient position, and surgical requirements which might necessitate controlled ventilation or muscle relaxation. This section will organize the numerous possible combinations into five techniques for maintaining the state of anesthesia (Table 10-5).

The first technique listed, *inhalation anesthesia with spontaneous ventilation,* utilizes nitrous oxide, one of the volatile anesthetics (halothane, enflurane, or isoflurane), and oxygen. This combination provides amnesia, unconsciousness, and analgesia, with only a small amount of muscle relaxation. The latter is often desirable, since the patient can breathe spontaneously through either a face mask or an endotracheal tube.

Other advantages of this inhalation technique are listed in Table 10-6. The predictability of amnesia is obviously important. Indeed, one of the great advantages of inhalation anesthesia (and one often taken for granted) is that, if enough volatile anesthetic is administered to maintain stable heart rate and blood pressure (i.e., autonomic stability), amnesia is certain. "Excellent controllability" means that altering the concentration of volatile anesthetic produces alterations in the depth of anesthesia. When the gas flows are turned off at the end of surgery, the patient awakens quite rapidly and does not experience significant postoperative respiratory depression from residual anesthetic. This rapid wakening increases patient safety.

The disadvantages and limitations of inhalation anesthesia with spontaneous ventilation are also listed in Table 10-6. These follow from the pharmacologic effects of the volatile anesthetics on the cardiovascular system, on respiration, and on smooth muscle (Chapter 6). Such effects limit the use of this technique in patients with severe cardiovascular or respiratory disease or in patients with increased intracranial pressure. Limitations to the use of volatile anesthetics in pregnant women are discussed in Chapter 14.

The lack of postoperative analgesia, besides being uncomfortable, places the pa-

**TABLE 10-5**
**Five Techniques for Maintaining a State of General Anesthesia**

1. Inhalation anesthesia with spontaneous ventilation.
2. Inhalation anesthesia with endotracheal intubation and controlled ventilation.
3. Inhalation anesthesia with endotracheal intubation, controlled ventilation, and drug-induced skeletal muscle paralysis.
4. Balanced anesthesia with endotracheal intubation, controlled ventilation, and drug-induced skeletal muscle paralysis.
5. Dissociative anesthesia with endotracheal intubation, controlled ventilation, and drug-induced skeletal muscle paralysis.

**TABLE 10-6**
**Inhalation Anesthesia with Spontaneous Ventilation**

| Advantages | Disadvantages | Patient Limitations |
|---|---|---|
| Amnesia and unconsciousness predictable | Requires an intact chest cavity | Intrathoracic surgery |
| Controllability excellent | Skeletal muscle relaxation poor | Intraabdominal surgery |
| Wakening rapid | Respiratory depression | Severe lung disease |
| Postoperative ventilation good | $CO_2$ retention | |
| Patient safety good | Cardiac depression with decreased cardiac output | |
| | Smooth muscle relaxation | |
| | Vasodilation | Hypovolemia |
| | Uterine atony | Labor and delivery |
| | Increased intracranial pressure | Intracranial surgery |
| | Postoperative analgesia poor | |

tient at risk for pain-induced increases in blood pressure, heart rate, and peripheral vascular resistance.

Inhalation anesthesia with spontaneous ventilation is useful for surgery on the extremities, head, neck, and structures near the body surface, especially in patients who are healthy and can tolerate moderate degrees of cardiovascular and respiratory depression. The lack of postoperative analgesia can be overcome by administering small doses of narcotics prior to waking the patient.

The other four techniques listed in Table 10-5 provide alternatives for those patients in whom inhalation anesthesia with spontaneous ventilation is undesirable.

The second technique is *inhalation anesthesia with endotracheal intubation and controlled ventilation.* Like the first method, it utilizes nitrous oxide, one of the volatile anesthetics, and oxygen. However, the patient is modestly hyperventilated by the anesthesiologist so that the level of carbon dioxide is maintained below that which stimulates spontaneous breathing. The anesthesiologist thus controls the patient's breathing by removing the stimulus to spontaneous ventilation. This technique is especially useful when carbon dioxide retention secondary to hypoventilation should be avoided. Controlled ventilation is necessary for anesthetized patients lying prone or in the jackknife position, and for surgery inside the chest cavitiy.

The third technique is *inhalation anesthesia with endotracheal intubation, controlled ventilation, and drug-induced skeletal muscle paralysis.* Like the previous two methods, it uses nitrous oxide, a volatile anesthetic, and oxygen, but it adds a neuromuscular blocking agent to provide muscle relaxation. The relaxation obtained is sufficient for intraabdominal surgery. The patient must be diligently and continously monitored for ventilator failure or mechanical disconnection (both potentially fatal). It may be necessary, at the end of surgery, to antagonize (or "reverse," in anesthesia jargon) the nondepolarizing neuromuscular blocker with anticholinesterase and antimuscarinic agents (Chapter 11).

The fourth technique involves the use of nitrous oxide, oxygen, a narcotic, a benzodiazepine, and a neuromuscular blocking agent. This combination produces a state of general anesthesia classically referred to as *balanced anesthesia* (amnesia, analgesia, and muscle relaxation). Advantages of this technique include minimal cardiac depression, minor effects on cardiac output and smooth muscle tone, and little or no increase in intracranial pressure (provided that $P_{CO_2}$ is kept below 40 mm Hg). Balanced anesthesia is therefore particularly useful for patients with heart disease, increased intracranial pressure, or hypovolemia, and for obstetric patients requiring general anesthesia. A major disadvantage of balanced anesthesia is that the narcotic may have depressant effects on respiration that may persist after surgery. In such instances, therefore, postoperative ventilation may be required. However, the availability of narcotics with short durations of action (fentanyl), narcotic antagonists (naloxone), and of mixed agonist-antagonist narcotics (nalbuphine and butorphanol) have helped alleviate this problem. With correct dosage and timing, balanced anesthesia seldom necessitates postoperative ventilation, and patients benefit from the post-operative analgesia.

The final technique, *dissociative anesthesia,* uses ketamine, nitrous oxide, oxygen, a neuromuscular blocking agent, endotracheal intubation, and controlled ventilation. Ketamine differs from narcotics and the volatile anesthetics in that ketamine usually increases heart rate, blood pressure, vascular resistance, and relaxes bronchial

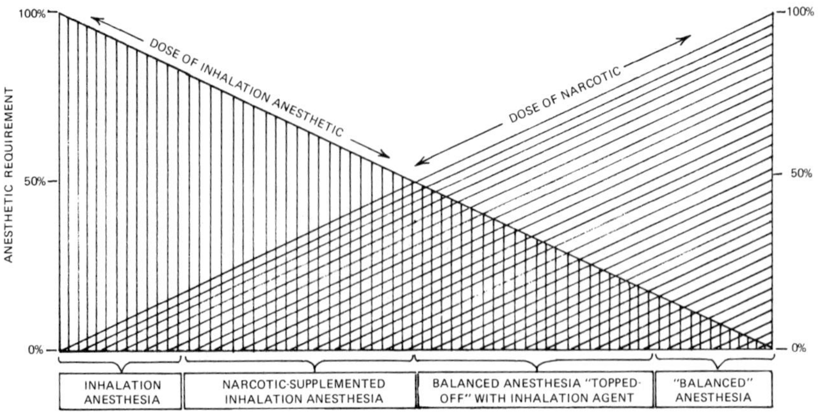


**Figure 10-1.** Illustration of the continuum of general anesthesia between the extremes of inhalation anesthesia (**left**) and balanced (nitrous-narcotic) anesthesia (**right**). In pure inhalation anesthesia, little or no narcotic is used. In pure balanced anesthesia, little or no inhalation agent is used. However, in many, if not most, anesthetics, the techniques are mixed. As the dose of either volatile agent or narcotic are decreased, the dose of the other is increased. The amount of $N_2O$ is usually held constant throughout this continuum.

smooth muscle. Dissociative anesthesia therefore has two primary uses: (a) for asthmatics, in whom bronchial relaxation is necessary, and (b) for hypovolemic patients, especially those in shock, in whom the maintenance of adequate blood pressure and organ perfusion is of primary importance.

Finally, it should be mentioned that there is often significant overlap between techniques. For example, narcotics are frequently administered to patients receiving inhalation anesthesia and, conversely, volatile anesthetics are frequently administered to "top-off" a balanced anesthetic technique and help maintain stability of autonomic responses. Thèrefore, as illustrated in Figure 10-1, there is a continuum between inhalation and balanced anesthesia. As the dose of volatile anesthetic decreases, the dose of narcotic increases. The experience, skill, and judgment of the anesthesiologist, together with the needs of the patient, determine the final combination achieved.

# Techniques of Regional Anesthesia

Table 10-7 lists six categories of regional anesthesia techniques and their major uses. This list begins with techniques requiring application of local anesthetic close to the site of surgery and proceeds to techniques requiring anesthetic application at sites nearer the CNS.

*Surface (topical) anesthesia* for sensory blockade of mucous membrane surfaces where absorption of the drug is good may be induced by topical application of an anesthetic solution. Such a technique is used to block sensory nerve endings on the cornea, the conjunctiva, and the mucous membranes of the nose, mouth, throat, vocal cords, larnyx, and trachea. Topical anesthesia of the nose, throat and mouth allows the conduct of tracheal intubation, broncoscopy (visual examination of the airway), and biopsies. Topical anesthesia of the urethra allows the performance of cystoscopies and certain other urologic procedures.

*Local infiltration* of anesthetic agents produces sensory blockade of nerve endings in the skin by blocking the subcutaneous branches of sensory nerves. The majority of minor surgical procedures, such as the removal of small tumors, incision and drainage of abscesses, and suturing of wounds, can be performed with local anesthesia. In addition, a combination of local infiltration and intravenous or nitrous oxide sedation may be used for more extensive operations, such as inguinal hernia repairs, breast biopsies, and placing hemodialysis shunts and cardiac pacemakers. The infiltration technique consists of making multiple injections of local anesthetic solution into the layers of tissue to be excised. Details on specific agents, their maximal doses, and their toxicities are discussed in Chapter 7.

The remaining regional anesthesia techniques involve the injection of local anesthetic at sites progressively further from the site of surgery. The technique of injecting a local anesthetic solution around nerve trunks leading to the surgical site is referred to as a *conduction* (*or nerve*) *block*. Such blocks can be performed on most major nerves and include those of the brachial plexus for surgery on the arm and hand (Figure 10-2); block of the branches of the trigeminal nerve for surgery on the teeth, jaws and face; block of the femoral and sciatic nerves (or their branches) for surgery on the leg and foot; and the block of the pudendal nerves for analgesia during delivery. Eriksson (1980) describes many of these blocks in detail.

The intravenous regional technique, the *Bier block*, is used to produce anesthesia below the elbow or knee. It is particularly useful when the surgical technique requires a bloodless field. The Bier block requires occlusion of the blood supply to an arm or

**TABLE 10-7**
**Regional Anesthesia Techniques**

| Technique | Use(s) |
|---|---|
| Surface (topical) anesthetic | Sensory block of mucous membranes |
| Local infiltration | Block of subcutaneous branches of sensory nerves |
| Conduction (nerve) block | Motor and sensory block by interrupting nerve conduction |
| Intravenous (Bier) block | Sensory block of upper and lower extremities |
| Peridural (epidural, caudal) block | Motor, sensory, and autonomic block of nerve roots and spinal cord |
| Subdural (spinal, saddle) block | Motor, sensory, and autonomic block of nerve roots and spinal cord |

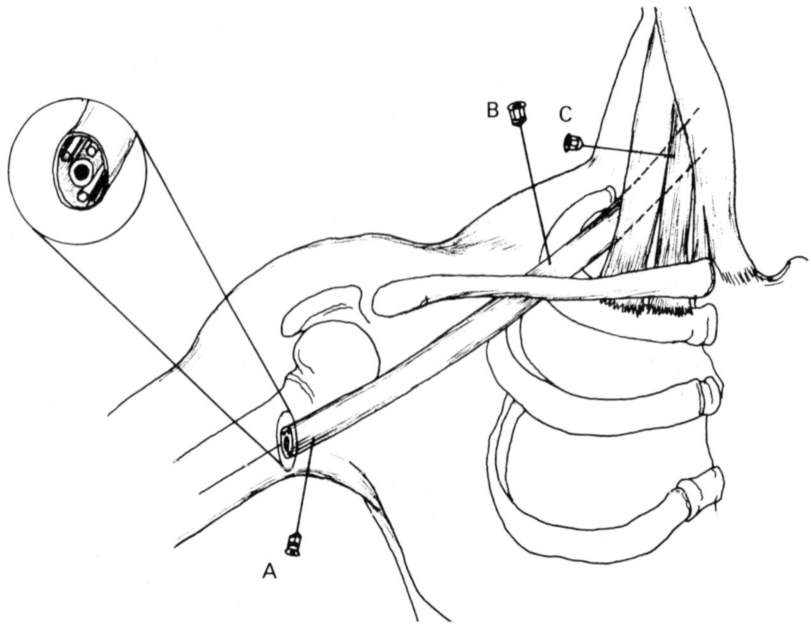


**Figure 10-2.** Illustration of the sites commonly used for blockade of the nerves innervating the upper extremity. **A**, Axillary block with the needle inserted into the neurovascular sheath surrounding the axillary artery and the median, radial, and ulnar nerves **B**, Supraclavicular block with the needle inserted above the clavicle at a point where the nerve fibers cross the first rib. **C**, Interscaline block with the needle inserted between the anterior and middle scalene muscles.

leg by a pneumatic tourniquet applied to the limb above the surgical site. A local anesthetic solution (such as lidocaine, 0.5%, 3 mg/kg) can then be injected intravenously, filling the collapsed veins of the limb. While the exact mechanism of anesthetic action is not clear, it is likely that the anesthetic diffuses out of the veins into the soft tissues and nerve endings of the limb, including those of the surgical site. The effect of the anesthesia is limited both by the time the circulation to the extremity can be safely occluded (≈ 1.5 hours) and by the length of time that a patient will tolerate the tourniquet pressure (≈ 1.0–1.25 hours). Following surgery, the tourniquet is deflated and circulation to the limb is restored. The anesthetic solution then circulates throughout the body and is metabolized. Toxic reactions may occur if the tourniquet is deflated too early or too rapidly, leading to an abrupt rise in the blood levels of the anesthetic (Chapter 7). To reduce the magnitude of the abrupt rise to peak blood level of drug, the tourniquet should not be deflated until at least 15 minutes after drug injection and, when deflating, intermittent reinflation should be used to slow systemic absorption. Inflation-deflation cycles of about 15–30 seconds should be used for about 3–4 minutes, and one should closely observe the patient for signs of systemic toxicity (Chapter 7).

The four regional techniques described thus far involve alteration of sensory pathways at sites between the spinal canal and the surgical site. The two remaining techniques, *peridural* and *subdural blocks,* require injection of the anesthetic solution into the spinal canal. As shown in Figure 10-3, a dural sheath within the canal encloses the spinal cord and the cerebrospinal fluid (CSF). The space between the dura and the vertebral body is called the *peridural space.* Typically quite small (2–5 mm wide), it contains blood vessels, fat, and the roots of nerves entering and leaving the spinal cord. When anesthetic is injected into the peridural space, the technique is referred to as *peridural anesthesia.* Such injection results in blockade of the motor,

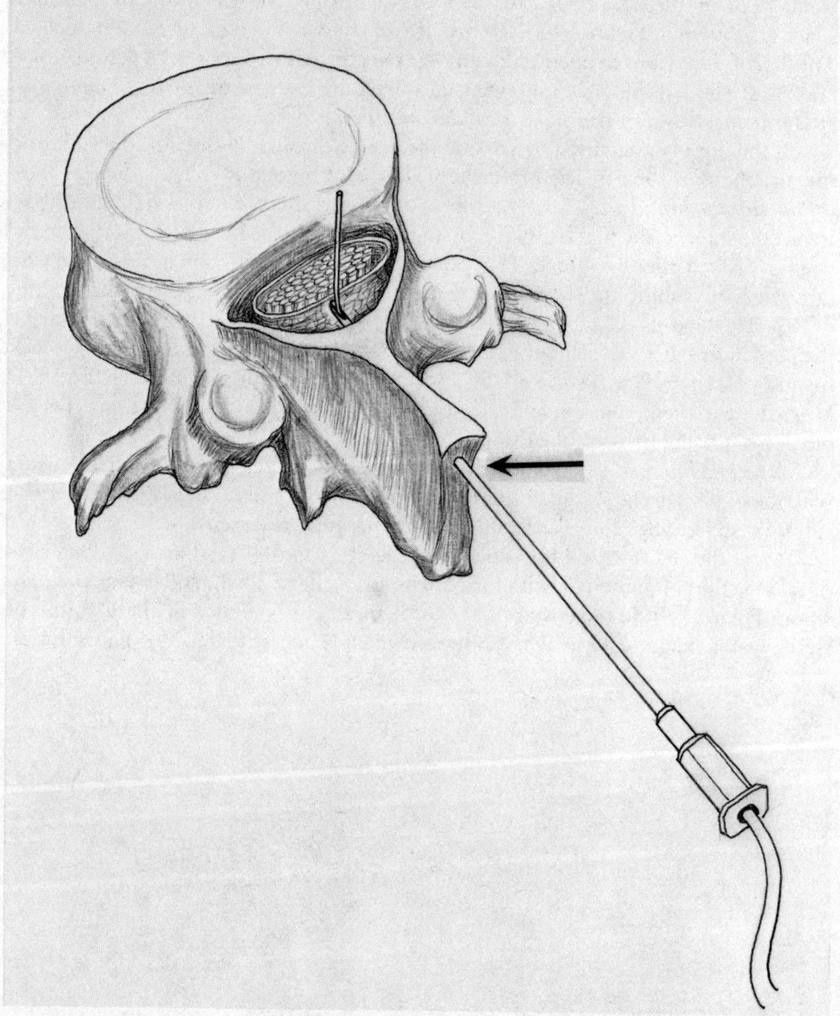

**Figure 10-3.** Illustration of an epidural catheter being passed through an introducer needle into the epidural space. At this point, the needle can be removed and the catheter taped in place. Note the interspinous ligaments between dorsal spines (**arrow**).

sensory, and autonomic neurons in those nerve roots in contact with the anesthetic solution.

Two types of peridural anesthesia are recognized, each requiring a different route of entry into the spinal canal. If entry is through the space between the dorsal spines of two adjacent spinal vertebra, the technique is referred to as *epidural anesthesia*. If entry to the peridural space is through the sacral hiatus, the technique is referred to as *caudal anesthesia* (Figure 10-4). Each technique can also be described as "one-shot" or as "continuous." In the former, once the needle has been placed within the peridural space, the anesthetic solution is injected and the needle is withdrawn. In the continuous peridural technique, after correct needle placement and injection of a test dose of anesthetic, a small catheter is passed through the needle into the peridural space (as shown in Figure 10-3), the needle withdrawn, and the catheter left in place. Through it, injections of anesthetic can be given repeatedly, even over a period of several days. These techniques employing a catheter are referred to as either *continuous epidural anesthesia* or *continuous caudal anesthesia*.

If the dura is punctured by passing the needle through it and into the CSF, and the anesthetic is then injected into the CSF, the technique is called *subdural anesthesia, subarachniod anesthesia*, or, more commonly, *spinal anesthesia* (Figure 10-5). In most instances, the block is placed with the patient in the lateral position, then the drug is injected after dilution in 10% dextrose to make the solution heavier than CSF (a *hyperbaric* solution). The patient is then turned supine after the needle is withdrawn. The level of the block is determined by dose and by patient position. Placing the patient in the Trendelenburg position (Figure 3.8**B**) moves the level of the block towards the chest. Placing the patient in reverse Trendelenburg position (Figure 3-8**A**) keeps the anesthetic solution in the lower portion of the spinal canal and prevents the block from rising to affect the thoracic nerves.

A *saddle block* is a spinal anesthetic in which the hyperbaric solution is injected with the patient in the sitting position. The solution descends to the caudal end of the subdural space, affording excellent rectal and perineal anesthesia.

An additional method for achieving anesthesia in the rectal area involves subdural injection of anesthetic with the patient prone, head down, and in jackknife position (Figure 3-9). In this instance, the local anesthetic is diluted in about 10 mL of sterile water (making a *hypobaric* solution which is lighter than CSF). This solution

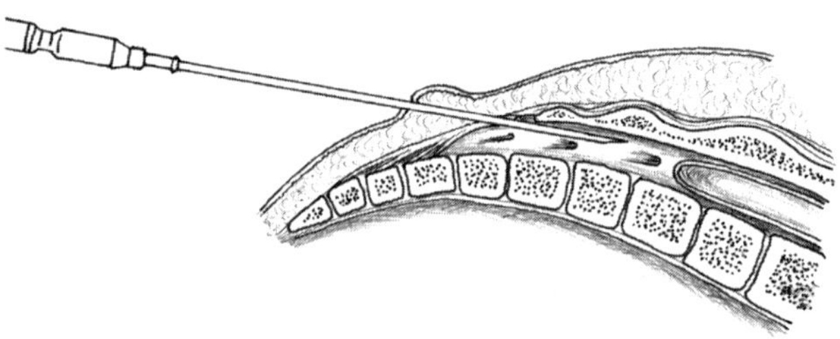

**Figure 10-4.** Illustration of a needle advanced through the sacrococcygeal ligament into the caudal canal. Note the tip located well below the caudal terminus of the dural sac.

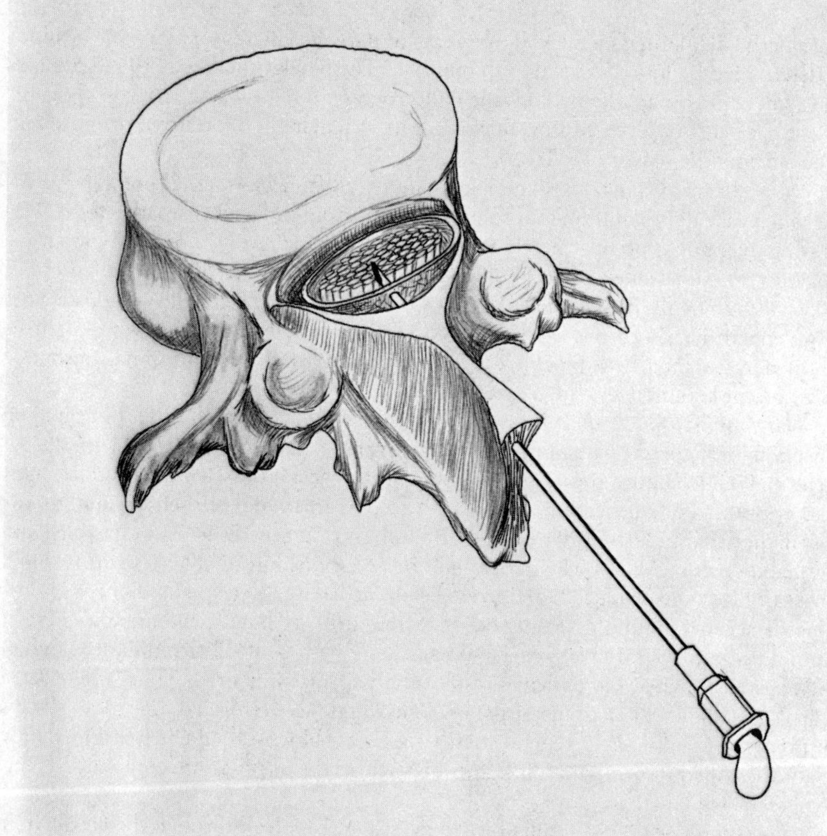

**Figure 10-5.** Placement of a needle within the dural sac. Note the free flow of CSF from the hub of the needle.

rises to the caudal end of the subdural space. Such a block is called *hypobaric spinal anesthesia*. It is frequently used for hemorrhoidectomies, for repair of perirectal fistulas, and for incision and drainage of perirectal abscesses.

## Comments on Spinal Anesthesia

Spinal anesthesia was introduced into medicine at the beginning of the twentieth century. It is technically relatively simple to perform and provides excellent analgesia and muscle relaxation for surgery below the umbilicus and, when combined with light general anesthesia, for surgery higher in the abdomen. It is, however, not without potential for major complications. Thus, despite its apparent simplicity, it should be attempted only by those either closely supervised or skilled in its use. Detailed descriptions of the techniques are presented by Murphy (1981b).

Injection of a local anesthetic into the subarachnoid space (usually at the L3-4 interspace) results in motor, sensory, and autonomic blockade of the nerve roots in contact with the solution. Dosage (usually 10–14 mg of 1% tetracaine) is reduced in the elderly, debilitated, acutely ill, or pregnant patient. The sensory level of the block is determined by loss of sensation to pinprick. The block is maximal 10–15 minutes after injection. Sympathetic blockade will progress to a level two or more segments above the sensory level. Motor blockade will terminate at a level two or more segments below the sensory level.

Side effects of spinal anesthesia are many: *Hypotension* is quite common and reflects the vascular dilatation that results from the drug-induced sympathectomy. Hydrating the patient preoperatively tends to reduce the magnitude of the hypotensive response to spinal anesthesia. Should systolic blood pressure fall more than about 20%, additional fluids, Trendelenburg position, and judicious use of vasoconstrictors (e.g., ephedrine, 5–10 mg IV) usually correct the problem. Patients who might be harmed by a sympathetic blockade are obviously not candidates for spinal anesthesia (e.g., recent hemorrhage, shock, etc.).

*High spinal blockade* can result from injection of too much drug, too rapid an injection, or incorrect patient position (e.g., hyperbaric solution injected with the patient in Trendelenburg position). Paralysis of intercostal muscles can produce signs and symptoms of suffocation and may be accompanied by both sensory and motor loss in the arms and hands. Phrenic nerve paralysis results in difficulty in speaking and an inability to move air. The patient will be conscious but unable to breathe. High levels of blockage produce more severe bradycardia, hypotension, and unconsciousness. If sensory or motor losses occur in the arms or hands, the anesthesiologist should begin preparations for general anesthesia with controlled ventilation, inducing anesthesia when the patient's respiration becomes impaired. Thus, whenever a spinal anesthetic (or any type of regional anesthetic) is performed, one must always be prepared to administer general anesthesia. These blocks should be performed only by those skilled in resuscitation in facilities where the appropriate equipment is immediately available.

*Postspinal headache* results from a persistent CSF leak through the needle hole in the dura. It is intense, postural, and persistent. An incidence of about 6% occurs in patients 20–25 years old, decreasing to less than 1% in patients over 50 years old. The etiology of such an age distribution is unclear. Conservative therapy consists of supine bed rest and copious intravenous and oral fluids. Refractory headaches respond to a "blood patch," which consists of epidural injection of 6–10 mL of autologous blood injected at the level of insertion of the spinal needle.

*Nausea and vomiting* are not infrequent, resulting not only from the spinal block but from preanesthetic medications, hypotension, and visceral traction. An antiemetic such as droperidol (0.25–0.5 mL IV) prophylactically before placing the spinal block is quite effective.

*Urinary retention* is frequently seen postoperatively, most commonly due to the blockade of the nerve supply to the bladder. Bladder distension or hypertension in the face of an adequate spinal level may indicate the need for catheter drainage of the bladder contents.

Other reported, *rare* side effects of spinal anesthesia include occular and auditory complaints (usually associated with spinal headaches), infection, abscesses, meningitis, arachnoiditis, cauda equina syndrome, transverse myelitis, and exacerbation of preexisting neurologic disease. Patients with the latter should probably receive a spinal anesthetic only when there are contraindications to general anesthesia.

Spinal anesthesia is contraindicated in patients with elevated intracranial pressure (danger of brainstem herniation) or bleeding defects (danger of intrathecal bleeding), and in patients taking anticoagulants. There is controversy over performing spinal anesthesia in patients on "minidose" heparin therapy or in patients who will be heparinized during surgery.

## Comments on Epidural Anesthesia

Epidural anesthesia resembles spinal anesthesia, but with several important differences. First, it is not as predictable as spinal anesthesia; it has a slower onset of blockade; it can be "spotty," leaving isolated areas nonanesthetized; and it produces greater disparity between motor and sensory loss. Second, it is technically more difficult to perform since locating the epidural space by "loss of resistance" is more subtle than locating the subdural space by return of CSF. Third, much larger doses of local anesthetic are needed, making the systemic toxic reactions more frequent and more serious.

The mechanism of neural blockade after epidural injection of a local anesthetic is not entirely clear, but appears to involve drug diffusion across the dura with anesthesia of nerve roots as they enter or exit the spinal cord. Thus, onset of anesthesia is slow but variable between drugs: chloroprocaine setting up faster than lidocaine, which sets up faster than bupivacaine. Details of individual drugs, doses, and dosage maximums can be found in the review by Murphy (1981b). Briefly, the major factors determining the spread and solidity of the block are the volume and the concentration of the solution and the presence or absence of epinephrine.

Side effects and complications of epidural anesthesia are important. *Accidental dural puncture* will produce in a large percentage of patients, a typical spinal headache (discussed earlier) due to the 16–18-gauge dural hole. Such a headache usually requires an epidural blood patch for resolution. Injection of an epidural dose of local anesthetic (e.g., lidocaine 1.5%, 15 mL) into the subarchnoid space (into CSF) will produce a total spinal anesthetic with cardiovascular depression, respiratory collapse, and loss of consciousness. Volume infusion, vasopressors, Trendelenburg's position, endotracheal intubation, and controlled ventilation may all be required until the anesthesia recedes. Injection of a 2–3 mL test dose of the local anesthetic and waiting 2–3 min before slowly injecting the full dose should help minimize the chances of a subdural anesthetic (2–3 mL into the CSF should produce signs of a rapid-onset spinal anesthetic).

*Intravenous injection* of an epidural dose of a local anesthetic (as can occur if the continuous epidural catheter migrates into an epidural vein) results in the rapid-onset of high blood levels of the drug. This produces systemic toxicity manifest by convulsions, hypoxia, and/or cardiovascular collapse. The latter has been an especially important concern with bupivacaine and etidocaine (Marx, 1984; Kotelko, et al., 1984.). Oxygen, CNS depressants (e.g., diazepam or thiopental), intubation, controlled ventilation, and inotropic support may all be necessary.

*Rapid absorption* of local anesthetic from the epidural space produces blood levels of the drug that can approach toxicity. Addition of epinephrine (1:200,000 or 5 µg/mL) to the anesthetic solution produces local vasoconstriction and reduces vascular absorption, lowering peak blood levels, and therefore reducing systemic toxicity. The addition of epinephrine also intensifies and prolongs the epidural block. Intravascular injection of epinephrine-containing solutions produces tachycardia, an effect that can be an aid in diagnosing migration of a catheter tip into an epidural vein with a resulting intravascular injection.

## Note

After reviewing the last pages, I hope that it has become clear to the reader that spinal or epidural anesthetics are not necessarily "safer" or less prone to complications than general anesthesia. Indeed, the potential complications of regional anesthesia, especially in the hands of an unskilled practitioner, can be much more serious. These are not benign anesthetics; considerable skill, experience, judgment, and vigilance are needed. It is erroneous to think that a patient would be "too sick" for a general anesthetic and only a "spinal" would work. In fact, occasionally, a properly conducted general anesthetic may be "safer."

## Anesthesia Choices: Case Studies

To conclude this survey of anesthesia techniques, I will discuss possible anesthetic choices for several hypothetical patients. This discussion will be divided into two parts: *routine anesthetics* for patients listed on a daily schedule of elective surgery, and *more difficult anesthetics* for high-risk or emergency patients. The objective is to explain the thought processes and choices we, as anesthesiologists, make in our daily work. After studying these cases, the student will see how an anesthesiologist might apply the information contained in the proceeding chapters into designing an anesthetic appropriate for any circumstance which might present itself. Please note that each patient could be managed successfully with a multitude of methods and that the techniques described represent those that the author prefers, although others might not.

### The "Routine" Daily Surgery Schedule

Table 10-8 is a schedule of elective cases for one operating room within a large surgical suite. I have been assigned to this room and will deliver anesthesia service for four patients.

The first patient, Mildred Jackson, is a 42-year-old woman scheduled for a colectomy. She weights 55 kg, is a nonsmoker, takes no drugs, has no allergies, and has normal laboratory values except for a decreased hematocrit, reflecting blood loss from a colon tumor. I consider all the techniques (Tables 10-5 and 10-7) that provide suitable operating conditions and then decide with the patient (during the preoperative visit [Chapter 1]) which of these techniques will be employed.

**TABLE 10-8**
**Hypothetical (Friday, August 1) Surgery Schedule for One Operating Room within a Surgical Suite**

| Time | Patient | Age (yr) | Location | Procedure | Surgeon | Anesthesiologist |
|---|---|---|---|---|---|---|
| 7:30 | Jackson, Mildred | 42 | 3 West | Colectomy | Dr. Johnson | Dr. Julien |
| 10:30 | Peterson, John | 32 | 4 South | Hemorrhoidectomy | Dr. Johnson | Dr. Julien |
| 12:00 | Phillips, Matthew | 62 | 3 East | Thoracotomy with tumor resection | Dr. Miles | Dr. Julien |
| 15:00 | Owens, Thomas | 47 | 2 North | Bunionectomy (right foot) | Dr. McDonald | Dr. Julien |

Of the regional anesthesia techniques, either an epidural or a subdural anesthetic would provide the necessary motor and sensory blockade of the nerve roots supplying the abdomen. A continuous epidural anesthetic would also provide postoperative analgesia since the catheter can be left in place postoperatively, and low doses and concentration of long-acting local anesthetics (e.g., 6–8 mL, 0.25% bupivacaine with 1:200,000 epinephrine, injected every 3 hours) provide excellent analgesia without motor paralysis.

Of the techniques for general anesthesia, inhalation anesthesia with either spontaneous or controlled ventilation probably would not provide adequate muscle relaxation for abdominal surgery; a neuromuscular blocking agent will be necesssary. Balanced anesthesia would provide excellent cardiovascular stability and postoperative analgesia. Dissociative anesthesia would provide analgesia, amnesia, and muscle relaxation, but might result in undesirable tachycardia, hypertension, and hallucinations. Finally, inhalation anesthesia with paralysis and controlled ventilation would be entirely satisfactory assuming she is in good physical condition and prefers a general anesthetic. The choice among these methods is made after evaluation of her nutritional, hydration, and electrolyte status, her cardiovascular status, and her desires.

Two techniques will be presented, either of which would be satisfactory for this patient, although other techniques could be used with equally good expectations. The first, general anesthesia, would use thiopental (3 mg/kg) for induction, accompanied by pancuronium (0.1 mg/kg) for muscle relaxation, both for endotracheal intubation and for relaxation of the abdominal musculature for surgery. Following intubation, anesthesia is maintained with 70% nitrous oxide, 30% oxygen, and 0.5%–1.0% enflurane or isoflurane. Morphine (0.1 mg/kg) is added during the surgery to provide postoperative analgesia. At the end of surgery, the pancuronium is "reversed" with neostigmine (0.05 mg/kg) and atropine (0.025 mg/kg).

The second technique uses a regional anesthetic to provide analgesia and muscle relaxation, combined with a "light" general anesthetic. Under diazepam sedation, an epidural catheter is placed at the L2-3 interspace and a 3 mL test dose of 1.5% lidocaine with 1:200,000 epinephrine is injected through the catheter. Three minutes later, after confirming that the drug did not enter the subarachnoid space, an additional 15 mL of the solution is injected. Following onset of the block, Mrs. Jackson is anesthetized with thiopental (3 mg/kg) and succinylcholine (1 mg/kg), the trachea intubated, and anesthesia maintained with 60% nitrous oxide, 40% oxygen, and sufficient halothane (about 0.2%) to permit spontaneous ventilation, and yet allow tolerance of the endotracheal tube. At the completion of surgery, the patient is extubated and analgesia maintained with bupivacaine (0.25%, 6–8 mL with 1:200,000 epinephrine) injected about every 3 hours for 24–48 hours, after which time the catheter is removed.

The second patient, John Peterson, is a 32-year-old male scheduled for a hemorrhoidectomy. Of the regional anesthesia techniques, a caudal, lumbar epidural, or a subdural block would be effective. Narrowing of those choices will depend upon the surgeon's and the patient's preferences and the position in which the patient will be put in for surgery. If he is to be in jackknife position (Chapter 3), either a caudal or a hypobaric spinal anesthetic would be a good choice. If the patient is to lie on his back with his legs elevated (lithotomy position), either a lumbar epidural or a hyperbaric spinal block would be satisfactory. All would provide postoperative analgesia for the duration of the block. Of the techniques for general anesthesia, inhalation anesthesia with controlled ventilation and endotracheal intubation would be necessary for surgery performed with the patient in jackknife position. Narcotic supplementation would provide postoperative comfort. After discussion with Mr. Peterson and with the surgeon (who states that the jackknife position will be used), I decide to use a hypobaric spinal anesthetic with diazepam sedation. The patient is positioned on the table, the lower back prepped, and a 25-gauge spinal needle inserted at the L3-4 interspace. A solution of 14 mg tetracaine with 0.2 mL of 1:1,000 epinephrine diluted in 10 mL of sterile water (a hypobaric solution) is slowly injected and the needle withdrawn. Increments of diazepam (2.5 mg) are used as needed for sedation.

The third patient, Matthew Phillips, is a 62-year-old man scheduled for thoracotomy and resection of a lung tumor. Mr. Phillips now weights 60 kg, having experienced a 15 kg weight loss over 15 months. He smokes two packages of cigarettes per day and drinks heavily. His hematocrit is slightly elevated, as are his liver enzymes. ECG reveals a right bundle branch block and mild S-T segment depression. Chest x-ray reveals a nodule in the left lower lobe. Arterial blood gases include: pH 7.38, $Po_2$62, and $Pco_2$48.

For this patient, general anesthesia is chosen. In addition to the routine monitors, the right radial and right internal jugular veins are cannulated for blood pressure and CVP monitoring. Since an induction dose of thiopental (4 mg/kg) might be poorly tolerated due to its possible cardiovascular depression in this rather frail patient, anesthesia is induced with diazepam (0.2 mg/kg) for sedation and amnesia, fentanyl (10μg/kg) for analgesia, ketamine (0.5 mg/kg) for amnesia and analgesia, and lidocaine (1 mg/kg) to decrease cough reflexes. After succinylcholine (1 mg/kg), the trachea is intubated and anesthesia is maintained with nitrous oxide (50%), oxygen (50%), and isoflurane sufficient to maintain stable vital signs. Pancuronium (1–2 mg) is used as needed for muscle relaxation. At the termination of surgery, the intercostal nerves near the incision are blocked with 0.5% bupivacaine with 1:200,000 epinephrine (2 mL per nerve).

Finally, Thomas Owens is a healthy 47-year-old man scheduled for a bunionectomy on his right foot. Surface anesthesia and local infiltration are thought to be insufficient, but any of the four remaining regional techniques (conduction block, intravenous regional block, peridural block, or subdural block) would provide suitable operating conditions. A block close to the site of surgery, in this case at the ankle, would be a reasonable choice (lidocaine, 1% without added epinephrine). Diazepam (2.5 mg increments) would provide sedation and relief of anxiety. If the patient does not desire a regional anesthetic, inhalation anesthesia with spontaneous ventilation would be satisfactory.

## Anesthesia for the High-risk or Emergency Patient

Emergency or critically ill patients are a challenge to the judgment, knowledge, skill, and stamina of the anesthesiologist. To illustrate approaches to complex cases, it will be useful to discuss here several hypothetical surgical patients who present difficult anesthesia problems. Again, the approaches described are the author's; as with any art or skill, another practitioner might weigh the factors in a given case slightly differently.

- ***Case Report #1:*** ASTHMA AND ANESTHESIA. *A 28-year-old female is scheduled for an elective laparoscopic tubal ligation. She is admitted on the morning of surgery to the outpatient surgical department and is first seen by myself an hour before the scheduled surgery. Her history reveals multiple environmental allergies (to dust, molds, and other allergens) and possible asthma (she has twice visited the emergency room because of respiratory difficulty, which was relieved by epinephrine). She takes aminophylline, 250 mg each morning, for prevention of asthma. A physical examination shows mild pulmonary wheezing at rest.*

ANESTHETIC MANAGEMENT. *An asthma attack during surgery is one of the most frightening events an anesthesiologist can encounter. Anesthesia requires maintaining an open airway and adequate alveolar ventilation. Even though an endotracheal tube allows gas exchange between the atmosphere and the trachea, acute bronchospasm will prevent tracheal gas from reaching the alveoli and will result in acute respiratory failure with possibly serious consequences. The patient's medical history strongly suggests reactive airway disease; her blood level of aminophylline is 4 μg/mL, a level below the thereapeutic level (10–20 μg/mL), and she has mild pulmonary wheezing. For these reasons, the elective surgery is postponed until her condition can be made more optimal for it.*

*After consultation with the surgeon, I initiate the following therapeutic plan: (a) since the patient has already been admitted to a hospital ward, sufficient aminophylline (≈ 5 mg/kg) is administered intravenously to achieve a therapeutic level in her blood. Because aminophylline causes cardiac stimulation, as well as bronchodilation, blood pressure and pulse are closely monitored; (b) she is discharged on an oral dose of aminophylline (750 mg/day) sufficient to maintain the therapeutic level. Three days later, a blood assay shows the aminophylline level to be 15 μg/mL.*

*She is readmitted as an inpatient the evening before the rescheduled surgery. Physical examination that evening shows blood pressure of 125/85 mm Hg, pulse of 90 beats/min, and regular heart rhythm. The lung fields are clear, even on forced expiration, and the remainder of the examination and the laboratory studies are normal. She is considered to be in her optimal state of health for the surgery planned. On the morning of surgery, aminophylline is continously administered intravenously at a rate of 0.9 mg/kg/hr.*

*The choice of anesthetic for a laparoscopic tubal ligation should take into account the factors discussed in Chapter 8. I might consider the regional techniques of epidural or subarachnoid blocks (Table 8-2), or any of the general anesthesia techniques employing a muscle relaxant, including those using a volatile inhalation anesthetic, or ketamine (Table 8-4). Note that ketamine produces increased sympathetic activity, which would be desirable in augmenting bronchial dilatation; but it may also have the undesirable effect of increasing blood pressure and heart rate, and emergence delirium may occur if higher doses are employed (2–4 mg/kg IV).*

*I might also avoid balanced anesthesia, since narcotics do not produce bronchial dilatation and may release histamine (especially morphine). The three volatile anesthetics dilate the bronchi and are good choices for maintaining general anesthesia in asthmatics. Halothane, however, sensitizes the heart to catecholamines, often leading to serious cardiac irregularities in patients on therapeutic doses of aminophylline. Enflurane and isoflurane produce this sensitization to a much lesser degree.*

*An appropriate general anesthetic technique, therefore, would be to induce anesthesia with ketamine (0.5–1.0 mg/kg) and diazepam (0.2 mg/kg); to deepen the anesthesia with isoflurane (1%–2% in oxygen) by mask, a step that would decrease laryngeal reflexes and further dilate the bronchi; and then to administer succinylcholine (1 mg/kg for muscle relaxation for tracheal intubation) and lidocaine (1 mg/kg to further decrease tracheal reflexes). Following intubation, anesthesia would be maintained with isoflurane, nitrous oxide, oxygen, and a muscle relaxant. After surgery, the patient is extubated while still relatively deeply anesthetized, in order to avoid postextubation bronchospasm and laryngospasm. An additional dose of lidocaine (1 mg/kg) might also be of use in reducing airway reactivity.*

*But I might desire to avoid general anesthesia with tracheal intubation, further reducing the possibility of bronchospasm during surgery. In addition, an awake patient can inform me about any breathing difficulties, which can be treated with β-adrenergic agents (Chapter 7), aminophylline, or other appropriate agents. I might therefore consider either an epidural or a subarachnoid regional anesthetic. In choosing between these two, the epidural technique does not involve dural puncture, effectively avoiding postoperative spinal headache. Thus, one might think that an epidural anesthesia would provide a good compromise between comfort and safety for this patient. Problems which might be encountered with an epidural include respiratory compromise due to steep Trendelenburg position, systemic absorption of the* $CO_2$ *that was insufflated into the abdomen, upward displacement of the diaphragm by the intraperitoneal gas, inadvertent high block, and a metabolic acidosis that could not be offset by hyperventilation since the patient's ventilation is spontaneous and not controlled. Thus, choice between general and regional anesthesia can be difficult with neither being ideal in this patient. Nevertheless a choice must be made and plans carefully laid to minimize adverse consequences.*

• ***Case Report #2:*** CAROTID ENDARTERECTOMY. *A 68-year-old male, who has recently had several small transient strokes resulting from atherosclerotic obstruction of his left carotid artery, is scheduled for a carotid endarterectomy (removal of the atheromatous lesion). Evaluation the evening before surgery reveals an alert patient with mild right-sided weakness. His past history shows heavy cigarette smoking (two packages a day for 50 years) and hypertension (now being treated with propranolol and hydrochlorothiazide). His blood pressure is 155/90 mm Hg, and his pulse rate is 65 beats/min. Laboratory studies show a hematocrit of 49%; BUN 15mg/dL; sodium 142 meq/L; and potassium 3.7meq/L. X-ray studies reveal a 90% occlusion of the left internal carotid artery. During the physical examination, his breath sounds are distant and no cardiac murmurs are noted.*

ANESTHETIC MANAGEMENT. *This patient's neurologic disorder is secondary to his atherosclerosis, and is likely associated with generalized atherosclerotic changes in other vascular beds, including the coronary arteries. He is therefore at risk, not only for cerebral attacks, but also for myocardial ischemia. Preparation for surgery should therefore include a thorough assessment of cardiovascular function, including pharmacologic control of hypertension. Intraoperative goals include the prevention of hypotension, and both cerebral and myocardial hypoxia, especially during the period in carotid surgery when the carotid artery will be clamped. It is therefore essential to maintain his blood pressure near normal levels. It is also necessary to prevent postoperative hypertension that might disrupt surgical closures, cause extensive bleeding into the neck, or result in increased cardiac workload and ischemia.*

*A carotid endarterectomy may be performed either under regional anesthesia in a sedated patient or under general anesthesia with controlled ventilation. The former technique involves a cervical plexus block, local infiltration of the tissues of the neck, and intravenous sedation. While this technique has several theoretical advantages over general anesthesia techniques, the drawbacks of anxiety, agitation, poor patient acceptance, and difficult airway access have placed it in disfavor in most medical centers. In addition, general anesthesia allows greater control of cerebral blood flow and cerebral metabolic rate, resulting in somewhat better cerebral perfusion and improved protection of both the brain and the heart to ischemic changes. Under general anesthesia, 50% oxygen is usually used in order to avoid cardiac or brain ischemia. Ketamine is undesirable since it produces hypertension, tachycardia, and increased perirpheral vascular resistance, all undesirable in patients with atherosclerotic lesions in the coronary arteries. The volatile anesthetics might also cause problems, since elderly, hypertensive patients often tolerate poorly the cardiovascular depression those drugs produce. A balanced anesthesia technique, supplemented by low doses of a volatile anesthetic, would be appropriate. Blood pressure decreases could be controlled with a vasoconstrictor such as phenylephrine (Chapter 8); blood pressure increases could be controlled with a vasodilator such as nitroprusside or nitroglycerin (Chapter 9), or with an increased dose of the volatile anesthetic.*

*Under general or local anesthesia, the patient should be monitored with an ECG capable of recording a V-5 tracing, to detect any cardiac ischemia. Blood pressure may be monitored with an indwelling radial artery catheter. Intravenous drips for treating both undesired hypotension (e.g., dopamine, dobutamine, isoproterenol, or phenylephrine) and hypertension (e.g., nitroprusside or nitroglycerin) should be prepared before surgery and kept readily available. In some hospitals, carotid stump pressure or EEG monitoring is conducted during the period of carotid occlusion.*

*After surgery, the patient should be monitored in an intensive care unit and his hypertension treated as needed with a combination of antihypertension drugs and analgesics. Oxygen is administered postoperatively to maintain an inspired concentration of about 40%.*

- ***Case Report #3:*** MULTIPLE TRAUMA WITH SUBDURAL HEMATOMA. *A 21-year-old male is taken to the emergency room after being hit by an automobile while riding a motorcycle. He has an open fracture of the left femur, and his scalp is extensively lacerated (he was not wearing a helmet!). His blood pressure is 170/100 mm Hg, his pulse is 110 beats/min, and his respirations are 24 breaths/min. X-rays confirm* *fractures of the femur and skull, but there are no neck fractures. A chest x-ray reveals a left pneumothorax. Bowel sounds are active and peritoneal lavage is negative for blood. Blood samples are sent for typing and cross-matching. A Foley catheter is inserted into the bladder and urine is clear. A large-bore intravenous catheter (14 gauge) is placed in the right antecubital vein. Under local anesthesia, a chest tube is placed into the left chest and connected to suction for resolution of the pneumothorax and reexpansion of the left lung. Although at first agitated and disoriented, the patient soon becomes sleepy, leading the emergency room physician to suspect intracranial hemorrhage. The neurosurgeon and the anesthesiologist are called.*

ANESTHETIC MANAGEMENT. *The need for emergency action precludes taking the patient's full history and making a complete physical examination. However, as conditions permit, family or friends can be asked about the patient's medical history, physical problems, drug and alcohol habits, allergies, and medications. His decreased level of consciousness suggests an expanding intracranial hematoma with a secondary increase in intracranial pressure. Action is taken to begin reducing the intracranial pressure by injecting mannitol and steroids, and the lesion is confirmed and localized by computerized axial tomography (CAT). Hyperventilation, which will also reduce intracranial pressure, can be started only after endotracheal intubation. Since the patient's blood pressure is stable, he breathes oxygen by facemask, and anesthesia is induced with a rapid-sequence injection of thiopental and succinylcholine, cricoid pressure, and endotracheal intubation. The rapid-sequence technique minimizes the likelihood that the patient, who is presumed to have a full stomach, will inhale gastric contents after losing his protective laryngeal reflexes. Thiopental was used since it lowers intracranial pressure, as well as induces unconsciousness. Controlled hyperventilation is begun, and I accompany the patient to x-ray for the CAT scan, and then to the operating room for a craniotomy.*

*In the operating room, a plastic catheter is placed in the patient's right radial artery for monitoring blood pressure and taking samples for blood-gas determinations. He remains anesthetized with drugs that lower intracranial pressure (barbiturates and lidocaine), supplemented with narcotics, nitrous oxide and a muscle relaxant. Arterial oxygenation ($PO_2$) is maintained at about 100 mm Hg and arterial carbon dioxide pressure ($PCO_2$) is kept below 28–30 mm Hg. The resulting hypocarbia is one of the most effective methods of reducing elevated intracranial pressure, assisted by the steroids and mannitol.*

*This patient is monitored during surgery for ECG, pulse, blood pressure, urine output, breath and heart sounds, and neuromuscular function. The intensive care unit is notified that he will need postoperative ventilatory support, direct blood pressure monitoring, and both monitoring and treatment of elevated intracranial pressure.*

• ***Case Report #4:*** ABRUPUTIO PLACENTA. *A 24-year-old female is pregnant (35 weeks) and has had a normal pregnancy until now. An hour ago, a massive discharge of blood issued from her vagina, and she was brought to the hospital. Her past medical history is unremarkable, showing no drug use, allergies, or prior hospital admissions.*

*Blood is drawn and sent for laboratory studies and for typing and cross-matching. In anticipation of a large blood loss, 10 units of packed cells, 5 units of fresh-frozen plasma, and 10 units of platelets are ordered. Her hematocrit upon admission is 27%; her blood pressure is 100/70 mm Hg, and her pulse is 125 beats/min. At this point, additional blood loss occurs, estimated at 800 mL. A 16-gauge intravenous line had been inserted earlier, and approximately 1.5 L of crystalloid ($D_5LR$) was infused. Her blood pressure is now 80/60 mm Hg, and her pulse is 125 beats/min. Abruptio placentae (placenta-uterus separation) is diagnosed and an emergency cesarean section is scheduled.*

ANESTHETIC MANAGEMENT. *When the patient arrives in the operating room, I place an additional 14-gauge intravenous catheter and crystalloids are administered through it, pending the arrival of blood. A blood pressure cuff and ECG are placed and the patient is prepared for general anesthesia. (Regional anesthesia, i.e., spinal or epidural block, is deemed inappropriate, since the hypotension resulting from sympathetic blockage would further compromise an already distressed vascular system.) During prepping and draping, the patient's right internal jugular vein is catheterized with a 16-gauge, 5¼-in catheter for monitoring CVP. As soon as blood is available, transfusion is begun through both the peripheral and the central venous catheters.*

*Following draping and a rapid-sequence induction with ketamine (1.0 mg/kg), succinylcholine (1.0 mg/kg), and cricoid pressure, the patient's trachea is intubated. Muscle relaxation is maintained with a continuous infusion of succinylcholine; analgesia and amnesia are continued with nitrous oxide, if it does not decrease the blood pressure, and additional doses of ketamine. Blood, crystalloids, fresh-frozen plasma, and platelets are administered as dictated by CVP, arterial blood pressure, urine output, and estimated blood losses.*

*Following delivery of the placenta, oxytocin (Pitocin) is administered intravenously to induce uterine contraction. After the surgery, CVP, blood pressure, urine output, and serial hematocrits guide further fluid therapy and blood product replacement.*

- **Case Report #5:** AMPUTATION OF GANGRENOUS TOES. *A 56-year-old hypertensive diabetic male is scheduled for amputation of three gangrenous toes on his left foot. He is well known to me from several prior vascular surgeries. During the preoperative visit, learn from previous records that he has received numerous anesthetics in the past, both general and regional, but has tolerated many of them only poorly. During previous general anesthesia, the use of a volatile inhalation agent was accompanied by wide fluctuations in blood pressure; a second instance of general anesthesia was complicated by a postoperative myocardial infarction; and spinal anesthesia was complicated by hypotension requiring a phenylephrine drip for correction. His diabetes has been under poor control, with blood sugar concentrations persistently above 300 mg/dL. My objectives in the present case include control of the diabetes as well as a safe and effective anesthetic.*

  ANESTHETIC MANAGEMENT. *The goals of diabetic management during anesthesia are controversial. One regimen attempts to prevent hypoglycemia at one extreme and ketoacidosis and hyperglycemia at the other, but it accepts blood sugars in the range of 100–250 mg/dL. Under this regimen, the patient would be fasted after midnight, and at 6* A.M., *an intravenous solution containing 5% dextrose would be started. Next, half of his usual morning dose of insulin is administered subcutaneously. The 5% dextrose solution is continued during surgery at a rate of approximately 125 mL/hr/70 kg body weight. Additional fluid needs are met with sugar-free solutions such as lactated Ringer's. If the surgery is prolonged, blood glucose can be monitored with a reagent strip; if blood glucose is above 250 mg/dL, insulin can be added to the intravenous fluid.*

*An alternative regimen aims to maintain blood glucose between 70–150 mg/dL. Under this regimen, 5% dextrose is administered at a rate of 50 mL/hr/70 kg body weight and insulin administered by an infusion pump. (The hourly insulin dose, in units per hour, is found by dividing plasma glucose, in milligrams per decaliters, by 150. Thus, a plasma glucose concentration of 150 mg/dL would require an infusion of 1 unit/hr.) Serial samples of blood are drawn and the infusion rate of insulin adjusted as appropriate. The infusion of the 5% dextrose solution is continued during surgery at a rate of 50 mL/hr/70 kg body weight, and all other fluids administered are sugar-free.*

*Any of the techniques of general or regional anesthesia could provide anesthesia for the toe amputation. However, since only the distal portion of one leg is involved, the ideal anesthetic would affect only that leg. A spinal or an epidural anesthetic might successfully anesthetize the leg, but would also effect the patient's sympathetic nervous system. A nerve block at either the hip or the ankle would be preferable. If an ankle block is chosen, the local anesthetic solution should not contain epinephrine, since the vasoconstriction it causes would further compromise the vascular system and restrict blood flow to the foot.*

• **Case Report #6:** EMERGENCY APPENDECTOMY. *A 10-year-old female is admitted after 3 days of nausea, vomiting, and abdominal pain. Her condition is initially evaluated in the emergency room, where her vital signs are: pulse, 118 beats/min; blood pressure, 100/80 mm Hg; and temperature, 39.0 C. Laboratory studies show hemoglobin, 12 g/dL; hematocrit, 42%; sodium 148 meq/L; potassium, 3.8 meq/L; and BUN, 18 mg/dL. Physical examination leads to a diagnosis of acute appendicitis and moderate dehydration. An emergency appendectomy is scheduled. A 16-gauge intravenous catheter is inserted and fluids are administered to correct the dehydration (see Chapter 11).*

ANESTHETIC MANAGEMENT. *For an appendectomy, a general anesthesia technique with muscle relaxation or a regional anesthesia technique, either spinal or epidural, might be used. A regional technique might be inappropriate for this patient, however, because of her youth and because of her preoperative dehydration. General anesthesia is therefore chosen. After preoxygenation, a rapid-sequence induction with thiopental (4 mg/kg), succinylcholine (1 mg/kg), and cricoid pressure are used, since she is presumed to have a full stomach. The anesthesia is then maintained with a volatile anesthetic, nitrous oxide, oxygen, and a nondepolarizing neuromuscular blocker. A blood pressure cuff, ECG monitor, and an esophageal stethoscope (for heart and breath sounds) are usually sufficient monitors. CVP and urine would be monitored only if severe volume depletion is suspected.*

*At the completion of surgery, the neuromuscular blocking agent is reversed with an acetylcholinesterase inhibitor (e.g., neostigmine), combined with an anticholingeric agent (e.g., atropine). The patient is then extubated and taken to the postanesthetic recovery room.*

- ***Case Report #7:*** LARYNGECTOMY AND RADICAL NECK DISSECTION. *A 65-year-old male is scheduled for surgical excision of a neck tumor. The patient, a slight man of 50 kg body weight, has smoked two packages of cigarettes daily for 50 years. His history includes a moderate to heavy pattern of alcohol use, productive morning cough, a 6-month history of increasing hoarseness, and 25-pound weight loss. Laryngoscopy has revealed a cancerous mass in the region of the vocal cords, with palpable lymph nodes in the neck.*

*The patient's only prior surgery was 5 years earlier, when he underwent an uneventful exploratory laparotomy and repair of a bleeding ulcer under general anesthesia. He has no known allergies and takes no medication.*

*His chest x-ray reveals an increased anterior-posterior diameter with flattened diaphragm. An ECG shows normal sinus rhythm, occasional premature ventricular contractions, nonspecific S-T segment changes, and a left bundle branch block. Laboratory studies show hematocrit, 48%; potassium, 4.2 meq/L; sodium, 144 meq/L; BUN, 15 mg/dL; prothrombin time, 12.0 seconds (control = 10.5 seconds); and partial thromboplastin time, 29 seconds (control = 32 seconds). Test of arterial blood gases show pH, 7.40;* $Po_2$*, 60;* $Pco_2$*, 46.*

*The surgeon's preoperative note indicates that the vocal cords were poorly seen under indirect laryngoscopy. The surgeon plans to start with direct laryngoscopy, followed by surgical resection and tracheostomy. I must take into account the following considerations: (a) intubation may be made difficult by the tumor mass; (b) during surgery, the airway will not be easily accessible to me, since the endotracheal tube and hoses will be covered by surgical drapes; (c) muscle relaxants may have to be avoided, since the surgeon may require intact neuromuscular transmission in order to identify nerves in the neck; (d) this patient likely has generalized atherosclerotic disease and may tolerate volatile anesthetics poorly; (e) because the patient is a chronic retainer of carbon dioxide, as indicated by his elevated* $Pco_2$*, he may need postoperative breathing assistance.*

ANESTHETIC MANAGEMENT. *Local anesthesia is impractical for the planned surgery; a general anesthetic is indicated. Since it may be necessary to avoid neuromuscular blocking agents, and since the patient retains carbon dioxide, a technique employing controlled ventilation is desirable. Inhalation anesthesia with controlled ventilation (Table 10-5) would ordinarily provide excellent operating conditions. However, the cardiac depression and the smooth-muscle relaxation produced by the volatile anesthetics may be tolerated poorly by this patient. Ketamine may also be a poor choice, since it could induce tachycardia, hypertension, and increased vascular resistance, all of which might result in cardiac ischemia. As a compromise, therefore, the patient is medicated with narcotics (e.g., morphine sulfate, 0.25–0.5 mg/kg IV), a benzodiazepine (e.g., lorazapam, 1–2 mg IV), 50% nitrous oxide in oxygen, and sufficient halothane to control increases in blood pressure.*

*Special considerations govern anesthesia induction in this patient. Loss of consciousness before intubation may result in collapse of the airway and inability to breathe; and landmarks may be distorted by the tumor mass. Therefore, intubation (after viewing the vocal cords) in an awake, sedated patient is indicated. To this end, the patient is sedated with intravenous narcotics and benzodiazepines, and the oropharynx and base of the tongue are sprayed with 4% lidocaine solution. The superior laryngeal nerves are blocked with an injection of 1%–2% lidocaine, and a percutaneous injection of 2% (4–5 mL) lidocaine is given through the cricothyroid membrane into the trachea. An attempt is made to view the larynx by direct laryngoscopy. If the vocal cords can be seen adequately and if laryngeal anesthesia is sufficient, the endotracheal tube is inserted. If the vocal cords cannot be seen, the nasal passages should be anesthetized with 4% cocaine and a well-lubricated endotracheal tube placed through the nose into the nasopharynx. Then an attempt to intubate the trachea blindly can be made. If this is not successful, a fiberoptic bronchoscope can then be passed through the endotracheal tube and between the vocal cords under direct vision (Patil et al., 1983). The endotracheal tube is then passed into the trachea over the bronchoscope, the latter withdrawn, and breath sounds verified bilaterally. The patient is then anesthetized with thiopental (1–2 mg/kg). Anesthesia is maintained with nitrous oxide (50%) and oxygen (50%) and with additional doses of narcotic or halothane as dictated by autonomic responses.*

*Monitoring equipment for this patient includes an esophageal stethoscope, an ECG monitor with V-5 lead, an axillary or rectal temperature probe, a blood pressure cuff, a radial artery catheter, and a Foley catheter for measuring urine output; and a hand or foot must be left in view for evalulation of skin color and nail-bed perfusion. If muscle relaxants are used, a nerve stimulator is useful. If CVP or pulmonary artery pressure measurements are desired, the appropriate catheter may be inserted (Chapter 4).*

*During surgery, special attention is directed towards fluid and blood replacement, as will be discussed in Chapter 11. As the surgery nears completion and the surgeon performs the tracheostomy, I deflate the cuff on the endotracheal tube and carefully pull back the tube to a point just above the site of insertion of the tracheostomy tube. Following insertion of the latter tube. I disconnect the anesthesia circle from the endotracheal tube and reconnect it to the tracheostomy tube. Following verification of bilateral breath sounds, the endotracheal tube can be removed.*

*After completion of surgery, the patient is transported to the intensive care unit, where his ventilation is mechanically assisted until he can breathe well enough to maintain a* $P_{CO_2}$ *close to his preoperative value of 46 mm Hg.*

## Readings and References

Bridenbaugh, P. 1978. Successful regional anesthesia: premedication and supplementation (lecture 112A). *Twenty-ninth Annual Refresher Course Lectures*, 1978 Meeting of the American Society of Anesthesiologists, Park Ridge, Ill.

Bromage, P.R. 1978. *Epidural analgesia*. Philadelphia: W.B. Saunders.

Cousins, M.J., and Bridenbaugh, P.O. 1980. *Neural blockade in clinical anesthesia and management of pain*. Philadelphia: J.B. Lippincott.

Eriksson, E. 1980. *Illustrated Handbook in Local Anaesthesia.* 2nd ed. Philadelphia: W. B. Saunders.
Greene, N. 1981. *Physiology of spinal anesthesia.* 3rd ed. Baltimore: Williams & Wilkins.
Henderson, J. J., and Nimmo, W. S. 1983. *Practical regional anaesthesia.* Boston: Blackwell Scientific.
Kane, R.E. 1981. Neurologic deficits following epidural or spinal anesthesia. *Anesth. Analg.* 60:150–61.
Kotelko, D.M.; Shnider, S.M.; Dailey, P.A., et al. 1984. Bupivacaine-induced cardiac arrhythmias in sheep. *Anesthesiology* 60:10–18.
Lee, J.A., and Atkinson, R.S. 1978. *Lumbar puncture and spinal analgesia.* 4th ed. Edinburgh: Churchill Livingstone.
Marx, G.F. 1984. Cardiotoxicity of local anesthetics—the plot thickens. *Anesthesiology* 60:3–5.
Mayumi, T., and Dohi, S. 1983. Spinal subarachnoid hematoma after lumbar puncture in a patient receiving antiplatelet therapy. *Anesth. Analg.* 62:777–79.
Moore, D.C. 1965. *Regional block.* 4th ed. Springfield, Mass.: C.C. Thomas.
Murphy, T.M. 1981a. Nerve blocks. In: *Anesthesia.* Miller, R.D., editor. New York: Churchill Livingstone, pp. 593–634.
———1981b. Spinal, epidural, and caudal anesthesia. In: *Anesthesia.* Miller, R.D., editor. New York: Churchill Livingstone, pp. 635–78.
Patil, V., Stehling, L., and Zauder, H. 1983. *Fiberoptic endoscopy in anesthesia.* Chicago: Year Book.
White, P.F. 1982. Comparative evaluation of intravenous agents for rapid sequence induction: thiopental, ketamine, and midazolam. *Anesthesiology* 57:279–84.
Winnie, A.P. 1983. *Plexus anesthesia.* Philadelphia: W.B. Saunders.
Winnie, A P. 1984. *Brachial plexus in anesthesia.* Philadelphia: W. B. Saunders.

# 11. Termination of Anesthesia: Postanesthesia Recovery

To reach the end of surgery with a patient awake, breathing adequately, showing stable vital signs, and pain free, requires considerable skill, knowledge of operative surgery, and an appreciation of the excretion characteristics of the drugs used (Stark, 1974).

Indeed, of all the skills required in anesthesia, perhaps the most challenging are those associated with a smooth transition between the operative and the recovery states. In the ideal case, the patient is relaxed and the vital signs are stable as the last suture is placed and the dressing applied; stopping the flow of anesthetic gases is followed by rapid awaking; extubation is accomplished by the time the drapes are removed; and the patient is moved to the recovery room pain-free and breathing easily.

Waking the patient too early may lead to difficulties in closing the incision, loosening of the sutures, or hemorrhaging from the wound edges. In orthopedics, movements before a cast is applied may result in displaced fractures, dislocation, or misalignment. In plastic surgery, premature movement may tear pedical flaps and delicate nerve and tendon realignments. In abdominal surgery, straining may increase intraabdominal pressure and disrupt closures.

At the other extreme, the patient awakens slowly after surgery, is slow to resume spontaneous breathing, and has such prolonged respiratory depression that continued assistance in ventilation is needed. In this chapter, therefore, we will review some of the considerations involved in a timely, safe, and smooth termination of general anesthesia, as well as factors relevant to postanesthetic recovery.

## Drug Review

As surgery nears completion, the anesthesiologist reviews the anesthesia record for those drugs that may cause problems at the termination of anesthesia.

## Barbiturates

After intravenous injection, thiopental reaches high concentrations in the brain, causing loss of consciousness, and is then rapidly redistributed throughout the body. With redistribution, the level of thiopental in the brain falls and rapid awakening occurs unless other drugs, such as anesthetic gases, are given to maintain unconsciousness. Therefore, even though thiopental is still present in the body, its concentration in the brain is so low that it should not impede the patient's awakening after even a brief surgical procedure. Yet, the low levels of thiopental that persist in the body impair judgment and fine motor skills for 1–2 days after anesthesia. Patients should therefore be instructed not to drive or operate machinery, not to drink alcoholic beverages, and not to make any major decisions requiring judgment or insight for at least 24 hours following its use.

## Succinylcholine

Succinylcholine is rapidly metabolized in plasma within 3–5 minutes by the enzyme plasma cholinesterase; neuromuscular function then returns. Therefore, succinylcholine rarely causes problems at the termination of anesthesia unless the patient has an abnormal plasma cholinesterase that metabolizes succinylcholine at a much slower rate or not at all. The incidence of such occurrence is about one in 1500 patients.

## Nitrous Oxide

Nitrous oxide is administered during surgery in concentrations of up to 70%. The drug is relatively insoluble in blood and is not stored in body tissues. It is excreted rapidly through the lungs, excretion being virtually complete within approximately 5 minutes after administration is stopped. It should not delay emergence from anesthesia.

Of importance in terminating nitrous oxide anesthesia is the concept of *diffusion hypoxia*. When anesthesia is stopped and the patient is ventilated with room air, the $N_2O$ excreted into the lungs mixes with air. Since the blood contains a large volume of a $N_2O$, there is a gradient for $N_2O$ to pass from blood into the lungs. This outpouring of $N_2O$ from blood to the lungs mixes with the air in the lungs, decreasing the alveolar oxygen concentration below 21% (the amount of $O_2$ in inspired air), resulting in hypoxia. This outflow of $N_2O$ has a rapid onset and usually only lasts for 5–10 minutes after termination of anesthesia. Hypoxia can be avoided by administering 100% oxygen during the first 5–10 minutes of recovery.

## Volatile Anesthetics

The volatile anesthetics, halothane, enflurane, and isoflurane, are eliminated fairly slowly from the body. During anesthesia large amounts accumulate in fat and muscle. Since these structures are relatively poorly perfused, they continue to accumulate volatile anesthetics during anesthesia. Indeed, during anesthesia lasting no more than several hours, body fat never completely saturates with volatile anesthetics. Thus, at the termination of anesthesia, their concentration in fat is still below that in blood, and fat continues to take up anesthetic until the concentration in blood falls below that in fat and the gradient reverses. It therefore takes several hours for volatile anesthetics in muscle and fat depots to diffuse back into blood for eventual elimination through the lungs.

To minimize the prolonged anesthesia resulting from their slow elimination from the body, the anesthesiologist gradually decreases the concentration of volatile anesthetics inspired during surgery, so that at the termination of anesthesia, their blood levels have decreased to the point where emergence will be rapid, despite the slow elimination of drug that has accumulated in body tissues.

## Nondepolarizing Neuromuscular Blockers

The nondepolarizing neuromuscular blocking agents, *d*-tubocurarine, pancuronium (Pavulon), metacurine (Metubine), gallamine (Flaxedil), atracurium (Tracrium), and vercuronium (Norcuron), block synaptic transmission on all skeletal muscles, including those involved in respiration. Therefore, the anesthesiologist must artificially ventilate patients medicated with these drugs until they are either eliminated from the body or their actions "reversed" by an acetycholinesterase inhibitor (Chapter 6).

With all but atracurium and vercuronium, waiting for drug elimination as a means to terminate neuromuscular paralysis is inefficient due to drug elimination half-lives that are markedly longer than the duration of most surgeries. These long-acting neuromuscular blocking drugs have half-lives of about 2.0 hours, values which can be even longer in patients with renal failure, liver or biliary disease, or hypothermia.

Since there are no practical ways to hasten the elimination of the neuromuscular blocking agents, the alternative is to administer an acetylcholinesterase inhibitor together with an antimuscarinic agent (atropine or glycopyrrolate). Properly done, administration of such a combination is followed within several minutes by resumption of neuromuscular transmission and the return of spontaneous breathing.

If a patient does not resume breathing after reversal, the anesthesiologist must consider whether the dose of the acetylcholinesterase inhibitor was adequate. There are other possibilities, too, such as residual volatile anesthetic, narcotic-induced respiratory depression, and decreased respiratory stimulation due to hyperventilation of the patient by the anesthesiologist during surgery. The following points should be considered:

1. Has enough time been allowed for the acetylcholinesterase inhibitor to antagonize the block? Peak effect may require as long as 15 minutes.
2. Was the neuromuscular blockade too intense to be antagonized? This question can be answered with the aid of a peripheral nerve stimulator (Chapter 5). If nerve stimulation before reversal elicits a muscle twitch at least 20% of that observed before paralysis, recovery of normal neuromuscular transmission usually

occurs within 10–15 minutes. If nerve stimulation fails to elicit a muscle twitch, the blockade is too intense to be antagonized and controlled ventilation should be continued by the anesthesiologist and administration of the reversal drugs delayed.

3. Respiratory acidosis exaggerates neuromuscular blockade, as does decreased body temperature. Thus, attempts to maintain acid-base balance and body temperature contribute to more effective reversal.
4. Certain antibiotics, if given concurrently with a nondepolarizing blocker, prolong the neuromuscular blockade. Such antibiotic-induced potentiation of neuromuscular blockade is poorly reversed by acetylcholinesterase inhibitors. Antibiotics that produce such an effect are most frequently of aminoglycoside group (e.g., neomycin, gentamycin, and kanamycin). If the use of these antibiotics is anticipated, doses of neuromuscular blocking drugs should be decreased.
5. Since the nondepolarizing neuromuscular blockers are all excreted by the kidneys to greater or lesser degrees, patients with kidney failure cannot excrete the drugs efficiently; and as a result, they experience prolonged neuromuscular blockade. Fortunately, in such patients, the acetylcholinesterase inhibitors also have prolonged action, and the blockade can still be satisfactorily antagonized. Gallamine and metacurine, both excreted unchanged by the kidneys, probably should be avoided in patients without renal function.

In summary, knowledge and experience are necessary for the proper use of neuromuscular blocking agents so that adequate surgical relaxation is obtained from doses that can be reversed by acetylcholinesterase inhibitors at the completion of surgery.

## Opiate Narcotics

The opiate narcotics produce analgesia and respiratory depression. These effects generally persist in the recovery room, where the analgesia is desirable and the respiratory depression can present problems. Sometimes a patient who has received narcotics fails to breathe spontaneously at the end of surgery. If adequate time has been allowed for the elimination of volatile anesthetics, and if any neuromuscular blockade has been adequately reversed (as determined by use of a nerve stimulator), the anesthesiologist should consider whether the narcotic is responsible for the patient's respiratory depression. If the narcotic is thought to be responsible, a narcotic antagonist can be cautiously administered. The most specific narcotic antagonist is naloxone (Narcan), which is used in doses of 0.1–0.4 mg IV in adults. It takes effect within 1–2 min, and if ventilation is not adequate within 5 minutes, additional doses can be administered. If adequate spontaneous breathing has not resumed after 0.4 mg, other causes of the problem should be sought while controlled ventilation is continued.

Naloxone's duration of action is in the range of 30–60 minutes and, since the effect of most narcotics lasts longer than that, respiratory depression can recur as the effect of naloxone decreases. Hence, if it is necessary to use naloxone to terminate narcotic-induced respiratory depression, the patient should be observed closely.

The routine use of naloxone to restore respiration should be avoided, since the drug also terminates the analgesic effects of narcotics, resulting in intense postoperative pain accompanied by tachycardia, hypertension, increased vascular resistance, and even pulmonary edema, all of which can be detrimental (Taff, 1983).

### Ketamine

The dissociative drug ketamine is useful for inducing anesthesia in hypovolemic and asthmatic patients, and for maintaining anesthesia in critically ill patients. The latter usually receive postoperative care in an intensive care unit, and frequently require continued controlled ventilation. In patients who receive ketamine as an induction agent only, the drug rarely contributes to respiratory depression after surgery, and seldom interferes with the resumption of spontaneous ventilation. Postoperative delirium and disorientation can, however, be a problem. Intravenous diazepam (Valium) or physostigmine (Antilerium) can often blunt these CNS effects.

### Benzodiazapines

The benzodiazepines, diazepam (Valium) and lorazepam (Ativan), are often administered intravenously as supplemental amnesic agents. These drugs have long durations of action, but their use seldom results in failure to resume spontaneous breathing at the termination of anesthesia. Prolonged drowsiness from the benzodiazepines should be expected since their half-lives are quite long (Chapter 6).

## Assessment for Extubation

As the surgical procedure nears completion, and if the patient has been hyperventilated by the anesthesisologist, the rate of mechanical ventilation should be slowed gradually until a normal level of carbon dioxide in arterial blood is achieved. The muscle relaxants are then reversed, as discussed previously, and spontaneous ventilation is reestablished.

The anesthesiologist next decides whether the endotracheal tube will be removed in the operating room or whether it will be left in place and removed later in the recovery room or intensive care unit. (For consideration affecting the decision, see next paragraph.)

If the patient is to be extubated in the OR, a final check is made of pulse, blood pressure, and spontaneous ventilation. The patient then breathes 100% oxygen for approximately 2 minutes. If a nasogastric tube is in place, the stomach is emptied by suction through the tube. The oropharynx is then gently suctioned and, if indicated, the trachea is cleared by suction through the endotracheal tube. If the trachea is suctioned, the lungs should be refilled with oxygen before the cuff is deflated and the endotracheal tube withdrawn. Following removal of the tube, the patient breathes 100% oxygen through a face mask. The adequacy of respiration is confirmed by observing the excursions of the bag on the anesthesia circle and by auscultating the lungs. One complication that can occur after extubation is spasm of the vocal cords (laryngospasm). It seldom has serious consequences if extubation is done after filling the lungs with oxygen. Then, even if spasm persists for 1–2 minutes, hypoxia seldom occurs. Intravenous lidocaine (1 mg/kg) before extubation appears to reduce the severity of most episodes of postextubation laryngospasm. More severe episodes may require succinylcholine paralysis and reintubation.

Once the anesthesiologist is convinced that spontaneous ventilation is adequate, the blood pressure cuff and the ECG electrodes can be removed and the patient transported to the recovery room, preferably in the lateral decubitus position. If a patient is taken intubated to the recovery room, the blood pressure cuff and ECG electrodes should remain until extubation has been completed. Certain surgical procedures may require the patient to be fully awake before extubation. Such is the case following head and neck procedures where significant swelling of oropharyngeal tissues may have occurred, where intraoral bleeding may occur, or when the jaws have been wired together. In such cases, awake extubation minimizes the likelihood of aspirating blood or vomitus.

## Postanesthetic Recovery

The responsibilities of the anesthesiologist do not cease when the patient leaves the OR, because the patient is considered to be at risk while in the recovery room. In essence, postanesthetic care consists of careful observation, intensive monitoring, and treatment of patients as they emerge from the drug-induced conditions of unconsciousness, respiratory depression, and altered sympathetic nervous function. Recovery room nursing is a specialized and demanding job, one often unappreciated by many medical personnel. Its development as a specialty is welcome.

The patient should be accompanied by the surgeon and the anesthesiologist to the recovery room. The nurse should immediately place the patient on oxygen and record blood pressure, pulse rate, and respiratory rate, because intraoperative monitors have been disconnected for several minutes during transfer from the OR. The anesthesiologist communicates the patient's name, age, surgical procedure, any complications during surgery, other significant medical problems, drugs administered during anesthesia, and the patient's general condition at the termination of anesthesia. Special attention should be paid to:

1. *The patient's breathing and level of consciousness.* It should be remembered that the stimulation the patient received during transfer to the recovery room may have increased the ventilation rate and level of consciousness, and that the removal of such stimulation may allow the patient to slip back into a state of depressed respiration and unconsciousness. Thus, ventilation must be assessed both at the time of admission and later during quiet recovery.
2. *The patient's fluid balance.* All fluids administered during surgery should be clearly listed on the anesthesia record, including crystalloids, colloids, and blood products (Chapter 12). The patient's urine output and blood losses, and an es-

timate of evaporative fluid losses (if the latter are believed considerable) should also be listed.

## Postanesthetic Complications and Their Treatment

### Hypotension

The time required for transfer from the OR to the recovery room is one of the most critical periods for the patient. Hypotension can occur unexpectedly, during transfer or at any time during recovery. Common causes of postoperative hypotension include: the residual effects of anesthetics and preoperative and intraoperative medications, unreplaced blood and fluid losses, changes in body position, cardiac arrhythmias, hypoxia, pulmonary emboli, acute hemorrhage, myocardial infarction, and electrolyte imbalance. Of these, unreplaced fluid and blood losses are most frequently encountered, but proper evaluation requires that other, less common, causes be excluded.

### Hypertension

Marked elevations in blood pressure are commonly observed in the recovery room. Hypertension can be expected if the patient is in pain. Other causes, less frequent, stem from three sources: (a) carbon dioxide retention, (b) fluid overload, or (c) bladder distension. The treatment of hypertension, by either the anesthesiologist or the surgeon, includes giving analgesics, improving ventilation, and increasing oxygenation. Hypertension must be corrected, because it places the patient at risk for cardiac or neurologic complications. If hypertension persists despite analgesics and adequate ventilation, consideration should be given to the use of antihypertension medications such as hydralazine (Apresoline).

### Hypoxia

Postoperative hypoxia, a shortage of oxygen in the tissues, is most frequently due to either airway obstruction or to hypoventilation as a residual effect of narcotics or neuromuscular blockers. Airway obstruction is most commonly caused by pharyngeal obstruction from a sagging tongue in a sedated patient, but may also be caused by laryngeal spasm or edema. Pharyngeal obstruction can be relieved by backward tilt of the head, by anterior displacement of the mandible, sometimes by placing the patient in the lateral decubitus position, and by the insertion of a nasal or oral airway. Other causes include pulmonary emboli, pneumothorax, intrapulmonary shunts, and decreases in cardiac output. Cyanosis, agitation, and delirium are all symptoms characteristic of hypoxia.

Airway obstruction is assessed by auscultating the lungs, by observing chest movements, and by feeling the flow of expired gases with the hand. The extent of any residual neuromuscular blockade can be measured by a nerve stimulator, or it can be estimated by asking the patient to hold his head off the bed, hold an arm upright, lift his legs, or grip the examiner's hand. Respiratory depression produced by narcotics is suspected when respiratory rate is slow, but increases when the patient is asked to take a breath.

Hypoxia is always treated with oxygen (give by face mask), narcotic antagonists, or additional doses of neostigmine (if muscle relaxants were completely reversed). Occasionally, it may have to be treated by reintubation and ventilatory assistance until the cause is diagnosed and corrected.

## Hypercarbia

Hypoxia is often accompanied by hypercarbia (retention of carbon dioxide), usually secondary to inadequate ventilation. If hypercarbia is suspected, arterial blood gases should be determined to confirm the diagnosis, and the use of narcotic antagonists should be considered. As with hypoxia, the patient may require reintubation and assisted ventilation.

## Vomiting

Patients recovering from general anesthesia may vomit in the recovery room. Vomiting is dangerous because, if some of the vomitus is inhaled, serious complications may follow, such as pneumonitis, destruction of lung tissue, pulmonary edema, and respiratory failure; the latter may be fatal. Patients should not be extubated, therefore, until they have recovered protective airway reflexes that will close the glottis; then, if vomiting occurs, the vomitus will not be inhaled. If inhalation of vomitus is suspected, the patient should be reintubated, the trachea cleared by suction, and the trachea lavaged with saline (10 mL) through the endotracheal tube; the suction and lavage cycle should be repeated until the aspirate clears. The patient should then be closely observed for several days for any sign of pulmonary complications (for discussion, see James and Modell, 1983).

## Shivering

Shivering in the recovery room during emergence from anesthesia is frequent, and can be severe. Such shivering can greatly increase oxygen consumption, resulting in hypoxia, hypercarbia, and acidosis. To minimize postoperative shivering, efforts should be made during surgery to minimize heat loss and to rewarm the patient in the recovery room.

## Pain

Most patients usually tolerate some degree of pain. But excessive pain leads to increased activity of the sympathetic nervous system, resulting in tachycardia and hypertension. Modest doses of analgesics (e.g., Fentanyl, 25 μg increments IV, or meperidine 25–50 mg IM) should be given to alleviate the pain, but it must be kept in mind that these same analgesics may depress ventilation.

### Delirium

Some patients, especially children and young adults, are restless or even severely agitated during emergence from general anesthesia. The combination of sedative drugs and postoperative pain appears to precipitate this agitation. Additional doses of sedatives, therefore, are usually ineffective, and may even cause additional disorientation. Although narcotics may be of benefit, time and patience are, in general, most beneficial. Hypoxia should first be excluded as a cause of delirium.

## Final Comment

Patients in the recovery room are still under the influence of anesthetics and are therefore at risk for a number of complications. Principles of recovery room care include anticipation of possible problems, early recognition of their onset, and immediate action to begin treating them and to call for assistance. In the recovery room, as in the operating room, there is no substitute for vigilance.

### *Readings and References*

Drain, C.B., and Shipley, S.B. 1979. *The recovery room.* Philadelphia: W. B. Saunders.

Freeley, T.W. 1981. The recovery room. In: *Anesthesia.* Miller, R.D., editor. New York: Churchill Livingstone, pp. 1335–60.

Israel, J. S., and Dekornfeld, T. J. 1982. *Recovery room care.* Springfield, Ill.: C. C. Thomas.

James, C. F., and Modell, J. H. 1983. Pulmonary aspiration. *Semin. Anesth.* 2:177–82.

Stark, D. C. 1974. *Practical points in anesthesiology.* Flushing, N.Y.: Medical Examination Publishing Company, p. 59.

Taff, R.H. 1983. Pulmonary edema following naloxone administration in a patient without heart disease. *Anesthesiology* 59:576–77.

# V

# SPECIAL ANESTHESIA CONSIDERATIONS

# 12. Fluids, Electrolytes, and Blood Products

The responsibilities of the anesthesiologist during surgery include more than administering drugs and anesthetics. Among other tasks, the fluid and electrolyte needs of the patient must be evaluated and appropriate intravenous fluids and blood products administered. Hence, the anesthesiologist must understand the principles of intravenous fluid therapy.

## Preoperative Evaluation

As part of the preoperative visit, the anesthesiologist evaluates the patient's state of hydration, the cellular contents of blood, and serum electrolytes.

The state of hydration can be estimated by evaluating the pulse, mucous membrane hydration, skin turgor, and urine output; and by noting the changes in blood pressure and pulse rate when the patient moves from a reclining to a standing position. If dehydration is suspected, replacement of fluids are initiated as early as possible before surgery. Patients at risk for preoperative dehydration include those with prolonged vomiting, those who have received presurgical bowel preps, those on diuretic therapy, those with neurologic weakness, and those with chronic malnutrition and poor oral intake.

The body is about 60% water. Thus, a 60 kg patient (132 lb) has about 36 kg (or 36 L) of water. Moderate dehydration might result from loss of 10% of the total body water (here 3.6 L, which should be replaced before surgery. The type of replacement fluid is determined by evaluating serum electrolytes, as discussed later.

Patients occasionally have excessive fluids, resulting from such causes as liver, kidney, or heart failure. If excessive fluid is suspected, chest x-rays should be evaluated and the lung fields auscultated. Fluid restriction, diuretics, or even dialysis may be indicated.

The cellular contents of blood are most easily evaluated by examining the complete blood count (CBC), with special attention paid to the hemoglobin concentration and the hematocrit. Patients with unexplained anemia should be closely evaluated; the cause of the anemia should be sought and treatment begun before surgery. It is important to note that a normal hemoglobin concentration or hematocrit does not rule out either a low blood volume or dehydration. An anemic patient who is dehydrated may have a normal CBC. But anemia need not indicate that blood volume is low; fluid overload can produce a low hemoglobin concentration or hematocrit.

Electrolyte concentrations are determined by laboratory evaluation of serum sodium, potassium, chloride, blood urea nitrogen (BUN), and creatinine. Normal values are: sodium, 136–142 meq/L; potassium, 3.5–5 meq/L; chloride, 100–106 meq/L; BUN, 8–25 mg/100 mL; and creatinine, 0.7–1.5 mg/100 mL. Higher values than these are consistent with a diagnosis of dehydration and a need for fluids with low ionic concentrations. If the patient has excessive fluid and serum electrolytes are reduced in concentrations, normal fluid and electrolyte balance is achieved by restricting fluids.

Preoperative fluid management of the critically ill patient will require multiple observations of the responses to administered fluid. Such a patient should have his or her bladder catheterized and the volume and specific gravity of urine measured hourly. CVP (Chapter 4) should be measured; a Swan-Ganz catheter can be used for this purpose and for measurement of left arterial pressure and cardiac output if decreased myocardial function is suspected. The lungs should be auscultated frequently for signs of pulmonary edema.

## Fluid Requirements during Surgery

Patients entering the OR have normally taken nothing orally for at least 8 hours. Patients with normal hydration prior to the period of fasting have a normal fluid balance maintenance requirement of about 2 mL/kg/hr; a 70 kg patient entering surgery would have a water deficit of approximately 1.1 L (2 mL/kg/hr × 70 kg × 8 hours). One-half of this deficit is usually administered intravenously during the induction of anesthesia, and the remainder given at a steady hourly rate, along with replacement fluids for surgical losses (discussed later).

A healthy patient with normal renal function can usually be given any of several commercially available fluid preparations containing dextrose and electrolytes. Five percent dextrose may be given in water ($D_5W$), in lactated Ringer's solution ($D_5LR$), in 0.2 normal saline ($D_5$0.2NS), or in 0.5 normal saline ($D_5$0.5NS). Obviously, if the patient's electrolyte levels are abnormal, or if the patient has a known abnormality in the response to electrolytes, the choice of solution or fluid replacement must take these conditions into account.

Evaporative losses can only be estimated. They can range from 4–12 mL/kg/hr, and they must be carefully evaluated and replaced. If only minimal surgical trauma is anticipated, an additional 4 mL/kg/hr of fluids is given. For moderate surgical trauma, additional fluids to replace evaporative losses are increased to 8–10 mL/kg/hr. For extreme surgical trauma (such as accompanies intraabdominal surgeries, total hip replacement, radical mastectomy, or thoracotomy), fluids to replace evaporative losses are increased to 10–12 mL/kg/hr.) Fluids given for replacement of evaporative losses are in addition to those given for replacement of measured blood losses.

Blood volume in an adult is about 70 mL/kg body weight. Thus, a 70 kg patient has a blood volume of about 4.9 L. During surgery, fluid needs are increased by observable blood losses (blood on sponges, on surgical drapes, in suction bottles, on the floor, etc.) and by evaporative fluid losses from exposed body surfaces and viscera. When blood losses exceed 10%–15% of blood volume (about 490 mL in this case), replacement with blood products is considered. The decision whether to transfuse blood is based on the preoperative hematocrit, measured and observed surgical blood losses, and anticipated additional blood losses. If losses beyond 10%–15% do not occur, and if the preoperative hematocrit was in normal range, the lost volume can be replaced with intravenous fluids rather than blood products.

Formulas for replacing blood loss with crystalloids vary from 2:1 to as high as 4:1 (lactated Ringer's solution:blood loss). When blood loss exceeds 15%–20%, replacement with blood products rather than with crystalloids is indicated.

While fluid deficits are frequently seen in surgical patients (preoperative dehydration, inadequate intraoperative replacement, unreplaced fluid losses, etc.), fluid overload can also occur either preoperatively or intraoperatively. One interesting example of surgeon-induced intraoperative fluid overload with important anesthetic implications occurs during transurethral resection of the prostate gland. In this surgery, large volumes of irrigating solution (often distilled water, since sugar- or ion-containing solutions affect the surgical cautery) are passed into the bladder in order to wash out blood and prostate particles and thus allow a clear view during the resection. Considerable quantities of water are absorbed into the open venous sinuses and can cause hypervolemia, decreased electrolyte concentrations, hemolysis, hypertension, and altered mental status with confusion and delirium ("water intoxication"). Giving a diuretic and stopping the surgery are both indicated.

## Blood Replacement during Surgery

When intraoperative transfusions are anticipated before surgery, an adequate supply of compatible blood should be readily available. Samples of donor and recipient blood are typed for ABO and Rh antigens, screened, and crossmatched to identify any antibodies in serum that might react with antigens on the donor's blood cells.

Since crossmatching is time-consuming, abbreviated testing formats can be followed in emergencies. Depending upon time constraints, the following kinds of donor blood, ranked from most to least desirable, may be administered: (a) type-specific, fully crossmatched, (b) type-specific, partially crossmatched, (c) type-specific, uncrossmatched, and (d) type O, Rh-negative uncrossmatched.

If possible, the use of type O, Rh-negative blood should be avoided unless that is the patient's own blood type; after receiving more than two units of type O, Rh-negative blood, a patient of a different blood type may suffer hemolysis of subsequently administered red cells of his own type. Blood losses can be replaced either with whole blood or with any of its components, including packed red cells, platelets, fresh frozen plasma, cryoprecipitate, or albumin.

The use of whole blood, except when strictly indicated, has been criticized as wasteful, since separating blood into its components allows several patients to benefit from a single unit of donor blood.

Whole blood is usually administered only for severe hemorrhage, when blood loss may lead to hypovolemic shock. In such circumstances, the blood should be as fresh as possible so that the levels of platelets (life span of 9–10 days) and certain labile clotting factors (V and VIII) will be adequate to insure blood clot formation at the sites of bleeding. In addition, as stored whole blood ages, the affinity of its red cells for oxygen gradually decreases, so that the red cells carry less oxygen to the tissues.

Surgical blood losses are often replaced with packed red cells. These contain the same amount of hemoglobin as whole blood, but much of the plasma, platelets, and clotting factors are separated out and remain available for other patients. If blood losses are not massive, the use of packed red cells is acceptable. When hypovolemia or clotting defects accompany blood loss, however, the additional administration of platelets, fresh-frozen plasma, cryoprecipitate, or serum albumin may be necessary.

Transfusion of platelets is indicated when platelet counts are low (below 50,000 cells/mm$^3$) and bleeding times prolonged. Low platelet counts are probably the major cause of hemorrhagic bleeding disorders in patients who have received multiple units of banked blood. Transfusion should be considered for patients with platelet counts below 50,000/mm$^3$ and for those whose laboratory tests show prolonged bleeding time, prothrombin time, or partial thromboplastin time. One unit of platelets will increase the platelet count from 7,000 to 10,000 cells/mm$^3$. Platelet half-life is about 8 hours.

Fresh frozen plasma (FFP) contains natural concentrations of the plasma proteins and the plasma clotting factors. Because it also contains natural levels of antibodies, it must be type-compatible with the patient's blood. Crossmatching is not needed. Each unit of FFP is prepared from a single donor and carries the same risks of hepatitis as a unit of whole blood.

Cryoprecipitate is a fraction of plasma rich in both fibrinogen and the antihemophilic factor (factor VIII). Cryoprecipitate is produced from a single donor by a freeze-and-thaw process, then pooled with cryoprecipitate from other donors and administered to hemophiliacs to facilitate clotting.

Human serum albumin is a commercial product containing the albumin from pooled donors. The product is filtered and pasteurized to inactivate any hepatitis virus. Unlike FFP, it contains no clotting factors, and is used primarily as a volume expander to treat hypovolemia from blood loss. Typing and crossmatching need not be performed. Serum albumin use is not advised in patients with severe anemia and in those who cannot tolerate a salt load (it is high in sodium). Serum albumin preparations are expensive, and their alleged overuse has been the subject of controversy.

Other available blood products include washed red blood cells, frozen red blood cells, platelet-poor whole blood, white blood cells, and artificial blood. Their use in more sophisticated blood component therapy is covered in more advanced textbooks on anesthesiology.

The complications of blood and blood product transfusions include circulatory overload, allergic reactions, infections, serum hepatitis, and hemolytic transfusion reactions. Transfusion reactions most frequently result from human error, either in the laboratory or in the operating room, and can lead to intravascular hemolysis, vascular collapse, and renal failure. All blood transfusions should be performed with care, and the first 100–200 mL should be given slowly as a "test dose" to allow early detection of the signs of a transfusion reaction (tachycardia, hypotension, hemoglobinurea, and increased bleeding). If a transfusion reaction is suspected, the transfusion should be stopped immediately. The remaining donor blood and a fresh sample of the patient's blood should be sent to the laboratory for evaluation, intravenous fluids and diurectics should be given in anticipation of renal failure, and circulatory collapse should be appropriately treated with fluids and vasopressors to insure adequate renal blood flow.

Viral hepatitis is a transfusion-related complication occurring in about 1%–3% of patients; icterus is the major clinical manifestation, while elevation in liver enzymes are the laboratory corrolates. Serologic evidence is available for diagnosis of hepatitis A or hepatitis B. By exclusion, negative serology in a patient with elevated liver enzymes is termed non-A, non-B (type C) viral hepatitis. All blood products, with the exception of pasteurized serum albumin, are capable of transmitting hepatitis virus.

Minor transfusion reactions are either fever-producing or allergic. Such reactions are characterized by urticaria, chills, and fever. Antihistamines such as diphenhydramine (Benadryl) may be of use.

## *Readings and References*

Brown, B.R., editor. 1983. *Fluid and blood therapy in anesthesia.* Philadelphia: F.A. Davis Co.

Ellison, N. 1983. Hemostasis: monitoring and treatment of deficiencies (lecture 107). *ASA annual refresher course lectures,* Park Ridge, Ill.

Fishbach, D.P., and Fogdall, R.P. 1981. *Coagulation: the essentials.* Baltimore: Williams & Wilkins.

Fogdall, R.P. 1983. Coagulation disorders and complications. *Semin. Anesth.* 2:143–52.

Giesecke, A.H. 1981. Perioperative fluid therapy-crystalloids. In: *Anesthesia.* Miller, R. D. editor. New York: Churchill Livingstone, pp. 865–83.

Miller, R.D., and Brzica, S.M. 1981. Blood, blood component, colloid, and autotransfusion therapy. In: *Anesthesia.* Miller, R.D., editor. New York: Churchill Livingstone, pp. 885–922.

Tannenbaum, S. 1983. Blood—which component and why? *Hosp. Physician* 19:41–55.

# 13. Anesthesia for Infants and Children

The conduct of anesthesia in infants and children requires constant awareness of their anatomic, physiological, and biochemical differences from adults. With attention to depth of anesthesia and fluid and electrolyte balance, as well as to anesthetic technique, even neonates can be subjected safely to relatively radical surgical procedures.

Attention must also be given to the psychological preparation of both the child and the parents in order to keep emotional stress to a minimum.

## Preoperative Considerations

The pediatric patient has most of the same worries as the adult patient, and a few that are unique to children. Pediatric patients may be completely naive or quite experienced as patients, but one cannot predict what role their experience or lack of it will play in their reaction to the hospital setting.

Hospitalization represents a great change in the normal routine of most children. The change alone may cause tremendous psychological stress, and the child's understanding, however vague, that something is wrong will magnify stress. Parental reaction to the hospitalization is sensed quite clearly by most children, and a calm, reassuring attitude in the parents will reduce stress in the child.

The anesthesiologist must establish mutual trust with the child and the parents. The apprehensions of the parents and the child should be addressed by the anesthesiologist. The trust relationship can be established most easily if the anesthesiologist conveys that the safety and comfort of the child are the chief concerns of all the medical personnel involved.

It is usually not necessary to order preoperative intramuscular drug injections for children. Those who have undergone many operations and have come to dread the preoperative injection often show great relief when told that they need not have one. If premedication is judged necessary, orally administered sedatives such as chloral hydrate (10–25 mg/kg) can be ordered. Alternatively, a barbiturate suppository (30 or 60 mg), such as pentobarbital (2–4 mg/kg), administered 45–60 minutes before surgery, provides excellent sedation. Both of the above techniques result in an onset of sedation about 15–20 minutes after drug administration. If more rapid onset of sedation is desired, a rectally administered solution of methohexital (Brevital) (20–30 mg/kg) provides profound sedation within about 5 min of administration. Methohexital should be used in this manner only in the presence of an anesthesiologist.

During the preoperative visit, the anesthesiologist reviews records of previous hospitilization, previous anesthetics, and the current chart; takes a medical history, usually from the parents; and performs a physical examination. The parents should especially be questioned about recent respiratory infections or fevers in the child, and any family history of adverse reactions to anesthetics. The child should be checked for congenital anomalies, especially those involving the mouth, upper airway, the heart, and the lungs.

On the morning of surgery, the child should be met in the holding area and reassured by the anesthesiologist. As a calming influence, a small child may be carried to the operating room in the arms of the anesthesiologist or the nurse. Once there, procedures should be explained in a simple way, and the child should be told more about any procedure or equipment that arouses interest. To minimize preoperative pain, the intravenous catheter is often not inserted until after the induction of anesthesia (discussed later).

## Anatomic and Physiologic Considerations

### Anatomy of the Upper Airway

Before inducing anesthesia in children, the anesthesiologist must recognize the differences in head and neck anatomy between children and adults. The important differences, which are particularly evident in neonates, are:

1. Infants have a relatively large head and short neck.
2. The tongue of the infant is relatively large and the mouth relatively small, compared with those of the adult.
3. The vocal cords of the infant are at about the level of cervical vertebrae 2 to 4 rather than at the adult levels of cervical vertebrae 5 to 6. In addition, the vocal cords of the infant slant, with the anterior point being lower than the posterior point when the infant is supine. In that position, the vocal cords appear to be directed away from the anesthesiologist rather than appearing vertical, as they do in adults.
4. The infant's epiglottis is relatively large, long, stiff, and U-shaped, making laryngoscopic viewing of the cords more difficult than in an adult. For this reason, infants are usually intubated with the aid of a straight blade on the laryngoscope

handle, rather than a curved blade. The straight blade is used to lift the epiglottis, affording a better view.

5. In infants, the narrowest portion of the airway is located at the level of the cricoid cartilage, which forms a complete ring around the trachea. Above the cricoid cartilage, at the vocal cords, the airway is wider. Therefore, an endotracheal tube barely small enough in diameter to pass between the vocal cords will exert excessive pressure on the soft tissues at the level of the cricoid cartilage, causing irritation, trauma, and swelling. All of these predispose the infant to postoperative respiratory difficulties. To minimize these problems, the anesthesiologist chooses a tube that will pass easily below the level of the cricoid cartilage, exerting only minimal pressure on the mucosa of the tracheal wall. The child's anatomy here contrasts with that of the adult, in whom the narrowest portion of the airway is at the level of the vocal cords. A cuffed endotracheal tube must be used in adults in order to prevent excessive leakage of anesthetic gases, while an uncuffed tube suffices for children under age 6–7 years.
6. The trachea of the infant is quite short, approximately 4 cm long from vocal cords to carina, necessitating accurate placement of the endotracheal tube. Breath sounds must be checked bilaterally several times during surgery, since even small movements of the head may result in the tube's passing below the carina into one of the mainstem bronchi. On the other hand, if the tube is not placed far enough below the vocal cords and if the head is then extended, the tube may pull out of the trachea, extubating the infant.

## Cardiovascular Physiology

Figure 13-1 shows important changes in cardiovascular parameters from birth to age 14 years. The normal pulse rate in the newborn averages 130–140 beats/min, decreasing to an average of 110 at 2 years, 100 at 4 years, and 90 at 8 years. Hence, in children under age 4 years, a heart rate below 100 beats/min is slow; a rate below approximately 130 would be slow for a neonate.

Systolic blood pressure at birth is approximately 65 mm Hg, with even lower levels observed in premature infants. By age 1 year, systolic pressure increases to approximately 80 mm Hg; by age 6 years, to 99 mm Hg. Since infants have a relatively high cardiac ouptut, their low systolic blood pressure results from low systemic vascular resistance, which does not increase to compensate for either hypovolemia or drug-induced reduction in cardiac output. Premature infants have a blood volume at birth of about 95–100 mL/kg body weight, while term newborns have a blood volume of about 85–90 mL/kg. By around 1 year of age, blood volume decreases to approximately 75 mL/kg and thereafter ranges between 70 and 75 mL/kg.

The hematocrit of the newborn averages 50%–60%, with an average hemoglobin concentration of approximately 17 g/100 mL of blood. By 3 months of age, hematocrit falls to about 30%–35%, with a hemoglobin concentration of approximately 12 g/100 mL of blood. By 2 years of age, hematocrit increases to about 40%, with a hemoglobin concentration of approximately 13.5 g/100 mL of blood, and these levels are relatively constant throughout the remainder of childhood.

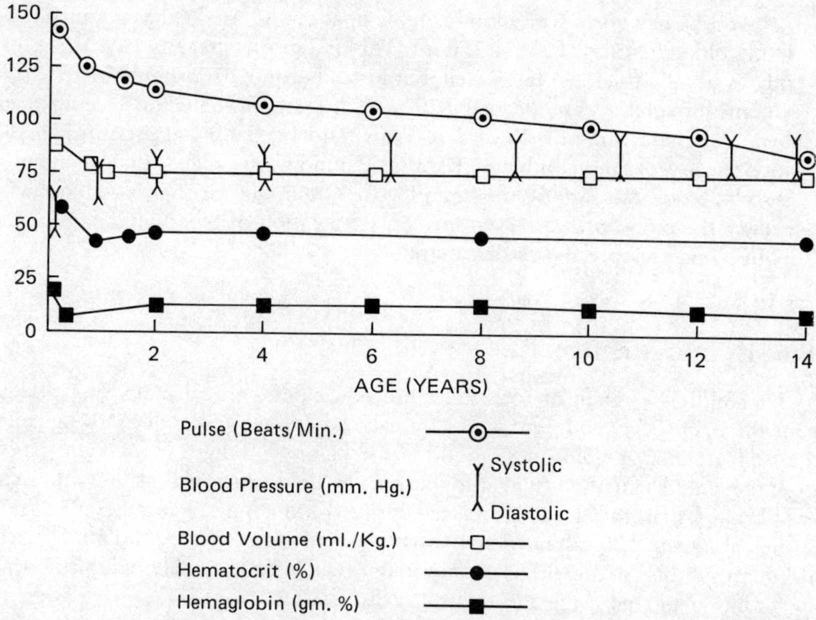


**Figure 13-1.** Cardiovascular parameters from birth to age 14 years. Units of measurement for the ordinate are listed below the figure for each of the five parameters graphed (see text for discussion).

With these cardiovascular parameters as background, two important guidelines in pediatric anesthesia can be stated:

1. *An unexpected decrease in a child's heart rate can be presumed due to oxygen deficiency until proven otherwise.* Children have a high metabolic requirement for oxygen, and oxygen deficiency can rapidly arise, producing a decrease in heart rate. This is in contrast to adult patients, who initially develop an increase in heart rate in response to hypoxia. Thus, the anesthesiologist's initial reponse to unexplained bradycardia in children should be ventilation with oxygen. Giving oxygen is especially important in newborns, since their physiological response to oxygen deficiency is an increased right-to-left shunt through the ductus arteriosus, which worsens the hypoxia. The bradycardia reduces cardiac output and causes hypotension, decreased tissue oxygenation, and further slowing of heart rate. Fortunately, giving oxygen rapidly restores pulse rate, cardiac output, and blood pressure.
2. *Low blood pressure in children, if not due to decreased heart rate, can be presumed due to low blood volume until proven otherwise.* In children, reductions in blood pressure are usually related to reductions in the circulating blood volume. Indeed, the adequacy of blood replacement can be quite accurately assessed by measuring the systolic blood pressure.

A 3 kg newborn, with blood volume of about 85 mL/kg, has a total circulating blood volume of about 250 mL. A blood loss as great as 10% (here, 25 mL) is usually tolerated fairly well, but losses beyond 10% should be replaced volume for volume. A blood loss of 20%–25% (here, 50–65 mL) is accompanied by a 50% reduction of both cardiac output and arterial blood pressure. Therefore, the loss of 50 mL of blood, less than 2 ounces, may reduce such an infant's systolic blood pressure from 60 mm Hg to 30 mm Hg. Greater blood loss will reduce the blood pressure even further. Restoration of blood volume restores both blood pressure and cardiac output.

### Fluid Requirements

For children weighing up to 20 kg, maintenance fluids are calculated at 4 mL/kg/hr for the first 10 kg, and 2 mL/kg/hr for each additional kilogram. A 30 kg child requires maintenance fluids of 80 mL/hr (4 mL/kg/hr × 10 kg + 2 mL/kg/hr × 20 kg). If the child has had no fluids for 7 hours, the fluid deficit will be 560 mL. As a general rule, half of this deficit is replaced during the first hour of anesthesia, so that, for such a patient, 280 mL plus the first hour's fluid requirement of 80 mL is given then, for a subtotal of 360 mL. To this amount is added additional fluid to compensate for blood and insensible fluid losses, as discussed in Chapter 12.

### Body Temperature

Compared with adults, neonates and small children have a large body surface area relative to their body weight, and they lack the subcutaneous fat deposits possessed by adults. They therefore lose body heat rapidly in a cool environment. Since heat loss also results from general anesthetics that dilate cutaneous blood vessels and disrupt central temperature-regulating mechanisms, anesthetizing a neonate or small child on an unwarmed surgical table in a cool operating room would produce a drastic fall in body temperature. Body temperature must be maintained, therefore, by increasing room temperature and by using warming pads or blankets, overhead thermal lamps, and warmed prepping and irrigating solutions.

Body temperature must be continuously monitored during surgery. Rectal temperature probes are most often used for this purpose (Chapter 5).

## Considerations during Surgery

### Anesthesia Apparatus

Anesthesia is usually supplied to larger children and adults through a semiclosed system with an anesthesia circle and a carbon dioxide absorber (Chapter 3). But with smaller children and infants, the hoses, valves, and carbon dioxide absorber of the anesthesia circle provide such resistance to breathing that they may result in respiratory distress. These smaller patients require a low-resistance, valveless, nonrebreathing system with low dead space, and such features are provided by the Jackson-Rees system with warmed and humdified fresh gas flow (Chapter 4).

### Induction of Anesthesia

General anesthesia can be induced in infants and small children in several ways. If an intravenous catheter has not been inserted before surgery, their high level of alveolar ventilation allows for induction with a mixture of oxygen, nitrous oxide, and a volatile anesthetic such as halothane. Induction time can be shortened by giving methohexital rectally (20–25 mg/kg), about 10 minutes before induction.

For older children, or in children fearful of the face mask, intravenous induction with a fast-acting barbiturate such as thiopental (3–5 mg/kg) is desirable. If it is advisable to avoid both inhalation and intravenous induction, ketamine (2–4 mg/kg) may be administered intramuscularly. For emergency surgery on a child with a full stomach, either intubation of the awake patient or a rapid-sequence induction with intravenous thiopental and succinylcholine will reduce the risks of vomiting and inhaling vomitus.

### Monitoring

Monitoring equipment for pediatric anesthesia must include, at a minimum, a precordial stethoscope, an appropriately sized blood pressure cuff, a Doppler flowmeter, a temperature probe, and an ECG. For major surgical procedures, other monitors may be needed, such as an arterial catheter, a CVP catheter, a Foley catheter, a peripheral nerve stimulator, and a percutaneous oxygen analyzer (see Chapter 5 for discussion of these devices).

## Pharmacologic Agents

### Succinylcholine

Succinylcholine, frequently used to facilitate endotracheal intubation, may induce severe bradycardia in infants that may lead to cardiac arrest. This can usually be prevented by giving atropine (0.02 mg/kg IV) before giving succinylcholine; the atropine dose should be repeated if bradycardia nonetheless occurs. To avoid using succinylcholine for intubation, the anesthesiologist can relax the vocal cords by spraying them with a lidocaine solution (total dose, 1–2 mg/kg) prior to intubation. This tech-

**TABLE 13-1**
**Pediatric Dosages of Anesthetic Drugs**

| Drug | Route | Dosage (mg/kg)* |
|---|---|---|
| Premedications | | |
| Chloral hydrate | Oral | 10–20 |
| Diazepam | Oral | 0.2–0.4 |
| Pentobarbital | IM† or rectal | 2–4 |
| Secobarbital | IM or rectal | 2–4 |
| Morphine | IM | 0.05–0.15 |
| Meperidine | IM | 1.0–1.5 |
| Atropine | IM | 0.01–0.02 |
| Hydroxyzine | Oral | 1–2 |
| Promethazine | Oral | 0.5 |
| Chlorpromazine | Oral | 0.5 |
| Induction agents | | |
| Methohexital | Rectal | 15–25 |
| Methohexital | IV | 1–2 |
| Thiopental | IV | 3–5 |
| Ketamine | IV | 1–2 |
| Ketamine | IM | 4–8 |
| Atropine | IV | 0.02 |
| Succinylcholine | IV | 1.0–1.5 |
| Succinylcholine | IM | 2 |
| Pancuronium | IV | 0.5–0.1 |
| Maintenance | | |
| Inhalation agents | | |
| Nitrous oxide | Inhalation | 50%–70%‡ |
| Halothane | Inhalation | 0.7%–1.5%‡ |
| Enflurane | Inhalation | 1.5%–2.5%‡ |
| Isoflurane | Inhalation | 1.0%–2.0%‡ |
| Analgesics | | |
| Morphine | IV | 0.2–0.5 |
| Fentanyl | IV | 1–5 μg/kg/hr |
| Meperidine | IV | 0.5–1.0 |
| Ketamine | IV | 1 mg/kg/hr |
| Neuromuscular blocking agents | | |
| Pancuronium | IV | 0.1 |
| *d*-Tubocurarine | IV | 0.3 |
| Gallamine | IV | 0.5–1.0 |
| Metocurine | IV | 0.15–0.25 |
| Relaxant reversal | | |
| Anticholinergic | | |
| Atropine | IV | 0.025 |
| Glycopyrrolate | IV | 0.004 |
| Cholinesterase inhibitor | | |
| Neostigmine | IV | 0.05 |
| Edrophonium | IV | 0.3–0.5 |

**TABLE 13-1**
**(Continued)**

| Drug | Route | Dosage (mg/kg)* |
|---|---|---|
| Narcotic reversal | | |
| Naloxone | IV | 0.005 |
| Naloxone | IM | 0.01 |
| Cardiovascular agents | | |
| Digoxin | Oral | 0.04 (total digitalizing dose) |
| Digoxin | Oral | 0.01 (daily maintenance dose) |
| Phenytoin | IV (slowly) | 1–2 |
| Lidocaine | IV | 1.0 |
| Lidocaine | IV drip | 0.5–1.5 mg/kg/hr |
| Propranolol | IV | 0.002 to total dose of 0.01 mg |
| Atropine | IV | 0.02 to total dose of 0.6 mg |
| Dopamine | IV drip | 2–20 μg/kg/min |
| Isoproterenol | IV drip | 0.2–1.0 μg/kg/min |
| Nitroprusside | IV drip | 1–5 μg/kg/min |
| Sodium bicarbonate | IV | 1–2 meq/kg |
| Calcium chloride | IV (slowly) | 10 mg/kg or 50 mg/100 mL of tranfused blood |
| Epinephrine | IV | 5–10 μg/kg |
| Miscellaneous | | |
| Dantrolene | IV | 3 mg/kg initially, repeat to total of 10 mg/kg |
| Dantrolene (prophylaxis) | Oral | 1 mg/kg q 4 h to total of 4 mg/kg |
| Dexamethasone | IV | 0.2 |
| Furosamide | IV | 0.2–0.5 |
| Mannitol | IV | 0.5–1.0 gm/kg |

*Unless otherwise specified.
†Intramuscular injections not advocated for children unless considered absolutely necessary because of the pain and anxiety associated with the injection.
‡Percentage of alveolar concentration.

nique often enables a smooth intubation with continued spontaneous ventilation and few complications.

## Nondepolarizing Neuromuscular Blocking Agents

The two most frequently used nondepolarizing neuromuscular blocking agents are pancuronium and *d*-tubocurarine. For pediatric anesthesia, pancuronium (0.05–0.1 mg/kg IV; see Table 13-1) is usually preferred, since it partially blocks the muscarinic receptors on the heart, producing a mild tachycardia. In contrast, *d*-tubocurarine can produce bradycardia and hypotension, due to the ganglionic blockade and the histamine release it can cause.

### Volatile Anesthetics

Despite the advent of the newer volatile anesthetic agents, isoflurane and enflurane, halothane remains satisfactory for the induction and maintenance of anesthesia in children. It relaxes the upper airways, and children awaken promptly when it is discontinued. Hepatitis associated with halothane has not been reported in children. Finally, halothane is significantly less expensive than the newer volatile agents, an important factor with a high-flow, nonrebreathing system such as the Jackson-Rees.

## Pediatric Outpatient Surgery

With increasing frequency, children are undergoing surgery as outpatients. Outpatient surgery is less psychologically upsetting to the child and less disruptive to normal family routine than is inpatient surgery. It also reduces the cost of medical care.

Children selected for outpatient surgery must be healthy, except for the condition requiring surgery, and must be free of upper respiratory infection. Those classified as ASA Class III (Chapter 1) are usually not considered for outpatient surgery. Appropriate candidates are those who require relatively minor procedures that will produce little postoperative pain and few physiological changes.

The outpatient is seen by the surgeon several days before the surgery, when a history is taken, a physical exam is given, and blood for laboratory studies is drawn. Ideally, child and parents are interviewed by the anesthesiologist the day before surgery; but more frequently, the interview is conducted only shortly before the operation.

The child must be fasted on the day of surgery, and any indication, however slight, that solids or liquids may have been ingested is sufficient cause to cancel the procedure.

Children undergoing surgery as outpatients are seldom premedicated. Because the anesthesiologist usually does not see the child until just before surgery, there is insufficient time for premedication to be ordered, administered, and to take effect before the surgery. Also, premedicating drugs usually have long durations of action; and if given just before surgery, they might delay postoperative wakening and hospital discharge. An exception is rectally administered methohexital, which can sedate a very aggitated child within a few minutes, and which does not unduly delay wakening. More recently, an oral suspension of meperidine, diazepam, and atropine has been reported to provide excellent results (Brzustowicz et al., 1984).

An inhalation technique for both induction and maintenance of anesthesia is a good choice for outpatients. With it, children waken rapidly, experience little postoperative delirium, and can usually be discharged within a few hours after surgery.

Outpatients should be kept in the recovery room for at least 1 hour, and in the hospital for at least 4 hours after surgery, to ensure that no complications follow the anesthetic or the surgery. Parents should be given the names and telephone numbers of the hospital, surgeon, and the anesthesiologist should questions or unexpected problems arise.

## Pediatric Dosages of Anesthetic Drugs

Table 13-1 lists suggested dosages of several drugs used in pediatric anesthesia. When reviewing this table, the reader should be aware of several important points. First, these are only estimates of doses that are effective in the majority of patients. Some patients will require doses higher than these; some will require doses lower than these. Second, this list does not carry any recommendation that one must use all of these drugs in an anesthesiology practice. Indeed, one can practice very well with only a small percentage of the drugs listed. Third, this list does not give any recommendation concerning precautions to be observed with individual drugs. Before a student or trainee uses any of these agents, the patient and the proposed use should be discussed with an experienced anesthesiologist. However, it is hoped that such a list will provide the reader with an appropriate range of dosage. With this knowledge, one then can modify doses as appropriate for the individual patient. Specific drugs are discussed at length throughout this text. Such discussions are listed under individual agents in the index.

### *Readings and References*

Beasley, J.M., and Jones, S. E. F. 1980. *A guide to paediatric anaesthesia.* Oxford: Blackwell.

Berry, F.A. 1983. Premedication and induction of the difficult child (lecture 234). *ASA annual refresher course lectures.* Park Ridge, Ill.

Brown, T.C.K., and Fisk, G.C. 1979. *Anaesthesia for children.* Oxford: Blackwell.

Brzustowicz, R.M.; Nelson, D.A.; Betts, E.K., et al. 1984. Efficacy of oral premedication for pediatric outpatient surgery. *Anesthesiology* 60:475–77.

Dierdorf, S.F., and Krishna, G. 1981. Anesthetic management of neonatal surgical emergencies. *Anesth. Analg.* 60:204–15.

Gregory, G.A. 1981. Pediatric anesthesia. In: *Anesthesia.* Miller, R.D., editor. New York: Churchill Livingstone, pp. 1197–1229.

Gregory, G.A., editor. 1983. *Pediatric anesthesia.* New York: Churchill Livingstone.

Hatch, D.J., and Sumner, E. 1981. *Neonatal anaesthesia.* Chicago: Year Book Medical Publishers.

Jackson-Rees, G., and Cecil Gray, T. 1981. *Pediatric anesthesia: trends in current practice.* Woburn, Mass.: Butterworth.

Levin, R.M. 1980. *Pediatric anesthesia handbook.* 2nd ed. Garden City, N.Y.: Medical Examination Publishing Company.

Mayer, B.W. 1981. *Pediatric anesthesia.* Philadelphia: J.B. Lippincott.

Maze, A., and Bloch, E. 1979. Stridor in pediatric patients. *Anesthesiology* 50:132–45.

Smith, R.M. 1980. *Anesthesia for infants and children.* 4th ed. St. Louis: C.V. Mosby Company.

Stehling, L.C. 1982. *Common problems in pediatric anesthesia.* Chicago: Year Book Medical Publishers.

Stehling, L.C., and Zauder, H.L. 1982. *Anesthetic implications of congenital anomalies in children.* New York: Appleton-Century-Crofts.

Steward, D.J. 1979a. *Manual of pediatric anesthesia.*New York: Churchill Livingstone.

———1979b. Premedication for the pediatric patient (lecture 101). *Thirtieth annual refresher course lectures.* 1979 Annual Meeting of the American Society of Anesthesiologists. Park Ridge, Ill.

# 14. Anesthesia for the Pregnant Patient

## Introduction

Managing anesthesia in the pregnant patient requires consideration of the welfare of the fetus, as well as of the mother. The anesthesiologist's aim is to provide relief from pain with minimal risk to both. This chapter will focus on the choice of anesthesia techniques for pregnant patients undergoing (a) labor with analgesia, (b) vaginal delivery, (c) elective cesarean sections, (d) emergency cesarean sections, and (e) nonobstetric surgery.

In recent years, some obstetrical patients have been seeking alternatives to drugs for analgesia during labor and vaginal delivery, choosing instead to employ such psychoanalgesic methods as natural childbirth, the Lamaze method, Le Boyer delivery, the Jackson method, the Bradley method, or hypnosis. Such techniques are generally adequate for about 20%–30% of pregnant women; for the remainder, drugs are still used for pain relief during both labor and delivery.

## Hemodynamic Changes in the Pregnant Patient

Cardiovascular and hemodynamic alterations in pregnancy are summarized in Figure 14-1.

During the first trimester, cardiac ouptut rises dramatically by 30%–40%. The increased output results from an average increase in heart rate of 15 beats/min and an increase in stroke volume of approximately 30%. During the second and third trimesters, the increase in cardiac output is maintained, except when the patient lies supine (on her back), in which position the pregnant uterus partially obstructs venous blood return to the heart through the inferior vena cava, and cardiac output falls. Otherwise, however, the increase in cardiac output is maintained throughout preg-

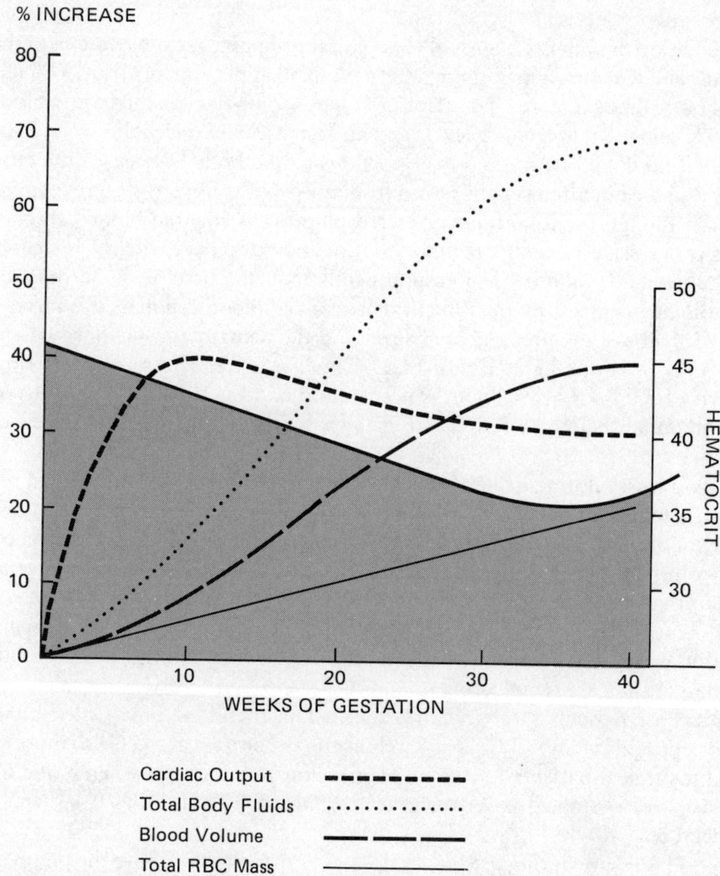


**Figure 14-1.** Cardiovascular and hemodynamic alterations during pregnancy. **Left ordinate,** Increases in cardiac output, total body fluid, blood volume, and total RBC mass. **Right ordinate,** Decrease in hematocrit that follows the relatively greater increase in blood volume over the increase of RBC mass (see text for details).

nancy, and is tolerated well, except by women with mitral stenosis, resulting in a fixed narrowing of the mitral valve of the heart. Those women experience congestive heart failure due to the inability of their heart to increase its stroke volume.

During uterine contractions in labor, cardiac output is further increased by both the periodic ejection of blood from the pregnant uterus into the central circulation and catecholamine liberation in response to pain. Cardiac output increases even more in the immediate postpartum period due to the transfer of uterine blood into the central circulation. Then, over a period of several weeks, cardiac output slowly returns to prepregnancy levels.

Retention of water is a normal concomitant of pregnancy, beginning in the first trimester and reaching a maximum at term with an approximate 60%–70% increase in total body fluids (Figure 14-1). This increase encompasses an increase in blood volume 40% above prepregnancy levels and an increase in extracellular water. Much of the added fluid collects in the lower portions of the body because of the effects of gravity and the impaired venous return from the pelvis caused by the pregnant uterus.

Even though the total number of red blood cells (the red blood cell mass) increases progressively during pregnancy, it does not keep pace with the increase in intravascular fluid volume. The resulting fall in hematocrit may be described as "physiologic anemia." By the time of delivery, red blood cell mass has increased to 20%–25% above the prepregnancy level and the hematocrit may have fallen from about 43% to about 33% (Figure 14-1). Thus, in a pregnant female at term, a hematocrit of 33% (or hemoglobin concentration of 11 g/100 mL) is considered normal, and values below these indicate maternal anemia, usually resulting from iron deficiency.

Blood losses during delivery approximate 300–500 mL for the vaginal delivery of a single fetus and 500–1000 mL for a cesarean section or for the vaginal delilvery of twins. But several factors help to compensate for the blood loss: (a) the increase in blood volume during pregnancy tends to offset it, as does (b) the transfer of uterine blood to the vascular system at the time of delivery, (c) postpartum uterine contraction decreases uterine bleeding, and (d) finally, the relative anemia of pregnancy assures that an excess of plasma over red cells will be lost, so that relatively more red cells than plasma are retained.

Obstetric patients rarely require transfusion, therefore, unless their blood loss exceeds approximately 1.5 L. Their circumstances contrast markedly to those of nonpregnant surgical patients for whom transfusion is considered when blood loss exceeds 10% of estimated blood volume (i.e., about 500mL in a 70 kg female; see Chapter 12).

Blood pressure during pregnancy does not normally rise above the prepregnancy level, despite the increases in stroke volume and cardiac output noted above. This fact implies that peripheral vascular resistance decreases during pregnancy. Elevated blood pressure should therefore be very carefully evaluated: it often indicates preeclampsia (a toxemia of pregnancy), a major cause of maternal morbidity (Wright, 1983).

Hypotension is similarly abnormal. If it occurs when the patient is supine, it may be a result of the supine hypotension syndrome, in which decreased venous return is caused by partial uterine obstruction of the inferior vena cava. Supine hypotension may be aggravated both by inhalation anesthetics and by regional anesthetic techniques that produce sympathetic block (subarachnoid or epidural anesthesia). Compression of the vena cava is usually diagnosed by monitoring the fetal heart rate and maternal blood pressure, and is easily treated by positioning the patient on her left side. If necessary, either ephedrine or fluids may be judiciously administered to increase blood pressure. (Ephedrine, of all vasoconstrictors, produces the least reduction in uterine blood flow.)

# Labor Analgesia

## Pain Pathways

Labor begins with the onset of uterine contractions, which become increasingly regular, frequent, and intense, progressing to a phase of relatively rapid cervical dilatation. With the completion of cervical dilatation, the first stage of labor ends. The second stage encompasses fetal descent, ending with delivery of the fetus.

Pain during the first stage results from the cervical dilatation. Pain impulses from the cervix travel with the sympathetic fibers and enter the spinal cord at the 10th, 11th, and 12th thoracic and the first lumbar spinal segments. Pain during the second stage of labor results from distention of the vagina and the stretching of the perineum. These pain impulses travel in the pudenal nerves and enter the spinal cord at the second, third, and fourth sacral segments.

## Pain Management

Analgesia during the first stage of labor may be provided by inhaled anesthetic gases, by various sedatives, narcotics, or ketamine given intravenously, or by regional use of local anesthetics. Of the inhaled agents, the safest and most satisfactory is self-administered nitrous oxide (35%–50%) in oxygen (50%–65%). This provides moderate analgesia for the awake, cooperative patient who is able to maintain protective airway reflexes. Such a patient is not likely to inhale vomitus, if vomiting occurs. An anesthesia machine or blender must be available for mixing the oxygen and nitrous oxide. If the patient becomes drowsy, uncooperative, or excited, the nitrous oxide concentration should immediately be lowered. Inadvertent overdosage leading to loss of protective airway reflexes is a major risk. Continuous monitoring and verbal contact with the patient are essential.

Of the intravenous agents, the opiate narcotics are the most effective; they provide both sedation and relief of pain. But the use of opiates for labor analgesia is a topic of much discussion; they reach the fetus and can produce changes in neonatal responsiveness and behavior in the first 48 hours of life. Such effects are of uncertain long-term significance and can be minimized by the use of short-acting opiates, administered in low doses early in labor. Narcotics, when used in doses sufficient to produce labor analgesia, also depress infant respiration to some degree. Benefits of opiates in labor include a reduction in pain and catecholamine levels, leading to increased uterine blood flow with increased fetal welfare. Therefore, the beneficial effects of a narcotic must be weighed against the possibly harmful effects. In general, the goal should not be to totally eliminate pain, but to reduce pain and to provide a degree of patient comfort; and any use of narcotics should reflect this goal.

Sedative-hypnotic drugs, such as the benzodiazepines and the barbiturates, are seldom used during labor. They do not relieve pain and are distributed to the fetus, producing prolonged depressent effects on the newborn. Ketamine can be used in low doses (0.1–0.2 mg/kg) to provide analgesia for labor and delivery.

Because both inhalation and injectable agents have drawbacks as labor analgesics, much effort has been directed to finding regional anesthesia techniques suitable for providing first-stage labor analgesia in a broad range of patients. Methods used have included paracervical block, paravertebral lumbar sympathetic block, subarachnoid block, lumbar epidural block, and caudal block. Of these methods, the last two have proved particularly useful.

Paracervical block is produced by injecting a local anesthetic solution into the outer rim of the cervix through the vagina. Although effective for analgesia in the first stage, this block is now used infrequently because of several limitations, the most important of which is reduced uterine blood flow resulting from high concentrations of local anesthetic in the uterine artery. The reduced blood flow leads to fetal acidosis and fetal bradycardia. Other limitations include a brief duration of action, inadequate analgesia for delivery (sensory nerve fibers from the perineum are not blocked), and risk of injecting the local anesthetic directly into the fetal head.

The paravertebral sympathetic block is also infrequently used, since it provides inadequate analgesia for delivery, it is technically difficult to place, and there is a relative lack of flexibility in controlling the duration or spread of the block.

The subarachnoid block (spinal or saddle block) can provide anesthesia for both labor and delivery, but it is usually administered during the second stage, shortly before delivery (to avoid compromise of expulsive efforts, both voluntary and involuntary). An additional limitation is the relatively high incidence of spinal headache (in up to 5% of patients) after its use (discussed further).

The two remaining regional techniques for labor analgesia, continuous lumbar epidural and continuous caudal anesthesia, are widely used. Because they employ indwelling catheters, they can provide analgesia over prolonged periods and can be continued after delivery. While either of these methods is adequate for labor analgesia and vaginal delivery, lumbar epidural anesthesia is often more satisfactory than caudal anesthesia for several reasons (a) in lumber anesthesia, the catheter is placed nearer the spinal cord segments T10 to L1, allowing more effective stage-one analgesia with lower doses of drug; (b) lumbar anesthesia is technically easier and anatomically more predictable than caudal anesthesia; (c) if an unplanned cesarean section becomes necessary, the lumbar approach provides sufficient anesthesia without exceeding safe quantities of local anesthetics.

## Anesthesia for Vaginal Delivery

There are three types of anesthesia for vaginal delivery: (a) conscious sedation and analgesia, (b) general anesthesia, and (c) regional anesthesia. Sedatives and analgesics, when used during labor, are frequently supplemented during delivery. The disassociative anesthetic, ketamine, used in very low doses (0.10–0.20 mg/kg IV), will produce analgesia in an awake patient without depressing the respiration, heart rate, or blood pressure of either the mother or the fetus. The cumulative dose of ketamine should not exceed 1 mg/kg since higher doses may cause maternal dreams, hallucinations, hypertension, and uterine hypertonus, as well as neonatal hypertonia and depression.

Regional anesthesia techniques used for delivery include lumbar epidural and caudal blocks, subarachnoid (saddle) block, pudendal nerve block, and local perineal infiltration. The subarachnoid block can be accompanied by a postspinal headache in a low percentage of all patients, with the highest incidence in pregnant patients. Postspinal headache seems to be due to persistent leakage of cerebrospinal fluid through the needle hole in the dura. It occurs in about 5%–6% of pregnant women receiving subarachnoid anesthetics through a 25- or 26-gauge needle, and in a higher percentage when a larger, 22-gauge, needle is used. The headache usually begins within 12–48 hours after the dural puncture, is postural, and may last as long as 7 days. Relief can often be gained from generous intravenous fluids, an abdominal binder (which increases pressure in the epidural space, decreasing flow of CSF into the space), and the maintenance of a supine position. Headaches resistant to such therapy can be treated by injecting 10 mL of the patient's own blood into the epidural space at the site of the dural puncture (epidural blood patch). Relief often follows within minutes of the injection, and the headache recurs in only a low percentage of patients.

General anesthesia with endotracheal intubation is now used rarely, because the mother is unconscious during delivery and the mother-newborn bonding associated with the birth process is delayed. In addition, the risks of vomiting and inhaling the vomitus are increased. Therefore, general anesthesia is used for vaginal delivery only when acute fetal distress occurs during the second stage of labor, and uterine relaxation induced by a general anesthetic may allow an operative vaginal delivery rather than an emergency cesarean section. For example, general anesthesia might be indicated for a breech delivery or for extraction of a second twin. All potent inhalation agents, such as halothane, provide uterine relaxation. Following delivery, injection of oxytocics and cessation of inhalation anesthesia allow postpartum uterine contraction.

## Anesthesia for Elective Cesarean Section

An elective cesarean section is one scheduled for a healthy woman not in labor who is admitted at term, usually for a repeat section. Such a patient may be offered a choice of either a general or a regional anesthetic. Most of these patients choose a regional anesthetic so that they can be conscious during the birth experience and, often, so their husbands can participate. Either a subarachnoid or a lumbar epidural anesthetic provides excellent analgesia and muscle relaxation, with relatively little effect on the newborn. If the patient strongly requests general anesthesia, she should be advised that she is at risk for aspiration of gastric contents and that this is a major cause of maternal morbidity and mortality. This results from dilation of the cardioesophageal sphincter, decreased gastric motility, and a prolonged gastric emptying time. Thus, pregnant patients are considered to have a full stomach at the time of anesthesia induction, even if they have not eaten for many hours. General anesthesia is therefore initiated with a rapid-sequence induction consisting of thiopental (4 mg/kg) and succinylcholine (1 mg/kg), cricoid pressure, and endotracheal intubation.

Anesthesia is maintained with nitrous oxide, oxygen, and succinylcholine until the child is delivered. Narcotics may be given to the mother after the umbilical cord is clamped. Awareness under general anesthesia is always possible, but the likelihood of its occurrence can be reduced by the use of either low concentrations of a volatile anesthetic or low doses of ketamine.

## Anesthesia for Emergency Cesarean Section

Emergency cesarean section may be either semiemergencies or true emergencies. In semiemergencies, cesarean section is usually chosen because of (a) a disproportionately large fetal head for the size of the pelvic outlet, or (b) a breech presentation in a woman pregnant for the first time. Both of these result in prolonged labor that fails to progress. Either regional or general anesthesia may be appropriate in these cases, and the patient may state a preference.

If a true emergency exists, however, general anesthesia is the technique of choice for cesarean delivery. True emergencies arise from either severe fetal distress or acute maternal bleeding. In either case, general anesthesia allows more rapid induction and depresses the mother's sympathetic nervous system much less than does blockade induced by either subarachnoid or epidural anesthetics. Thus, with general anesthesia, the infant is delivered sooner and a satisfactory maternal blood pressure is more easily maintained. The rapid induction with thiopental, followed by succinylcholine and maintained with 50% nitrous oxide, oxygen, and low concentrations of a volatile anesthetic, is most frequently used. However, in the presence of hemorrhage and maternal hypotension, ketamine (0.5–1.0 mg/kg) may be substituted for the thiopental.

## Anesthesia for Nonobstetric Surgery in the Pregnant Patient

About 50,000 pregnant women receive anesthetics for nonobstetric surgery each year in the U.S. Although few data are available, the risks to the pregnant mother from such anesthesia are probably no greater than those to the nonpregnant woman of similar age undergoing surgery for the same reason. Theoretically, the fetus could be jeopardized by such anesthesia. Several considerations must be weighed, therefore, before nonobstetrical surgery is scheduled for the pregnant patient.

The question of drug teratogenicity (drug induction of birth defects) must be carefully considered. In animals, fetal abnormalities have been caused by barbiturates, phenothiazines, antianxiety drugs (meprobamate and the benzodiazepines), and the narcotic analgesics. In humans, evidence for teratogenicity is strongest for the antianxiety drugs. Obstetric anesthesiologists judge that, although not proved to be teratogenic in humans, it is wise to avoid antianxiety agents, especially in the first 3 months of pregnancy.

The teratogenic potential of inhalation anesthetics is unclear. In animals, long-term exposure to nitrous oxide, halothane and, more recently, isoflurane (Mazze et al., 1984) increases the incidence of fetal deaths and congenital abnormalities. Statistical studies have shown higher than normal occurrence of congenital defects, stillbirths, and spontaneous abortions in the offspring of both female operating room personnel and wives of male operating room personnel. Chronic exposure of operating room personnel to trace amounts of anesthetic gases has been suggested as a possible cause. Limited surveys of women who received an anesthetic during pregnancy have *not* demonstrated the teratogenicity of inhalation anesthetics. But because relatively few women have been surveyed, these data are not conclusive.

There is no evidence that anesthetics cause premature labor, though the possibility has been investigated. Indeed, the volatile inhalation agents decrease uterine tone and inhibit uterine contractions. The evidence available, although not conclusive, makes it prudent to defer elective operations until after delivery. If an operation is judged essential, it should be delayed until the second or even the third trimester, if possible, because the fetus is most vulnerable to possible teratogenic effects early in development. Any surgical procedure in the first trimester is considered an emergency; if it is not an emergency, it should be delayed.

If an operation cannot be deferred without severe risk to the mother, surgery may have to be performed in the first trimester. Regional anesthesia should be used if possible, since local anesthetics have not been shown to be teratogenic. A subarachnoid block usually is chosen, since it requires less drug than do other regional nerve blocks. Other regional blocks, such as a supraclavicular or axillary block for emergency surgery on the arm, might occasionally be indicated, however.

First-trimester patients who must have surgery should not be premedicated and should not receive antianxiety drugs during the surgery. To win a patient's cooperation and help her achieve self-control, the anesthesiologist may need to explain to her carefully and compassionately why it is necessary to avoid mood-altering drugs. The anesthesiologist should strive to relieve her anxiety through a demonstration of concern for her and for her child.

If a general anesthetic is absolutely necessary (as for emergency intracranial surgery), anesthesia should be managed with the agents and techniques discussed in Chapter 10. To prevent the compression of the inferior vena cava that can occur in the supine position, the patient should be supported in the left lateral tilt position by placing a roll under her right hip. Fetal heart rate should be monitored during the surgery, but such monitoring may not be possible during the first trimester.

Finally, all women of childbearing age who are contemplating elective surgery should be asked whether they may be pregnant before the surgery is scheduled. If doubt exists, a preoperative pregnancy test can be ordered.

## *Readings and References*

Albright, G.A. 1978. *Anesthesia in obstetrics*. Menlo Park, Calif.: Addison-Wesley.

Blass, N.H. 1983. Non-obstetric surgery in the pregnant patient (lecture 135). *ASA annual refresher course lectures*. Park Ridge, Ill.

Bonica, J.J. 1969. *Obstetric analgesia and anesthesia*. Philadelphia: F. A. Davis Co., vols. 1 and 2.

Crawford, J.S. 1978. *Principles and practice of obstetric anaesthesia.* 4th ed. Oxford: Blackwell.

Datta, S., and Alper, M.H. 1980. Anesthesia for cesarean section. *Anesthesiology* 53:142–60.

James, F.M., and Wheeler, A.S. 1982. *Obstetric anesthesia: the complicated patient.* Philadelphia: F.A. Davis, Co.

Mazze, R.I.; Wilson, A.I.; Rice, S.A, et al. 1984. Effects of isoflurane on reproduction and fetal development in mice. *Anesth. Analg.* 63:249.

Moir, D.D. 1980. *Obstetric anesthesia and analgesia.* 2nd ed. London: Bailliere Tindall.

Pedersen, H., and Finster, M. 1979. Anesthetic risk in the pregnant surgical patient. *Anesthesiology* 51:439–51.

Ralston, D.H., and Shnider, S.M. 1978. The fetal and neonatal effects of regional anesthesia in obstetrics. *Anesthesiology* 48:34–64.

Shnider, S.M. 1970. *Obstetrical anesthesia.* Baltimore: Williams & Wilkins.

Shnider, S.M., and Levinson, G. 1979. *Anesthesia for obstetrics.* Baltimore: Williams & Wilkins.

———. 1981. Obstetric anesthesia. In: *Anesthesia.* Miller, R.D., editor. New York: Churchill Livingstone, pp. 1133–73.

Skaredoff, M.N., and Ostheimer, G. W. 1981. Physiologic changes during pregnancy: effects of major regional anesthesia. *Region. Anesth.* 6:28–40.

Symposium on Current Trends in Obstetric Analgesia. 1979. *Br. J. Anaesth.* 51:1S–66S.

Wright, J.P. 1983. Anesthetic considerations in preeclampsia-eclampsia. *Anesth. Analg.* 63:590–601.

# Appendix A Supplemental Anesthesia Readings

## Anesthesia Textbooks

Atkinson, R.S.; Rushman, G.B.; and Lee, J.A. 1982. *A synopsis of anesthesia*. 9th ed. Bristol: John Wright and Sons, Ltd.

Churchill-Davidson, H.C. 1978. *A practice of anesthesia*. Philadelphia: W.B. Saunders.

Collins, V.T. 1976. *Principles of anesthesiology*. 2nd ed. Philadelphia: Lea and Febiger.

Cullen S.C., and Larson, P. 1974. *Essentials of anesthetic practice*. Chicago: Year Book Medical Publishers.

Dripps, R.D.; Eckenhoff, J.E.; and VanDam, L.D. 1982. *Introduction to anesthesia*. 6th ed. Philadelphia: W.B. Saunders.

Gray, T.C.; Nunn, J.F.; and Utting, J.E. 1908. *General anesthesia*. 4th ed. London: Butterworths, vols. 1 and 2.

Lebowitz, P.W. editor. 1982. *Clinical anesthesia practice of the Massachusetts General Hospital*. 2nd ed. Boston: Little, Brown and Co.

Miller, R.D. editor. 1981. *Anesthesia*. New York: Churchill Livingstone, vols. 1 and 2.

Quimby, C.W. 1979. *Anesthesiology: a manual of concept and management*. 2nd ed. New York: Appleton-Century-Crofts.

Snow, J.C. 1982. *Manual of anesthesia*. 2nd ed. Boston: Little, Brown and Co.

Stark, D.C.C. 1980. *Practical points in anesthesiology*. 2nd ed. Garden City, N.Y.: Medical Examination Publ. Co.

*Wylie and Churchill-Davidson's A practice of anesthesia*. 5th ed. 1984. Churchill-Davidson, H.C., editor. Chicago: Year Book Medical Publishers.

Yao, F.-S.F., and Artusio, J.F. *Anesthesiology: problem oriented patient management*. Philadelphia: J.B. Lippincott.

## Anesthesia Journals

*Anesthesia and Analgesia,* Journal of the International Anesthesia Research Society. Published monthly by Elsevier Science Publishing Company, New York.

*Anesthesiology,* Journal of the American Society of Anesthesiologists, Inc. Published monthly by J. B. Lippincott, Philadelphia.

*British Journal of Anaesthesia.* Published monthly by MacMillan, Hampshire, England.

*The Canadian Anaesthetists' Society Journal.* Published bimonthly by the Canadian Anaesthetists' Society, Toronto, Canada.

*Obstetric Anesthesia Digest,* G. F. Marx, editor. Published quarterly by Elsevier Science Publishing Company, New York.

*Regional Anesthesia,* Journal of the American Society of Regional Anesthesia. Published quarterly by J.B. Lippincott, Philadelphia.

*Seminars in Anesthesia,* R. L. Katz, editor. Published quarterly by Grune & Stratton, Inc., New York.

## Anesthesia Subspecialty Textbooks*

Campkin, T.V., and Turner, J.M. 1980. *Neurosurgical anesthesia and intensive care.* London: Butterworths.

Cottrell, J.E., and Turndorf, H. 1980. *Anesthesia and neurosurgery.* St. Louis: C.V. Mosby Company.

Gothard, J.W.W., and Branthwaite, M.A. 1982. *Anaesthesia for thoracic surgery.* Boston: Blackwell Scientific Publishers.

Kaplan, J.A. 1979. *Cardiac anesthesia.* New York: Grune & Stratton.

Kaplan, J.A. 1983. Cardiovascular pharmacology. In: *Cardiac anesthesia.* New York: Grune & Stratton, vol. 2.

Kaplan, J.A. 1983. *Thoracic anesthesia.* New York: Churchill Livingstone.

Snow, J.C. 1982. *Anesthesia in otolaryngology and opthalmology.* 2nd ed. New York: Appleton-Century-Crofts.

Zauder, H.L. 1980. *Anesthesia for orthopaedic surgery.* Philadelphia: F.A. Davis Co.

## Respiratory Physiology

Comroe, J.H. 1974. *Physiology of respiration.* 2nd ed. Chicago: Year Book Medical Publishers.

Hedley-White, J.; Burgess, G.E.; Feeley, T.W., et al. 1976. *Applied physiology of respiratory care.* Boston: Little, Brown and Co.

Nunn, J.F. 1977. *Applied respiratory physiology.* 2nd ed. London: Butterworths.

*Except pediatric and obstetric anesthesia, both discussed in Chapters 13 and 14.

West, J.B. 1979. *Respiratory physiology: the essentials.* 2nd ed. Baltimore: Williams & Wilkins.

## Miscellaneous Anesthesia Topics

Brown, B.B., editor. 1982. *Anesthesia and the obese patient.* Philadelphia: F.A. Davis Co.

Brown, B.B., editor. 1978. *Outpatient anesthesia.* Philadelphia: F.A. Davis Co.

Eckenhoff, J.E. 1979. *Controversy in anesthesiology.* Philadelphia: W.B. Saunders.

Hershey, S.G., editor. 1983. *Refresher courses in anesthesiology.* Philadelphia: J.B. Lippincott, vol. II.

Katz, J.; Benumof, J.; and Kadis, L.B. 1981. *Anesthesia and uncommon diseases.* 2nd ed. Philadelphia: W.B. Saunders.

Mathieu, A., and Kahan, B.D. 1975. *Immunologic aspects of anesthesia and surgical practice.* New York: Grune & Stratton.

Orkin, F.K., and Cooperman, L.H. 1982. *Complications in anesthesiology.* Philadelphia: J.B. Lippincott.

Patil, V.; Stehling, L; and Zauder, H. 1983. *Fiberoptic endoscopy in anesthesia.* Chicago: Year Book Medical Publishers.

Peters, J.D.; Fineberg, K.S.; Kroll, D.A., et al. 1983. *Anesthesiology and the law* . Ann Arbor, Mich.: University of Michigan Health Administration Press.

Pratila, M.G., and Pratilas, V. 1978. Anesthetic agents and cardiac electromechanical activity. *Anesthesiology.* 39:338–60.

Ream, A.K., and Fogdall, R.P. 1982. *Acute cardiovascular management: anesthesia and intensive care.* Philadelphia: J.B. Lippincott.

Scurr, C., and Feldman, S., editors. 1982. *Scientific foundations of anesthesia.* Chicago: Year Book Medical Publishers.

Steen, P.A., and Michenfelder, J.D. 1979. Neurotoxicity of anesthetics. *Anesthesiology* 50:437–53.

Stoelting, R.K., and Dierdorf, S.F. 1983. *Anesthesia and co-existing disease.* New York: Churchill Livingstone.

Symposium on Anaesthesia and the Eye. *Br. J. Anaesth.* 53:641–703.

Tschirren, B. 1980. *Anesthetic complications.* Chicago: Year Book Medical Publishers.

Vickers, M.D., editor. 1982. *Medicine for anaesthetists.* 2nd ed. Boston: Blackwell Scientific Publishers.

Volpitto, P.P., and VanDam, L.D., editors. 1982. *The genesis of contemporary American anesthesiology.* Springfield, Ill.: C.C. Thomas.

Watkins, J., and Salo, M. 1982. *Trauma, stress and immunity in anesthesia and surgery.* Woburn, Mass.: Butterworths.

Wilkinson, P.L.; Ham, J.; and Miller, R.D. 1980. *Clinical anesthesia: case selections from the University of California, San Francisco.* St. Louis: C.V. Mosby Company.

# Appendix B
# Dosage Calculation Charts for Autonomic Agonists and Vasodilators

### TABLE B-1
### Calculator for Dopamine Dosage, 200 mg in 250 mL (800 μg/mL)
("single strength")

| Pounds | 77 | 88 | 99 | 110 | 121 | 132 | 143 | 154 | 165 | 176 | 187 | 198 | 209 | 220 | 231 | 262 |
|---|---|---|---|---|---|---|---|---|---|---|---|---|---|---|---|---|
| Kilograms | 35 | 40 | 45 | 50 | 55 | 60 | 65 | 70 | 75 | 80 | 85 | 90 | 95 | 100 | 105 | 110 |
| **Desired Dopamine Dosage (μg/kg/min)** | | | | | | | | | | | | | | | | |
| 1 | 3 | 3 | 3 | 4 | 4 | 4 | 5 | 5 | 6 | 6 | 6 | 7 | 7 | 7 | 8 | 8 |
| 2 | 5 | 6 | 7 | 7 | 8 | 9 | 10 | 10 | 11 | 12 | 13 | 13 | 14 | 15 | 16 | 17 |
| 3 | 8 | 9 | 10 | 11 | 12 | 13 | 15 | 16 | 17 | 18 | 19 | 20 | 21 | 22 | 24 | 25 |
| 4 | 10 | 12 | 14 | 15 | 17 | 18 | 20 | **21** | 22 | 24 | 26 | 27 | 28 | 30 | 32 | 33 |
| 5 | 13 | 15 | 17 | 19 | 21 | 22 | 24 | 26 | 28 | 30 | 32 | 34 | 36 | 37 | 37 | 41 |
| 6 | 16 | 18 | 20 | 22 | 25 | 27 | 29 | 32 | 34 | 36 | 38 | 41 | 43 | 45 | 47 | 50 |
| 7 | 18 | 21 | 24 | 26 | 29 | 31 | 34 | 37 | 39 | 42 | 45 | 47 | 50 | 53 | 55 | 58 |
| 8 | 21 | 24 | 27 | 30 | 33 | 36 | 39 | 42 | 45 | 48 | 51 | 54 | 57 | 60 | 63 | 66 |
| 9 | 24 | 27 | 30 | 34 | 37 | 40 | 44 | 47 | 51 | 54 | 57 | 61 | 64 | 68 | 71 | 74 |
| 10 | 26 | 30 | 34 | 37 | 41 | 45 | 49 | 53 | 56 | 60 | 64 | 68 | 71 | 75 | 79 | 83 |
| 11 | 29 | 33 | 37 | 41 | 45 | 49 | 54 | 58 | 62 | 66 | 70 | 74 | 78 | 83 | 87 | 91 |
| 12 | 31 | 36 | 40 | 45 | 49 | 54 | 58 | 63 | 67 | 72 | 76 | 81 | 85 | 90 | 94 | 99 |
| 13 | 34 | 39 | 44 | 49 | 54 | 58 | 63 | 68 | 73 | 78 | 83 | 88 | 93 | 98 | 102 | 107 |
| 14 | 37 | 42 | 47 | 52 | 58 | 63 | 68 | 74 | 79 | 84 | 89 | 95 | 100 | 105 | 110 | 116 |
| 15 | 39 | 45 | 51 | 56 | 62 | 67 | 73 | 79 | 84 | 90 | 96 | 101 | 107 | 113 | 118 | 124 |
| 16 | 42 | 48 | 54 | 60 | 66 | 72 | 78 | 84 | 90 | 96 | 102 | 108 | 114 | 120 | 126 | 132 |
| 17 | 45 | 51 | 57 | 64 | 70 | 76 | 83 | 87 | 96 | 102 | 108 | 115 | 121 | 127 | 134 | 140 |
| 18 | 47 | 54 | 61 | 67 | 74 | 81 | 88 | 94 | 101 | 108 | 115 | 122 | 128 | 135 | 142 | 149 |
| 19 | 50 | 57 | 64 | 71 | 78 | 85 | 93 | 100 | 107 | 114 | 121 | 128 | 135 | 143 | 150 | 157 |
| 20 | 52 | 60 | 67 | 75 | 82 | 90 | 97 | 105 | 112 | 120 | 127 | 135 | 142 | 150 | 157 | 165 |

Flow Rate (microdrops/min* or mL/hr)

*Note:* Highlighted dose (21 drops) is "starting dose" for 70 kg patient (calculated as 0.3 times body weight in kilograms; see Table 8.5, p. 138).

*Based on 60 microdrops equal to 1 mL or 13.33 μg/drop.

## TABLE B-2
## Calculator for Dopamine Dosage, 400 mg in 250 mL (1.6 mg/mL)
("double strength")

Rows: Desired Dopamine Dosage (μg/kg/min). Values: Flow Rate (microdrops/min* or mL/hr)

| Pounds | 77 | 88 | 99 | 110 | 121 | 132 | 143 | 154 | 165 | 176 | 187 | 198 | 209 | 220 | 231 | 262 |
|---|---|---|---|---|---|---|---|---|---|---|---|---|---|---|---|---|
| Kilograms | 35 | 40 | 45 | 50 | 55 | 60 | 65 | 70 | 75 | 80 | 85 | 90 | 95 | 100 | 105 | 110 |
| 1 | 1 | 1 | 2 | 2 | 2 | 2 | 2 | 3 | 3 | 3 | 3 | 3 | 4 | 4 | 4 | 4 |
| 2 | 3 | 3 | 3 | 4 | 4 | 4 | 5 | 5 | 6 | 6 | 6 | 7 | 7 | 7 | 8 | 8 |
| 3 | 4 | 4 | 5 | 6 | 6 | 7 | 7 | 8 | 8 | 9 | 10 | 10 | 11 | 11 | 12 | 12 |
| 4 | 5 | 6 | 7 | 7 | 8 | 9 | 10 | 10 | 11 | 12 | 13 | 14 | 14 | 15 | 16 | 17 |
| 5 | 7 | 7 | 9 | 9 | 10 | 11 | 12 | 13 | 14 | 15 | 16 | 17 | 18 | 19 | 20 | 21 |
| 6 | 8 | 9 | 10 | 11 | 12 | 13 | 15 | 16 | 17 | 18 | 19 | 20 | 21 | 22 | 24 | 25 |
| 7 | 9 | 10 | 12 | 13 | 14 | 16 | 17 | 18 | 20 | 21 | 22 | 24 | 25 | 26 | 28 | 29 |
| 8 | 10 | 12 | 13 | 15 | 16 | 18 | 19 | 21 | 22 | 24 | 25 | 27 | 28 | 30 | 31 | 33 |
| 9 | 12 | 13 | 15 | 17 | 18 | 20 | 22 | 24 | 25 | 27 | 29 | 30 | 32 | 34 | 35 | 37 |
| 10 | 13 | 15 | 17 | 19 | 21 | 22 | 24 | 26 | 28 | 30 | 32 | 34 | 36 | 37 | 39 | 41 |
| 11 | 14 | 16 | 18 | 21 | 23 | 25 | 27 | 29 | 31 | 33 | 35 | 37 | 39 | 41 | 43 | 45 |
| 12 | 16 | 18 | 20 | 22 | 25 | 27 | 29 | 31 | 34 | 36 | 38 | 40 | 43 | 45 | 47 | 49 |
| 13 | 17 | 19 | 22 | 24 | 27 | 29 | 32 | 34 | 37 | 39 | 41 | 44 | 46 | 49 | 51 | 54 |
| 14 | 18 | 21 | 24 | 26 | 29 | 31 | 34 | 37 | 39 | 42 | 45 | 47 | 50 | 52 | 55 | 58 |
| 15 | 20 | 22 | 25 | 28 | 31 | 34 | 37 | 39 | 42 | 45 | 48 | 51 | 53 | 56 | 59 | 62 |
| 16 | 21 | 24 | 27 | 30 | 33 | 36 | 39 | 42 | 45 | 48 | 51 | 54 | 57 | 60 | 63 | 66 |
| 17 | 22 | 25 | 29 | 32 | 35 | 38 | 41 | 45 | 48 | 51 | 54 | 57 | 60 | 64 | 67 | 70 |
| 18 | 24 | 27 | 30 | 34 | 37 | 40 | 44 | 47 | 51 | 54 | 57 | 61 | 64 | 67 | 71 | 74 |
| 19 | 25 | 28 | 32 | 36 | 39 | 43 | 46 | 50 | 53 | 57 | 61 | 64 | 68 | 71 | 75 | 78 |
| 20 | 26 | 30 | 34 | 37 | 41 | 45 | 49 | 52 | 56 | 60 | 64 | 67 | 71 | 75 | 79 | 82 |

*Based on 60 microdrops equal to 1 mL or 26.66 μg/drop.

## TABLE B-3
## Calculator for Isoproterenol and Epinephrine Dosage, 1.0 mg in 250 mL (4 μg/mL)

Rows: Desired Isoproterenol Dosage (μg/kg/min). Values: Flow Rate (microdrops/min* or mL/hr)

| Pounds | 77 | 88 | 99 | 110 | 121 | 132 | 143 | 154 | 165 | 176 | 187 | 198 | 209 | 220 | 231 | 262 |
|---|---|---|---|---|---|---|---|---|---|---|---|---|---|---|---|---|
| Kilograms | 35 | 40 | 45 | 50 | 55 | 60 | 65 | 70 | 75 | 80 | 85 | 90 | 95 | 100 | 105 | 110 |
| 0.01 | 5 | 6 | 7 | 8 | 8 | 9 | 10 | 11 | 11 | 12 | 13 | 14 | 14 | 15 | 16 | 17 |
| 0.02 | 11 | 12 | 14 | 15 | 17 | 18 | 20 | **21** | 23 | 24 | 26 | 27 | 29 | 30 | 32 | 33 |
| 0.03 | 16 | 18 | 20 | 23 | 25 | 27 | 30 | 32 | 34 | 36 | 39 | 41 | 43 | 45 | 48 | 50 |
| 0.04 | 21 | 24 | 27 | 30 | 33 | 36 | 39 | 42 | 46 | 48 | 52 | 54 | 58 | 61 | 64 | 67 |
| 0.05 | 27 | 30 | 34 | 38 | 42 | 45 | 49 | 53 | 57 | 61 | 65 | 68 | 72 | 76 | 80 | 83 |
| 0.06 | 32 | 36 | 41 | 45 | 50 | 54 | 59 | 64 | 68 | 73 | 77 | 82 | 86 | 91 | 95 | 100 |
| 0.07 | 37 | 42 | 48 | 53 | 58 | 64 | 69 | 74 | 80 | 85 | 90 | 95 | 101 | 106 | 113 | 117 |
| 0.08 | 42 | 48 | 55 | 61 | 67 | 73 | 79 | 85 | 91 | 97 | 103 | 109 | 115 | 121 | 127 | 133 |
| 0.09 | 48 | 55 | 61 | 68 | 75 | 82 | 89 | 95 | 103 | 109 | 116 | 122 | 130 | 136 | 143 | 150 |
| 0.10 | 53 | 61 | 68 | 76 | 83 | 91 | 98 | 106 | 114 | 121 | 129 | 136 | 144 | 151 | 159 | 167 |

*Based on 60 microdrops equal to 1 mL or 0.066 μg/drop.

**TABLE B-4**
**Calculator for Dobutamine Dosage, 250 mg in 250 mL (1 mg/mL)**
("single strength")

Desired Dobutamine Dosage (μg/kg/min) by row; Flow Rate (microdrops/min* or mL/hr) in cells

| Pounds | 77 | 88 | 99 | 110 | 121 | 132 | 143 | 154 | 165 | 176 | 187 | 198 | 209 | 220 | 231 | 262 |
|---|---|---|---|---|---|---|---|---|---|---|---|---|---|---|---|---|
| Kilograms | 35 | 40 | 45 | 50 | 55 | 60 | 65 | 70 | 75 | 80 | 85 | 90 | 95 | 100 | 105 | 110 |
| 1 | 2 | 2 | 3 | 3 | 3 | 4 | 4 | 4 | 4 | 5 | 5 | 5 | 6 | 6 | 6 | 7 |
| 2 | 4 | 5 | 5 | 6 | 7 | 7 | 8 | 8 | 9 | 10 | 10 | 11 | 11 | 12 | 13 | 13 |
| 3 | 6 | 7 | 8 | 9 | 10 | 11 | 12 | 13 | 13 | 14 | 15 | 16 | 17 | 18 | 19 | 20 |
| 4 | 8 | 10 | 11 | 12 | 13 | 14 | 16 | 17 | 18 | 19 | 20 | 22 | 23 | 24 | 25 | 26 |
| 5 | 10 | 12 | 13 | 15 | 17 | 18 | 19 | **21** | 22 | 24 | 25 | 27 | 28 | 30 | 31 | 33 |
| 6 | 13 | 14 | 16 | 18 | 20 | 22 | 23 | 25 | 27 | 29 | 31 | 32 | 34 | 36 | 38 | 40 |
| 7 | 15 | 17 | 19 | 21 | 23 | 25 | 27 | 29 | 31 | 34 | 36 | 38 | 40 | 42 | 44 | 46 |
| 8 | 17 | 19 | 22 | 24 | 26 | 29 | 31 | 34 | 36 | 38 | 41 | 43 | 46 | 48 | 50 | 53 |
| 9 | 19 | 22 | 24 | 27 | 30 | 32 | 35 | 38 | 40 | 43 | 46 | 49 | 51 | 54 | 57 | 59 |
| 10 | 21 | 24 | 28 | 30 | 33 | 36 | 39 | 42 | 45 | 48 | 51 | 54 | 57 | 60 | 63 | 66 |
| 11 | 23 | 26 | 30 | 33 | 36 | 40 | 43 | 46 | 49 | 53 | 56 | 59 | 63 | 66 | 69 | 73 |
| 12 | 25 | 29 | 32 | 36 | 40 | 43 | 47 | 50 | 54 | 58 | 61 | 65 | 68 | 72 | 76 | 79 |
| 13 | 27 | 31 | 35 | 39 | 43 | 47 | 50 | 55 | 58 | 62 | 66 | 70 | 74 | 78 | 82 | 86 |
| 14 | 29 | 34 | 38 | 42 | 46 | 50 | 55 | 59 | 63 | 67 | 71 | 76 | 80 | 84 | 88 | 92 |
| 15 | 31 | 36 | 40 | 45 | 49 | 54 | 58 | 63 | 67 | 72 | 76 | 81 | 85 | 90 | 94 | 99 |
| 16 | 34 | 38 | 43 | 48 | 53 | 58 | 62 | 67 | 72 | 77 | 82 | 86 | 91 | 96 | 101 | 106 |
| 17 | 36 | 41 | 46 | 51 | 56 | 61 | 66 | 71 | 76 | 82 | 87 | 92 | 97 | 102 | 107 | 112 |
| 18 | 38 | 43 | 49 | 54 | 59 | 65 | 70 | 76 | 81 | 86 | 92 | 97 | 103 | 108 | 113 | 119 |
| 19 | 40 | 46 | 51 | 57 | 63 | 68 | 74 | 80 | 85 | 91 | 97 | 103 | 108 | 114 | 120 | 125 |
| 20 | 42 | 48 | 54 | 60 | 66 | 72 | 78 | 84 | 90 | 96 | 102 | 108 | 114 | 120 | 126 | 132 |

*Based on 60 microdrops equal to 1 mL or 16.66 μg/drop.

## TABLE B-5
## Calculator for Dobutamine Dosage, 500 mg/250 mL (2 mg/mL)
("double strength")

| Pounds | 77 | 88 | 99 | 110 | 121 | 132 | 143 | 154 | 165 | 176 | 187 | 198 | 209 | 220 | 231 | 262 |
|---|---|---|---|---|---|---|---|---|---|---|---|---|---|---|---|---|
| Kilograms | 35 | 40 | 45 | 50 | 55 | 60 | 65 | 70 | 75 | 80 | 85 | 90 | 95 | 100 | 105 | 110 |
| Desired Dobutamine Dosage (μg/kg/min) | | | | | | | | Flow Rate (microdrops/min* or mL/hr) | | | | | | | | |
| 1 | 1 | 1 | 1 | 1 | 2 | 2 | 2 | 2 | 2 | 2 | 3 | 3 | 3 | 3 | 3 | 3 |
| 2 | 2 | 2 | 3 | 3 | 3 | 4 | 4 | 4 | 4 | 5 | 5 | 5 | 6 | 6 | 6 | 7 |
| 3 | 3 | 4 | 4 | 5 | 5 | 5 | 6 | 6 | 7 | 7 | 8 | 8 | 9 | 9 | 9 | 10 |
| 4 | 4 | 5 | 5 | 6 | 7 | 7 | 8 | 8 | 9 | 10 | 10 | 11 | 11 | 12 | 13 | 13 |
| 5 | 5 | 6 | 7 | 8 | 8 | 9 | 10 | 10 | 11 | 12 | 13 | 13 | 14 | 15 | 16 | 16 |
| 6 | 6 | 7 | 8 | 9 | 10 | 11 | 12 | 13 | 13 | 14 | 15 | 16 | 17 | 18 | 19 | 20 |
| 7 | 7 | 8 | 9 | 10 | 12 | 13 | 14 | 15 | 16 | 17 | 18 | 19 | 20 | 21 | 22 | 23 |
| 8 | 8 | 10 | 11 | 12 | 13 | 14 | 16 | 17 | 18 | 19 | 20 | 22 | 23 | 24 | 25 | 26 |
| 9 | 9 | 11 | 12 | 13 | 15 | 16 | 18 | 19 | 20 | 22 | 23 | 24 | 25 | 27 | 28 | 30 |
| 10 | 10 | 12 | 14 | 15 | 16 | 18 | 19 | 21 | 22 | 24 | 25 | 27 | 28 | 30 | 31 | 33 |
| 11 | 12 | 13 | 15 | 16 | 18 | 20 | 21 | 23 | 25 | 26 | 28 | 30 | 31 | 33 | 35 | 36 |
| 12 | 13 | 14 | 16 | 18 | 20 | 22 | 23 | 25 | 27 | 29 | 31 | 32 | 34 | 36 | 38 | 40 |
| 13 | 14 | 16 | 18 | 19 | 21 | 23 | 25 | 27 | 29 | 31 | 33 | 35 | 37 | 39 | 41 | 43 |
| 14 | 15 | 17 | 19 | 21 | 23 | 25 | 27 | 29 | 31 | 34 | 36 | 38 | 40 | 42 | 44 | 46 |
| 15 | 16 | 18 | 20 | 22 | 25 | 27 | 29 | 31 | 34 | 36 | 38 | 40 | 43 | 45 | 47 | 49 |
| 16 | 17 | 19 | 22 | 24 | 26 | 29 | 31 | 34 | 36 | 38 | 41 | 43 | 46 | 48 | 50 | 53 |
| 17 | 18 | 20 | 23 | 25 | 28 | 31 | 33 | 36 | 38 | 41 | 43 | 46 | 48 | 51 | 54 | 56 |
| 18 | 19 | 22 | 24 | 27 | 30 | 32 | 35 | 38 | 40 | 43 | 46 | 49 | 51 | 54 | 57 | 59 |
| 19 | 20 | 23 | 26 | 28 | 31 | 34 | 37 | 40 | 43 | 46 | 48 | 51 | 54 | 57 | 60 | 63 |
| 20 | 21 | 24 | 27 | 30 | 33 | 36 | 39 | 42 | 45 | 48 | 51 | 54 | 57 | 60 | 63 | 66 |

*Based on 60 microdrops equal to 1 mL or 33.33 μg/drop.

## TABLE B-6
## Calculator for Phenylephrine Dosage, 10 mg in 250 mL (40 μg/mL)

| Pounds | 77 | 88 | 99 | 110 | 121 | 132 | 143 | 154 | 165 | 176 | 187 | 198 | 209 | 220 | 231 | 262 |
|---|---|---|---|---|---|---|---|---|---|---|---|---|---|---|---|---|
| Kilograms | 35 | 40 | 45 | 50 | 55 | 60 | 65 | 70 | 75 | 80 | 85 | 90 | 95 | 100 | 105 | 110 |
| Desired Phenylephrine Dosage (μg/kg/min) | | | | | | | | Flow Rate (microdrops/min* or mL/hr) | | | | | | | | |
| 0.1 | 5 | 6 | 7 | 8 | 8 | 9 | 10 | 11 | 11 | 12 | 13 | 14 | 14 | 15 | 16 | 17 |
| 0.2 | 11 | 12 | 14 | 15 | 17 | 18 | 20 | **21** | 23 | 24 | 26 | 27 | 29 | 30 | 32 | 33 |
| 0.3 | 16 | 18 | 20 | 23 | 25 | 27 | 30 | 32 | 34 | 36 | 39 | 41 | 43 | 45 | 48 | 50 |
| 0.4 | 21 | 24 | 27 | 30 | 33 | 36 | 39 | 42 | 46 | 48 | 52 | 54 | 58 | 61 | 64 | 67 |
| 0.5 | 27 | 30 | 34 | 38 | 42 | 45 | 49 | 53 | 57 | 61 | 65 | 68 | 72 | 76 | 80 | 83 |
| 0.6 | 32 | 36 | 41 | 45 | 50 | 54 | 59 | 64 | 68 | 73 | 77 | 82 | 86 | 91 | 95 | 100 |
| 0.7 | 37 | 42 | 48 | 53 | 58 | 64 | 69 | 74 | 80 | 85 | 90 | 95 | 101 | 106 | 113 | 117 |
| 0.8 | 42 | 48 | 55 | 61 | 67 | 73 | 79 | 85 | 91 | 97 | 103 | 109 | 115 | 121 | 127 | 133 |
| 0.9 | 48 | 55 | 61 | 68 | 75 | 82 | 89 | 95 | 103 | 109 | 116 | 122 | 130 | 136 | 143 | 150 |
| 1.0 | 53 | 61 | 68 | 76 | 83 | 91 | 98 | 106 | 114 | 121 | 129 | 136 | 144 | 151 | 159 | 167 |

*Based on 60 microdrops equal to 1 mL or 0.66 μg/drop.

### TABLE B-7
### Calculator for Nitroprusside Dosage, 50 mg in 250 mL (200 μg/mL)

("single strength")

| Desired Nitroprusside Dosage (μg/kg/min) | Pounds | 77 | 88 | 99 | 110 | 121 | 132 | 143 | 154 | 165 | 176 | 187 | 198 | 209 | 220 | 231 | 262 |
|---|---|---|---|---|---|---|---|---|---|---|---|---|---|---|---|---|---|
| | Kilograms | 35 | 40 | 45 | 50 | 55 | 60 | 65 | 70 | 75 | 80 | 85 | 90 | 95 | 100 | 105 | 110 |
| | 0.1 | 1 | 1 | 1 | 1 | 2 | 2 | 2 | 2 | 2 | 2 | 3 | 3 | 3 | 3 | 3 | 3 |
| | 0.2 | 2 | 2 | 3 | 3 | 3 | 4 | 4 | 4 | 5 | 5 | 5 | 5 | 6 | 6 | 6 | 7 |
| | 0.3 | 3 | 4 | 4 | 4 | 5 | 5 | 6 | 6 | 7 | 7 | 8 | 8 | 9 | 9 | 10 | 10 |
| | 0.4 | 4 | 5 | 5 | 6 | 6 | 7 | 8 | 8 | 9 | 10 | 10 | 11 | 12 | 12 | 13 | 13 |
| | 0.5 | 5 | 6 | 6 | 7 | 8 | 9 | 9 | 10 | 11 | 12 | 13 | 13 | 14 | 15 | 16 | 16 |
| | 0.6 | 6 | 7 | 8 | 9 | 10 | 11 | 12 | 13 | 14 | 15 | 16 | 16 | 17 | 18 | 19 | 20 |
| | 0.7 | 7 | 8 | 9 | 10 | 11 | 12 | 13 | 15 | 16 | 17 | 18 | 19 | 20 | 21 | 22 | 23 |
| | †0.8 | 8 | 9 | 10 | 12 | 13 | 14 | 15 | 17 | 18 | 19 | 21 | 22 | 23 | 24 | 25 | 26 |
| | 0.9 | 9 | 11 | 12 | 13 | 14 | 16 | 17 | 19 | 21 | 22 | 23 | 24 | 26 | 27 | 29 | 30 |
| | 1.0 | 11 | 12 | 13 | 15 | 16 | 18 | 19 | **21** | 23 | 24 | 26 | 27 | 29 | 30 | 32 | 33 |
| | 2.0 | 21 | 24 | 28 | 30 | 32 | 36 | 38 | 42 | 46 | 48 | 52 | 54 | 58 | 60 | 64 | 66 |
| | 3.0 | 32 | 36 | 40 | 45 | 48 | 54 | 57 | 63 | 69 | 72 | 78 | 81 | 87 | 90 | 96 | 99 |
| | 4.0 | 42 | 48 | 54 | 60 | 64 | 72 | 76 | 84 | 92 | 96 | 104 | 108 | 116 | 120 | 128 | 132 |
| | 5.0 | 53 | 60 | 68 | 75 | 83 | 90 | 95 | 105 | 115 | 121 | 130 | 135 | 145 | 150 | 160 | 165 |
| | 6.0 | 64 | 72 | 82 | 90 | 96 | 108 | 114 | 126 | 138 | 144 | 156 | 162 | 174 | 180 | 192 | 198 |
| | 7.0 | 74 | 84 | 95 | 105 | 112 | 126 | 133 | 147 | 161 | 168 | 182 | 189 | 203 | 210 | 224 | 231 |
| | 8.0 | 85 | 96 | 109 | 121 | 128 | 144 | 152 | 168 | 184 | 192 | 208 | 216 | 232 | 240 | 256 | 264 |

Flow Rate (microdrops/min* or mL/hr)

*Note:* Doses from 0.1–1.0 μg/kg/min presented in 0.1 increments. From 1.0–8.0 μg/kg/min presented in 1.0 increments. To obtain fractional doses above 1 μg/kg/min, add the appropriate number of drops for each. For example, 2.4 μg/kg/min for a 60 kg patient gives 43 drops/min (i.e., 36 drops for 2 μg/kg/min and 7 drops for 0.4 μg/kg/min).

*Based on 60 microdrops equal to 1 mL or 3.3 μg/drop.

†Starting dose = 1.0 μg/kg/min = 21 drops for 70 kg patient.

## TABLE B-8
## Calculator for Nitroprusside Dosage, 100 mg in 250 mL (400 μg/mL)
("double strength")

| Pounds | 77 | 88 | 99 | 110 | 121 | 132 | 143 | 154 | 165 | 176 | 187 | 198 | 209 | 220 | 231 | 262 |
|---|---|---|---|---|---|---|---|---|---|---|---|---|---|---|---|---|
| Kilograms | 35 | 40 | 45 | 50 | 55 | 60 | 65 | 70 | 75 | 80 | 85 | 90 | 95 | 100 | 105 | 110 |
| Desired Nitroprusside Dosage (μg/kg/min) | Flow Rate (microdrops/min* or mL/hr) | | | | | | | | | | | | | | | |
| 0.1 | 0.5 | 1 | 1 | 1 | 1 | 1 | 1 | 1 | 1 | 1 | 1 | 1 | 1 | 2 | 2 | 2 |
| 0.2 | 1 | 1 | 1 | 1 | 2 | 2 | 2 | 2 | 2 | 2 | 3 | 3 | 3 | 3 | 3 | 3 |
| 0.3 | 2 | 2 | 2 | 2 | 2 | 3 | 3 | 3 | 3 | 4 | 4 | 4 | 4 | 5 | 5 | 5 |
| 0.4 | 2 | 2 | 3 | 3 | 3 | 4 | 4 | 4 | 5 | 5 | 5 | 5 | 6 | 6 | 6 | 7 |
| 0.5 | 3 | 3 | 3 | 4 | 4 | 4 | 5 | 5 | 6 | 6 | 6 | 7 | 7 | 8 | 8 | 8 |
| 0.6 | 3 | 4 | 4 | 4 | 5 | 5 | 6 | 6 | 7 | 7 | 8 | 8 | 9 | 9 | 10 | 10 |
| 0.7 | 4 | 4 | 5 | 5 | 6 | 6 | 7 | 7 | 8 | 8 | 9 | 10 | 10 | 11 | 11 | 12 |
| †0.8 | 4 | 5 | 5 | 6 | 7 | 7 | 8 | 8 | 9 | 10 | 10 | 11 | 11 | 12 | 13 | 13 |
| 0.9 | 5 | 5 | 6 | 7 | 7 | 8 | 9 | 10 | 10 | 11 | 11 | 12 | 13 | 14 | 14 | 15 |
| 1.0 | 5 | 6 | 7 | 7 | 8 | 9 | 10 | 11 | 11 | 12 | 13 | 14 | 14 | 15 | 16 | 17 |
| 2.0 | 11 | 12 | 14 | 15 | 17 | 18 | 20 | 21 | 23 | 24 | 26 | 27 | 29 | 30 | 32 | 33 |
| 3.0 | 16 | 18 | 20 | 22 | 25 | 27 | 29 | 32 | 34 | 36 | 38 | 41 | 43 | 45 | 48 | 50 |
| 4.0 | 21 | 24 | 27 | 30 | 33 | 36 | 39 | 42 | 45 | 48 | 51 | 54 | 57 | 60 | 64 | 66 |
| 5.0 | 26 | 30 | 34 | 37 | 41 | 45 | 49 | 53 | 56 | 60 | 64 | 68 | 71 | 75 | 79 | 83 |
| 6.0 | 32 | 36 | 41 | 45 | 50 | 54 | 59 | 64 | 68 | 73 | 77 | 82 | 86 | 91 | 95 | 100 |
| 7.0 | 37 | 42 | 48 | 52 | 58 | 63 | 69 | 74 | 79 | 85 | 90 | 95 | 100 | 106 | 111 | 116 |
| 8.0 | 42 | 48 | 54 | 60 | 66 | 72 | 78 | 85 | 90 | 97 | 102 | 109 | 114 | 121 | 127 | 133 |

See *Note,* Table B-7.
*Based on 60 microdrops equal to 1 mL or 6.6 μg/drop.
†Starting dose.

## TABLE B-9
## Calculator for Nitroglycerin Dosage, 50 mg in 250 mL (200 μg/mL)

| Pounds | 77 | 88 | 99 | 110 | 121 | 132 | 143 | 154 | 165 | 176 | 187 | 198 | 209 | 220 | 231 | 262 |
|---|---|---|---|---|---|---|---|---|---|---|---|---|---|---|---|---|
| Kilograms | 35 | 40 | 45 | 50 | 55 | 60 | 65 | 70 | 75 | 80 | 85 | 90 | 95 | 100 | 105 | 110 |
| Desired Nitroglycerin Dosage (μg/kg/min) | Flow Rate (microdrops/min* or mL/hr) | | | | | | | | | | | | | | | |
| 0.1 | 1 | 1 | 1 | 1 | 2 | 2 | 2 | 2 | 2 | 2 | 3 | 3 | 3 | 3 | 3 | 3 |
| 0.2 | 2 | 2 | 3 | 3 | 3 | 4 | 4 | 4 | 5 | 5 | 5 | 5 | 6 | 6 | 6 | 7 |
| 0.3 | 3 | 4 | 4 | 4 | 5 | 5 | 6 | 6 | 7 | 7 | 8 | 8 | 9 | 9 | 10 | 10 |
| 0.4 | 4 | 5 | 5 | 6 | 6 | 7 | 8 | 8 | 9 | 10 | 10 | 11 | 12 | 12 | 13 | 13 |
| 0.5 | 5 | 6 | 6 | 7 | 8 | 9 | 9 | 10 | 11 | 12 | 13 | 13 | 14 | 15 | 16 | 16 |
| 0.6 | 6 | 7 | 8 | 9 | 10 | 11 | 12 | 13 | 14 | 15 | 16 | 16 | 17 | 18 | 19 | 20 |
| 0.7 | 7 | 8 | 9 | 10 | 11 | 12 | 13 | 15 | 16 | 17 | 18 | 19 | 20 | 21 | 22 | 23 |
| 0.8 | 8 | 9 | 10 | 12 | 13 | 14 | 15 | 17 | 18 | 19 | 21 | 22 | 23 | 24 | 25 | 26 |
| 0.9 | 9 | 11 | 12 | 13 | 14 | 16 | 17 | 19 | 21 | 22 | 23 | 24 | 26 | 27 | 29 | 30 |
| 1.0 | 11 | 12 | 13 | 15 | 16 | 18 | 19 | **21** | 23 | 24 | 26 | 27 | 29 | 30 | 32 | 33 |
| 2.0 | 21 | 24 | 28 | 30 | 33 | 36 | 39 | 42 | 46 | 48 | 52 | 54 | 58 | 60 | 64 | 66 |
| 3.0 | 32 | 36 | 40 | 45 | 50 | 54 | 59 | 63 | 69 | 72 | 78 | 81 | 87 | 90 | 96 | 99 |
| 4.0 | 42 | 48 | 54 | 60 | 66 | 72 | 78 | 84 | 92 | 96 | 104 | 108 | 116 | 120 | 128 | 132 |
| 5.0 | 53 | 60 | 68 | 75 | 83 | 90 | 98 | 106 | 115 | 121 | 130 | 135 | 145 | 150 | 160 | 165 |
| 6.0 | 64 | 72 | 82 | 91 | 100 | 109 | 118 | 127 | 136 | 145 | 154 | 164 | 173 | 180 | 190 | 200 |
| 7.0 | 74 | 85 | 95 | 106 | 117 | 127 | 138 | 148 | 159 | 170 | 180 | 191 | 201 | 210 | 223 | 233 |
| 8.0 | 85 | 97 | 109 | 121 | 133 | 145 | 158 | 170 | 182 | 194 | 206 | 218 | 230 | 240 | 255 | 266 |

See *Note,* Table B-7.
*Based on 60 microdrops equal to 1 mL or 3.33 μg/drop.

# Index